Traveller and on *Woman's Hour*

Praise for Heal Me

'[Buckley] writes with wit and compassion about her odyssey, but the book is at its best when it explores the failings of the male-dominated healing system, where those with serious conditions are dismissed as hysterical. A timely, worrying and extremely important book'   *Observer*

'*Heal Me* is both a searingly honest first-hand account of Buckley's journey, both spiritual and physical, and an insightful, deeply researched story of pain from the multiple perspectives of medical science, psychology and faith. An absolute must-read on the subject, what's laid bare here about our understanding of and attitudes to chronic pain is alternately sobering and inflammatory'   *Independent*

'This book shouldn't be entertaining and yet … her global rollercoaster journey turns out to be as compulsive as any thriller. Her brave book is a reminder never to give up hope'   *The Lady*

'Buckley's account of her illness is elegant, with apposite literary references. As a welcome bonus, she is bitingly funny in her descriptions of the shortcomings of the medical profession, as well as her unnerving encounters with alternative therapists … The message from her story is uplifting' *The i*

Julia Buckley is a journalist from Cornwall whose work has appeared in the likes of *National Geographic Traveller*, CNN, the *Independent* and the *Sunday Times*, where she is assistant travel editor.

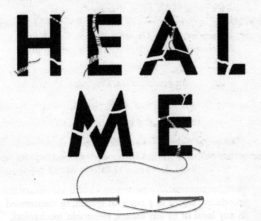

HEAL ME

IN SEARCH OF A CURE

JULIA BUCKLEY

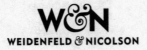

WEIDENFELD & NICOLSON

For everyone who needs a Kevin

This paperback edition first published in 2019
First published in Great Britain in 2018 by Weidenfeld & Nicolson
an imprint of The Orion Publishing Group Ltd
Carmelite House, 50 Victoria Embankment
London EC4Y 0DZ

An Hachette UK Company

1 3 5 7 9 10 8 6 4 2

Copyright © Julia Buckley 2018

The moral right of Julia Buckley to be identified as
the author of this work has been asserted in accordance with
the Copyright, Designs and Patents Act of 1988.

ISBN (paperback) 978 1 4746 0152 8
ISBN (ebook) 978 1 4746 0153 5

Typeset at The Spartan Press Ltd,
Lymington, Hants

Printed and bound by CPI Group (UK) Ltd,
Croydon, CR0 4YY

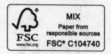

www.orionbooks.co.uk

Contents

Woman is a pain that never goes away
Menander, ancient Greek playwright

It was anger that did write it
Jane Anger, 16th-century feminist

May 2013

It was a year to the day since my life had ended and I was lying in the California desert, being serenaded by a celestial choir.

I couldn't see the angels but their conductor, Charmayne, assured me they were there. Charmayne herself was no angel – she was as earthly as you could get. Somewhere in her fifties, her grey hair tumbled towards her buttocks in wild corkscrews. She wore a maxidress in the scorching desert heat, but not one with any shape or form to it, nor one that demanded a waist-defining belt; Charmayne's maxidress was magnificently sack-like.

She had glasses with clunky NHS frames and milk-bottle lenses despite being eight time zones and three decades beyond NHS glasses. Her face was pristine, entirely unblemished by makeup. As she talked – her voice doing arpeggios from a childlike soprano to a gruff tenor and back again – it felt as if she had one eye on you and one on the universe.

She was raw humanity, unencumbered by gender and all its confines. Charmayne wouldn't have known what a bingo wing was if I'd flapped mine in her face; I bet she'd never counted calories or corseted herself in Spanx. I had never seen a woman so confident, so comfortable in herself, so unapologetic for what she was. She was untrammelled femininity, Mother Earth crossed with a Haight-Ashbury flower child, and I was in awe.

I was less in awe of the celestial choir, though. Although I couldn't see it, I could hear it, and it wasn't what I'd expected. I'd been hoping for transcendent, bell-like tones – Gregorian chants sung by a Mickey Mouse chorus. But the celestial choir, as channelled by Charmayne, seemed angry.

'Aaawoooooaaaarrrrgghhhhhh,' they snarled. 'Owww-whoowwwww,' they howled. They made the throaty gurgles of the cold and mildly intoxicated signalling politely that they'd like to go inside. They growled like spectral hounds and barked like furies. Unless that was Charmayne's dog barking – he was helping with the choir session, too. It was difficult to tell with my eyes screwed shut.

I said I'd lost my life exactly a year earlier, but I hadn't died. No, it was far worse – or so it felt back then, at least. I'd developed chronic pain. Not that 'developed' is the right word, with its implications of a gradual onset and time to adjust. Instead, my pain hit suddenly, rearing up from the depths of my body and mugging me at work one uneventful Tuesday morning. One minute I was reaching for a coffee; the next, my right arm was being ravaged by a fireball. But instead of a real fireball, it was my nervous system short-circuiting and electrocuting itself over and over again, and because there was no real fire, it was impossible to snuff out. Every short circuit flipped another fuse, until the circuit breaker burned out, and it began to spread.

Most people think they know pain. Everyone's done something: broken a limb, been stung by a wasp, recovered from an operation or rammed a baby through their birth canal. But chronic pain is different. It isn't just pain that lingers; it's pain that dominates. It swaddles you in its gloom and slips blinkers on you until everything you see, and everything you experience, is filtered through that pea soup of pain.

The vast majority of chronic pain conditions are not only incurable but also untreatable. They don't respond to drugs, and science hasn't – yet – located a central fuse box to repair.

So people with chronic pain not only live with pain; they're told that this is it until death they do part. It is a diagnosis that dehumanises your body as much as it eviscerates your spirit. And it's made worse because, if there's no obvious physical explanation for it – as is the case with most types of chronic pain (diseases like arthritis aside) – people think, consciously or not, that you're making it up.

Three GPs, eight consultants, three physiotherapists, one nurse and two psychologists had tried to rout my pain in the first year of its existence. All had failed, though each had laid their failure at my door, not theirs. There's no physical reason for it, they said; or, there's kind of a physical reason but not enough of a physical reason to correspond to your level of pain. Maybe, some of them ventured, possibly, do you think ... could it be in your head?

Of course it's in my head, I wanted to scream. I hadn't studied science past GCSE, but even I knew that pain comes from your head. When you fall off a cliff and break your leg, the leg doesn't hurt intrinsically; it sends chemical messages and electrical impulses to the brain, which the brain sifts through and parses as pain. The pain in your leg isn't coming from the broken bone poking through your bloodied shin; it's coming from your head. That doesn't make it any less real, though. Pain is pain.

I would say this to the doctors, and they would agree with me, and talk about how they were very sympathetic to my plight and deeply troubled I was still off work but that, sadly, science has yet to map the brain efficiently and unfortunately, awfully, chronic pain is, so far – sorry! – untreatable. They would usher me out of the room with a sympathetic hand-shake and an offer to come back 'if anything changed', and a week later I'd get a copy of their letter to my GP repeating what they had already told 'this lovely lady'. Sometimes, they recommended he prescribe her antidepressants.

The months ticked by, and the pain stayed the same. As did I – the pain had smothered me in aspic and jammed the pause button on my life. I couldn't work, I couldn't write, I couldn't travel on public transport, I couldn't see my friends. I couldn't wear clothes with buttons, I couldn't chop vegetables, I couldn't do the washing up. I couldn't, half the time, even wash my hair.

I couldn't read because the pain refused to let me hold even the lightest paperback; I couldn't watch TV because it would stalk through my body if I stayed in one place for more than a few minutes. All I could do was cry, which I did a lot; scream, which I did well beyond the point at which my neighbours stopped acknowledging me; and fear for the future, which I did until the evening after the eighth consultant had discharged me, and it dawned on me that I didn't actually have a future, because to have a future, you had to have a life.

The most reasonable option would be to kill myself, that much was clear; but I knew that doing that would kill my mother. I had already moved back in with her, to my childhood room in Cornwall with its pink carpet from 1986 and walls pockmarked with ancient Blu Tack. Yes, it was humiliating to join the statistic of thirtysomethings living with their parents, but if I had someone cooking, cleaning and helping to dress me, at least I would avoid scurvy and trench foot.

So partly for my mother's sake, and partly because I'd always delighted in proving people wrong, I decided that day not to kill myself. Instead, I resolved, I would dedicate what remained of my life to finding a miracle. I would read every book, try every therapy and visit every quack, guru and Jesus clone I could.

Which is where Charmayne came in.

I found her in Joshua Tree, a town in the Mojave Desert teetering on the edge of the tectonic plate that looms above the Coachella Valley – an area I'd long considered my spiritual home, though Joshua Tree would later come to eclipse it. Bordering the eponymous national park with its cacti stretching their bushy arms in the air and beckoning to their creator, Joshua Tree had been a hippy magnet for decades.

4

There was a retreat centre specialising in tough vipassana meditation. Up the road was the Integratron, a huge white dome in the middle of the desert which was supposedly a communication point with aliens. I'd driven through Joshua Tree several times back when I had a life, and had noted that it was a place of personal freedom, an escape from societal norms. Some of the men demonstrated this through the casting out of their razors; some of the women, their bras.

I rented a cabin in the middle of the desert for a week. The shower was outside, on a bed of rocks. Inside, the cabin paired a composting toilet with inefficient air conditioning. I nearly left on the spot.

I went to the retreat centre, but they told me snippily that it was closed for a private event. I asked about healing, and one of the receptionists said she'd call me back with a list of therapists. Instead, she called me that evening and offered to give me an illicit massage herself. I couldn't say no – that was a forbidden word on my journey. You never know who's going to be your saviour.

It definitely wasn't her.

She told me that she'd worked out some time ago that the key to all back problems lay in the 'fanny', as she called it – or buttocks, as I realised, with no small relief, she meant. The massage consisted of ramming her fingers into my 'fanny' and twisting really hard, in a claustrophobic booth of a strip-mall tanning salon. Ram, twist, repeat. Ram, twist, repeat. It was a long hour.

A week passed in Joshua Tree without event. I meditated on my aversion to the compost toilet; I lay outside, treating the desert as a sauna with a view. Saunas were good for me, all those doctors who'd failed to heal me had said, because they relax the muscles. It was true: the sun scorched through my flesh and into my sinews. It was like rubbing Deep Heat onto the joints themselves, and for the first time in a year, the pain eased a little. The fire was still kindling in my arm, and a carving knife was still lodged in my armpit, but the rest of my body felt warm and buoyed – a hot bath minus the prune fingers.

Other than the 40-degree heat, there had been something else keeping me in the cabin, and that was the shower gel and shampoo the owners had left for me – made with clary sage at a Joshua Tree 'apothecary', according to the label. It smelled of cleansing and new beginnings, and I wanted some to remind me of my time in the desert when I didn't hurt so much, because I knew that the minute I returned to a damp English summer, my joints would mutiny. So I found the apothecary – the Grateful Desert, it was called – and as I took the shower gel from a wall full of essential oils and herbal blends, I asked if they had anything for nerve or joint pain.

She steered me towards an oily tincture of St John's Wort that had been harvested by the light of the full moon under the stars of Joshua Tree. It was a body rub to aid insomnia, she said, but it worked by relaxing the muscles, so it would probably help. 'But what you really need,' she said, handing me a business card, 'is Charmayne.'

The business card had a picture of a forked stick on it, the name 'Charmayne', and a phone number. She watched me trace my finger over the stick.

'She's a dowser,' she said.

Vicky was from the Deep South and hadn't really been into alternative medicine before she moved to Joshua Tree, but Charmayne, she assured me, was the real deal. 'She's in a higher dimension,' she said. 'She's a god-given healer.'

'What does she do?' I asked.

'She's just Charmayne,' said Vicky. And then on cue, a loud noise – somewhere between a grunt, a gurgle and a roar – exploded from somewhere round the back of the Grateful Desert.

Vicky said: '*That's* Charmayne.'

The noise increased. There was squealing, more grunting, howling and bellowing. It sounded equally painful for giver and receiver.

'Are you cool with the noises?' asked Vicky.

'Does she always do that?' I said.

'No, it's different for every person,' said Vicky, explaining that Charmayne used sound therapy to do her healing.

I had tried sound therapy before. It had involved gongs and sounding bowls, and once a guy had gone off-piste and serenaded me with a sitar. Devil grunts had not been part of the equation.

But no one said a miracle would be pleasant – something I would repeat to myself again and again in the years to come – and anyway the clary sage had led me here. Maybe Charmayne would howl me back to health. Maybe she would be Virgil to my Dante, guiding me through the groans of hell and purgatory. Maybe I would emerge to see the stars once more.

I asked if she had any appointments the following day.

'Charmayne doesn't really do appointments,' said Vicky. 'Can you hang on till she's finished with this one, and talk to her yourself?'

I went next door to the wholefood cafe, and ordered an ice cream smoothie, then a muffin. Comfort eating was the one pleasure left to me, along with, possibly, shopping. Shopping for muumuus to conceal my ballooning body for my California trip had been an oddly gripping distraction from the pain. (Distraction therapy, as it happens, is a central tenet of pain management on the NHS.)

I sat outside the cafe and watched the entrance of the Grateful Desert. Parked outside was a jankety old car, covered entirely – bonnet, sides, boot, roof, door handles – in stickers. 'Coexist,' said one, its letters largely composed of Stars of David, stars-and-crescents, and crosses. 'Obama08,' said another. 'Barack Obama is not a foreign socialist giving out free healthcare,' ranted a third. 'That would be Jesus.'

Welcome to California.

The door swung open and a young woman staggered out, looking far too physically fragile to make any kind of guttural squawks. I raced inside.

I knew Charmayne instantly. There was something biblical about her. I could imagine her out in the desert, calling in the wilderness amongst the Joshua trees (named, by the way, by the Mormon settlers because their heaven-stretched arms reminded them of the prophet).

'You found her!' Vicky grinned. 'She came from England for you,' she told Charmayne.

Charmayne looked me up and down, but not in a way that anyone had looked me up and down before. She was appraising my aura, not my body.

'What you wanna do?' she said, in a voice that was at once girly and gruff. The voice of a siren.

'Can I have some healing please?' I asked.

Charmayne stepped up to me – she came up to my armpit, but then I'm extremely tall – and squinted.

'Hmm,' she grunted, and whipped a pendulum out of her pocket. She held it out between us and cocked her head to one side. We stared as it shivered in the air.

'Huh,' she said. 'I think tomorrow afternoon.' The pendulum began to bounce from side to side, picking up speed.

'Three o'clock,' she announced, and stuffed the pendulum back in her pocket. 'Do you know what I do? Are you cool with noises?'

I tried not to think of the noises, but I smiled involuntarily.

'I think so,' I said. 'But I'm awkward and English so if I laugh or anything, that will definitely be the only reason why. Is that okay?'

'Sure,' she said. 'See you tomorrow.' I felt her hot stare follow me out through the door.

I turned up at three the next day; the car with all the stickers rolled up 10 minutes later ('She doesn't do time like us,' Vicky had reassured me). Charmayne ambled over to the passenger door and fiddled with something on the seat. It was Rolly, her labrador – he was a healer too. Rolly led us into an oversized cupboard at the back of the shop, where there was a photo of another labrador on a small table ('Susie – Rolly is her, reincarnated,' Charmayne told me

8

afterwards), a chair and a massage bed. Charmayne squatted on the floor and I took the chair.

'What are we clearing?' she asked, and I told her about the arm and the pain and asked her to make it stop.

'Sure,' she said, and settled herself on the floor, legs crossed. 'Let's go.'

Then the noises started.

Vicky had told me that the sounds were different for everyone, and I'd been holding out for something a little more palatable. Perhaps the fragile young woman from yesterday had had deep-rooted issues, I'd reassured myself. But no.

'Houuuuarrrrrghhhhhh,' spat Charmayne, channelling norovirus. 'Graaaaaaaooooooohhhhh. Euuuaaaaarrrrrh. Eurrgh. Eurrghh. *Eurrghhh.*' After a few minutes, she stopped for a swig of water.

'Doing alright?' she asked.

'I think so,' I said.

'Hey, you need this. They say it's good for you,' she said.

'Who's "they"?' I realised I hadn't asked.

Charmayne rolled her eyes at me, but sympathetically.

'The celestial beings,' she said, took a gasp of breath and bayed like a wolf, as Rolly looked on impassively. I scrunched my eyes shut.

The celestial beings sang to me for nearly an hour and a half. From the noises they made, anyone would have thought they were performing an exorcism, but according to Charmayne they were just 'clearing stuff'. Only twice did she refer to the 'stuff' they might be clearing – once, as she'd asked me to recount how the pain had started, and the second time, when she asked whether something had happened to me between the ages of seven and eight.

Not that I'm aware of, I told her. I didn't tell her that a few years back, for work, I'd interviewed a medium, and he too had referred to a traumatic event between the ages of seven and eight. Perhaps that's an age that's lost to most people, one between infancy and the memorable, older part of childhood. Perhaps everyone forgets what they were doing between the ages of seven and eight, so mediums and psychics and people who prey on the gullible refer to this period as standard. Or perhaps I really had blocked out something traumatic. Trauma, I would learn three years later from a Harvard professor, is the main predictor of chronic pain.

Either way, the celestial beings were out to clear it.

At the end of the session, Charmayne asked how I felt. 'Not sure,' I said. I was still in pain, but then I'd been sitting on a wooden chair for an hour and a half. My maximum 'sitting tolerance' had last been calculated by my NHS pain management team at four and a half minutes, and that was with a cushion. This had been an experience so unlike any other that I had a feeling I'd need to leave it a day or two to process.

I asked to settle up and she pointed at an envelope stuffed with dollar bills on the floor.

'Just put what you feel like in there,' she said, and left the cupboard. Rolly watched me add $30 to the envelope – not much, but I hadn't asked for 90 minutes in the first place – and ushered me out.

Charmayne came bounding up. 'How you feeling?' Her face was shining. She was a goddess – so different to everyone who'd gone before her. I couldn't bear to admit I was still in pain.

'I'm not quite sure yet,' I told her. 'A little better, I think? But I think I need to let it settle before I know for certain.'

'That definitely helped,' said Charmayne. 'Man, you had so much to clear! They were going on and on. We should do it again.'

'Ah,' I said, feigning bitter disappointment. 'I'd love to, but I'm leaving tonight. I fly back to England tomorrow.' (This was a lie. I was leaving Joshua Tree that night, but I was flying home in six days' time.)

'We can do it over the phone,' announced Charmayne.

I couldn't think of anything I'd rather do less than lie on the pink carpet at my mum's house and listen to Charmayne bellowing down the phone at me.

'That would be lovely,' I said. 'But I couldn't pay you over the phone.'

Then Charmayne said a wonderful thing. 'Honey, I'm not doing this to get paid,' she said. 'I'm doing this to try and help you. And I think it will help.'

Before Charmayne, the only person who had said they wanted to help me had been a neurologist I had seen privately. He had declared himself shocked by the effect my pain had had on my life, horrified that a journalist such as I could no longer work (he wasn't the first doctor who instantly took me more seriously on learning my profession), and appalled that nobody had properly investigated me before. He had commissioned a raft of tests, and dispatched me with a handshake and a promise. 'We will get to the bottom of this,' he had said, looking me straight in the eye. 'I won't let you down.'

Finally someone understood. Finally someone was going to unbuckle my blinkers and unwrap my swaddling bands.

We did the tests: MRIs, brain scans and nerve conduction studies, which seemed to involve sticking needles in various bits of my body, electrocuting me through them, and measuring how loud I screamed. At my second appointment, he told me that my arm showed some nerve damage, but not enough to explain the extent of the pain. There wasn't enough damage to operate on, he was afraid, but the good news was that the nerve was already showing signs of recovery.

No, he was afraid he didn't know why it didn't *feel* like it was recovering, six months after the injury, but he would prescribe me some neurological painkillers in the meantime.

The third time I saw him, I reported that the pills had eased the pain a little, but that they had entirely snuffed out my brain. I could no longer hold a conversation, dictate a one-line email, remember the previous line of a book, or work out why I'd walked into the room I'd just walked into.

'Ah, yes,' he sighed. 'Unfortunately pregabalin works on the entire brain, rather than locally. It's entirely natural to have side effects.'

I told him that the side effects were so debilitating that even if it had conquered the pain, I couldn't keep taking pregabalin. Even were I physically fine, I said, I wouldn't be able to go back to work while I was pharmaceutically lobotomised.

Also, I said, ever since I had started the pills, I had been experiencing particularly vivid suicidal urges.

'That's impossible,' he said. 'Pregabalin was originally developed as an antidepressant. I mean, it's not completely unheard of for a drug to have the opposite effect than is intended, but it's pretty much impossible. You're suicidal because you're depressed.'

In *The Yellow Wallpaper*, a 19th-century semi-autobiographical novella by feminist Charlotte Perkins Gilman, the protagonist – anonymous, as all we patients are – is confined to bed on the orders of her doctor husband after suffering a 'temporary nervous depression'. The lack of stimulus makes her iller, but he tells her she is getting better, over and over again.

'You really are better, dear, whether you can see it or not,' he says. 'I am a doctor, dear, and I know.'

She goes insane.

I'm not depressed, I told the neurologist. I know my body. I know it's the medicine.

'It's okay to be depressed, Julia,' he said. 'Let's increase your dose by six times. I'd like to see if it makes a difference.'

I saw him once more, after my GP had taken me off the pregabalin because its listed side effects did, it turned out, include suicidal urges (it wasn't originally an antidepressant, either). This time, he shook his head sadly, and told me he thought I'd be better served by a pain specialist rather than him. There was really nothing that he, a neurologist, could do.

He had said he wouldn't let me down, that he would help me.

And now here was Charmayne saying the same thing.

'I think we should work together over the phone,' she was

saying. 'Forget the money. We'll see each other again one day – if you're that bothered about it, pay me then.'

I took her number and promised to call. Driving off, I wondered whether at last I had found the person who was going to cure me. The treatment was so implausible – Charmayne was so implausible – that there had to be something to it. This whole episode – the Joshua trees, the hippies, the trail from composting toilet to clary sage to the Grateful Desert to Charmayne – it had to mean something. It had to signal a turning point. Look! I was winding my way down the side of the tectonic plate, and the carving knife that had spent the past 12 months buried in my armpit was barely registering the turns of the steering wheel. Perhaps this could be it. Please let this be it.

The knife was back by the time I got to Palm Springs, but it had been an hour's drive – that was to be expected. Charmayne wasn't Jesus. It wouldn't be instantaneous. I would see how I felt in the morning.

The pain was still there in the morning. And the morning after that. By the time I flew home, six days later, it was worse.

PERFECT STORMS

Pain has no tomorrows

Alda Merini (1931-2009: mental health patient, asylum inmate, poet)

John Smith steps on a nail.

His nociceptors – sensory receptors in his foot – are stimulated by the pressure. They release a chemical, which shoots up the A-delta nerve fibres to their siblings in his spinal cord. SOS, they say. Something bad is happening.

The nociceptors in the spinal cord react instantly. They contract his muscles to remove him from the harm, and John Smith jerks his foot away.

He still doesn't know he's stepped on a nail.

That's where the C fibres come in.

The C fibres are a more considered version of the A-delta fibres. Where the A-deltas react instantly, neurotically, the C fibres take a little more time. First, they establish whether damage has occurred. If it has, they ping another message up to the nociceptors in the spinal cord, and from there to the brain. Don't panic, but something's happened, they say. Not sure what, but you should probably take a look.

That's when John Smith knows he's stepped on a nail.

To him, of course, the process is instantaneous. John Smith thinks he made that mortifying, unmanly yelp the instant he stepped on the nail because it hurt so much, but he didn't. He's just slow to catch up. He had to wait for his brain.

Because it's John Smith's brain that decides whether or not he's in pain. Think of it as a reality TV show, a search for a star: the brain is head judge, the body mere acolyte. It's his brain, and his brain alone, that gets the final say over whether the pressure on his foot from this nail gets through to Bootcamp, where it will get a makeover and officially become an all-singing, all-dancing Injury.

The makeover is swift. Once his brain has decided John Smith has been injured, it unleashes its rebranding team. It instructs the autonomic nervous system to carpet-bomb him with stress hormones like adrenaline and cortisol. It tells his heart to pump faster, and makes his blood pressure rise to give him the best chance at either fight or flight.

Once John Smith is over the immediate impact – sitting down with a cup of tea to steady those shaking hands – the autonomic nervous system takes a back seat. His immune system takes the wheel, inflaming the spot where the nail hit to do useful stuff like upping blood flow to the area and increasing sensitivity, ensuring he takes care of the injury. In other words, it makes it hurt. This is acute pain, and it's there to protect him. It alerts him to tissue damage, and reminds him not to step on that part of his foot.

If all goes to plan, John Smith will recover from his injury within six to 12 weeks. Over that time, the brain will constantly have been requesting reports on the progress of his foot, and will eventually sign off on it, rubber-stamp it healed. John will go back to taking his full weight on his foot. He'll probably have a faint, residual fear of stepping on another nail, because his primitive limbic system, or 'monkey brain', is wired to remember stressful events; but unless the wound has left a scar, in another three months he won't even remember the precise spot where the nail went in.

Nine times out of 10, this full recovery takes place. But if John Smith was born under an unlucky star – if he's one of us, the doomed 10 per cent – that one small step on the nail will become one giant leap into purgatory.

Chronic pain usually, if not always, starts with acute pain. There's a genuine injury – John Smith really did impale his foot on that nail – but even though the immune system does its stuff, the wound heals and the swelling goes down, it still hurts.

If he's the kind of person who gets on with things, he'll

shrug and limp stoically on, trying to ignore it. If he's the type to be on first-name terms with his GP's receptionists, he'll book an appointment. The doctor will most likely take a look, note that the injury has healed, and tell John to take some ibuprofen and give it a bit longer. If it's still painful in a month or two, a particularly diligent GP might say, feel free to come back.

Both approaches are disastrous.

Science says that the longer you've been in pain, the less likely your chances of getting out of it. In a process called neuroplasticity, the nervous system begins to reset itself: pain pathways are strengthened, normal ones left to atrophy. Neurologically, you're already misfiring – that's why you're still in pain – but the longer you misfire, the more thoroughly your nervous system is brainwashed into thinking that this is your normal state. It's racing around muddy B roads, completely oblivious to the fact that, before the diversion of the injury, it was easier to take the dual carriageway. Then, it starts off-roading. Then, it starts laying down new tarmac. If you don't reroute it soon, the original motorways grass over completely.

But because chronic pain presents as acute pain, it's hard to diagnose in the crucial, early stages. Remember that scene in *Total Recall* where Arnold Schwarzenegger morphs into a little old lady in order to get through security and onto the shuttle to Mars? Chronic pain does a pitch-perfect rendition of genuine, acute pain. At first, you can't tell the difference. But then, it gets stuck on repeat – like Schwarzenegger's old lady hologram, senselessly echoing herself over and over again. It's only then that you realise there's something more sinister behind it, and that that something wants to destroy you. But by then it's too strong to do anything about it. After all, Schwarzenegger always wins.

Because of its similarity to acute, protective pain, most pain is not defined as chronic until it's passed the two or three month stage. By that point, it's already too late.

I've always wished I had stepped on a nail. Stepping on a nail is at least a tangible injury, one that comes with added risks like tetanus, one that everyone can understand must hurt. Unfortunately for me, my injury was as trivial as it was unfathomable. I reached for a cup of coffee.

It's a tale I know by heart, now, because I've recited it hundreds of times, giving blow-by-blow accounts to specialists, recounting it to alternative therapists, explaining it to disbelievers and picking through it furiously, my bitter mantra, wondering why I didn't do things differently.

It was Tuesday 15 May 2012, and I was at work in a hipster office on Shoreditch High Street. I'd arrived armed with coffee, energy-boosting juice plus porridge that morning, because it was going to be a long day. I was counting down to the holiday of a lifetime: two and a half weeks in Cambodia and Vietnam.

Instead of doing what I'd done on every single holiday of my working life, which was to spend half the time working and the other half stressing because I was on holiday and I was working, I had spent the past few weeks coming in a little earlier, leaving a little later, and wasting a little less time on Facebook. And it had worked – at this rate, I'd have finished everything before I left. There were just a couple more deadlines to power through.

I was working for an American website, so my editors were based in New York. That sunny morning, I turned on the computer to find an email from one of them, Dana, which had come in overnight. It was a new deadline – the sales team had signed a cruise company, and I had to write previews of two cruises, even though I had never been on a cruise, immediately.

I scanned the itinerary of the first – a Mediterranean cruise around Italy, France and Spain. I knew most of the ports; it would be easy.

I banged it out, leaving my coffee to get cold.

As I looked at the second itinerary – a wine cruise around France – I became aware that my arm was hurting. But then, my arm was always hurting; I'd had problems with it since I was a teenager. I'd been given extra time for my A Levels and dictated my finals. Over two decades, I'd seen countless doctors, had myriad scans and undergone numerous treatments, both medical and alternative. Nothing had cured it, but nobody seemed too bothered by it, and regular physio and massage had kept it under control since I'd started working. My arm always hurt, sometimes more, sometimes less. Treating it ate into my salary, and colleagues made jibes about my late arrival after physio every week, but that was just how things were.

This time, looking at the wine cruise itinerary, I was aware that the pain wasn't cramping as usual, but tingling, as if there were fire ants sprinting up and down, from my fingertips to my armpit. Especially in my armpit.

Whatever. My arm hurt. That was just how things were.

My neck was hurting, too, but again, that's what my neck tended to do. Aching necks are a typical side effect of a sedentary lifestyle, and I was sedentary, and lazy on top of it. The previous week my neck had ached so much one afternoon that it had felt like my head was trying to saw itself off from the inside. It was so painful that my eyesight had started to blur, and I'd asked Becky, who sat opposite me, whether her neck was killing her too. She'd looked up, thought for a moment, and cupped it with her hand.

'Yeah, I suppose it does ache a bit,' she'd said. See, Julia? Everyone's necks ached. Mine just ached more than Becky's because I was lazy, unfit, unmotivated. I'd regretted taking this job from day one – I'd prostituted myself, ditching real journalism in favour of the free hotel stays that came with marketing reviews – and the boredom was making me more aware of my neck.

My arm was burning. My neck was aching. That was just how things were.

I hammered out the wine cruise piece in one go. It was 11am, and the froth had melted into my untouched cappuccino, leaving brown scum bubbles on the inside of the cup. Still drinkable, I decided – still caffeinated, at least. I leaned back in my ergonomic-by-numbers chair and reached forward for the cup, my body going one way, my arm the other. As I did so, a shard of awareness that Something Had Happened swam up into my consciousness, and I knew instinctively that it was life-changing, but I quickly swallowed that knowledge back down.

My right arm was on fire from the inside. The ants had gone; by now, it felt like someone had laid out lines of petrol up and down, back and forth and round every inch of every sinew, then sparked a match in my neck. It burned, billowing up and down my arm and ricocheting between my collarbone and each and every fingertip. There was another, separate fire – a bonfire this time – kindling under my right shoulder blade, and a carving knife had lodged in my armpit. Above the carnage, my neck appeared to have gone under a lorry.

I whispered to Becky: 'I think something's happened.'

I stood up. I wobbled past the desks of unsmiling advertising types, with whom we shared an office. I locked myself in the unisex toilet and stared at the blank blackboard on the wall. I wanted to cry, but the adrenaline had vacuumed my tear ducts. So I made a cup of tea instead.

I took the mug back to my desk and said to Becky, 'I think I'm going to have to go home, but I'd better wait for Dana to get in.' My voice was wavering, but possibly because my office nemesis – who, a couple of weeks earlier, had taken me on one side and admonished me for arriving late every Thursday after physio – was busy throwing death stares at me. What if they thought I was making it up?

I waited for Dana to materialise in New York, and as I waited, I did more work on autopilot, typing with my left hand. My right side may have been on fire, but the rest of me – including my mind – was entirely numb. I was scared of being taken for a pre-holiday shirker, so I held out until 5pm before I emailed Dana to say that something had happened, that I appeared to have injured my arm and neck, and I was in a lot of pain, and I was so sorry but I was going to have to go home earlier than usual, after a mere eight hours at my desk. Her reply came quickly. 'We're all struggling here,' it read. 'But if you feel you need to take off early, I can't stop you.'

RSI, said the locum GP the next morning, signing me off for two weeks with immediate effect. 'But how are you going to meet your deadlines?' wailed my other boss. So I carried on working – for four weeks after my injury, in the end, even through my holiday (I was in too much pain to travel around on my trip of a lifetime by then, so I just stayed on a friend's airbed in Phnom Penh).

This is where my mantra stops because every time I tell my story, this is where I start to cry and shake with rage: at the fate that Tuesday dealt me, at my mindless, kamikaze actions, at the doctor who discharged me with nothing more than a sicknote, at the employers who let me work when rest might have let it recover. However many times I say it, write it, explain it, excuse it, promise myself it wasn't my fault, I can't turn back the clock. All those little things came together in a perfect storm.

I'm not so unusual, by the way. There are more of us than you'd think.

———

John Smith's foot still hurts.

It's been three months since he stepped on that nail, and six weeks since the wound healed. Yet the foot is still too tender to take his weight.

He returns to the doctor, who establishes there's no physical reason for the foot to still hurt. Then the doctor – let's assume it's a he – will say one of two things. He might say, 'You're getting older, John, aches and pains just happen,' and send him on his way (this is what happened to me when I first saw a doctor about my pain). If John Smith's doctor does that – if another few months are wasted, waiting it out – he will effectively have handed down a life sentence of pain to John. Healthy neural motorways will start grassing over, and the new network of pain-slurried B roads and farm tracks will become the de facto way for his nervous system to get around.

But if the doctor is a good one, and has experience of chronic pain (which not enough doctors do, despite it affecting up to half the UK population at any one time,[1] and back pain being the second most common reason for taking time off work), he'll suspect it could be Schwarzenegger lurking behind that sweet old lady face, and swing into action. He might start John off with some physiotherapy, which won't help his misfiring nervous system, but will at least keep the foot mobile and strong, to avoid atrophying muscles causing their own, acute problems.

He might commission some kind of scan, which will almost certainly be useless, but will at least reassure John that there's nothing physically wrong. This is important because the mind can play a large part in pain, in the same way that the day you find a lump in your whatever, you immediately know it's cancer, and you suddenly start experiencing all the other symptoms you might possibly feel if it were, until the doctor confirms it's just a cyst, or a rib, or an allergic reaction, and all of a sudden you feel fine again. Equally, he might refer him to a specialist, just to confirm there's nothing sinister at play.

The most helpful thing the GP could do at this stage is to start John on various types of painkillers. Although this sounds like a cop-out – and though it's often intended as such – it can actually be a breakthrough. Once it's ingrained, chronic pain rarely responds to drugs, but if you can break the circuit, even for an instant, your fuse box will sometimes reboot itself: a switch will be tripped, the nervous system will remember its original pathways, and reopen the motorways. In his landmark book *Pain: The Science of Suffering*, Patrick Wall explains that sometimes, even a couple of weeks of pain relief can be enough to break the cycle. That book was written in 1999 and Wall, who died soon after, had long been regarded as the world expert on pain; yet in the two years that I was bouncing from doctor to doctor over a decade later, the only person ever to discuss this approach with me was a 'pain specialist' anaesthetist – and even then, it was me who brought it up, a year after my injury, having read the book.

If John Smith's doctor is a superb GP who knows about chronic pain, doesn't give a hoot about going over budget and laughs in the face of NHS targets – rather like the one I ended up with, my hero who we'll call Dr Good – he might refer him for some kind of pain management. This sounds good, and proactive – and in theory, it is. It's probably one of the best things a GP can do in today's system. But there's a colossal problem with it. Pain management, as practised by the NHS, is palliative, not curative. It starts with the assumption that John Smith is, and will forever remain, fucked.

Pain management courses aren't easy to get on to. First, your GP has to refer you – usually with a pleading, UCAS-style application explaining why you deserve your place on the course, and vowing you will be a diligent student. Then comes the wait, which may include an introductory session and even interviews – I had two – to check both your dedication and your psychological pliability. Only then will the specialists running the show decide whether to accept you.

Every pain management course is slightly different, but the majority focus on two disciplines: pacing and Cognitive Behavioural Therapy. Pacing is genuinely critical – it's the idea that, by staying below your pain threshold, lurking just out of its range, you'll gradually be able to increase your limits without increasing the pain. It's a frustrating, exhausting and relentlessly boring way to live – imagine timing your sitting tolerance, then setting an alarm to sound every two minutes, chivvying you to get up and move – but this way, the theory goes, you'll gradually become more active, comfortably.

The theory behind CBT is that, like bacteria, thoughts feed on each other and multiply. Positive begets positive, negative begets negative. Say John Smith accidently puts his whole weight on his foot one morning, and is rewarded with a sudden shot of pain. 'Ow!' he might think. 'This pain gets worse by the day. It's been three months and I still can't walk properly. When is it going to end? What if it never ends? What if I'll never run that half-marathon? What if I can't drive any more? I'll lose my job. I'll lose my wife. My friends will abandon me. I'll die alone, a cripple, and in pain.'

This is called catastrophising. By the time he's finished catastrophising, says CBT, John Smith will be awash in an orgy of negativity; his pain engorged, and he more aware of it. And that will be his first step off the correct path and into a shadowy wood, and next thing he knows he'll be standing in front of a gate saying, 'Abandon all hope ye who enter here,' and it will be game over.

Whereas, CBT reasons, if John Smith thinks positive things about that extra shot of pain – if he thinks, 'Gosh, that hurts – but then, let's not forget, I haven't let my foot take my weight in three months. No wonder! Who's to say it won't feel better in five minutes, or even tomorrow, and ooh I smell cake, my wife must be baking for me, for she is the best wife in the world' – his mind will be taken off the pain.

Human beings are wired to worry – you can thank your limbic system for that. But if John Smith can condition himself to think positive, and to fire off that Pavlovian response every time he feels pain, he won't notice it as much.

If CBT sounds like common sense, that's because, however much psychologists try to intellectualise it, it is. Maybe it's different for other illnesses – I know people who swear by it for anxiety – but when it comes to pain management, the central tenets of CBT are pretty much identical to those of positive thinking, the law of attraction, cosmic ordering, and every other New Age talking therapy that most doctors despise and NICE (which rules on NHS funding) certainly wouldn't shell out for. And yet, these same doctors insist on programming us with CBT. It works for 80 per cent of patients, they claim. That seems low, in a way. Surely common sense should help us all?

What CBT ignores, though, is that sometimes it's cathartic to wallow in self-pity for a bit. Sometimes it helps – really helps – to cry it out. Equally, CBT fails to take into consideration that sometimes you can spend so long desperately trying to think positive about a certain situation that you completely overlook what might be a practical solution to it. Thinking positive is helpful, usually; but sometimes, it just smears a sugary glaze over reality and fixes you there. CBT may make the 80 per cent cheery little automatons, but it might also block them from seeing a solution.

But then, that's the whole problem with pain management. 'Management' assumes there is no cure. 'Management' assumes you're never going to get better. 'Management' assumes that 'coping' (my course was actually called COPE) is as good as it's ever going to get. Pain management courses take a group of vulnerable, unhappy people, and tell them that they'll never get their lives back but not to worry too much, because if they only try and turn that smile upside down, it might not seem quite as bad.

This is how the NHS chooses to attack chronic pain: not by running patients through a list of system-rebooting drugs, not on long-term physiotherapy and not by getting to the bottom of underlying causes, but by handing millions of pounds over to psychologists to tell sick people that they'll never get well but never-mind-let's-try-and-think-positive. If they did that with cancer, or diabetes, or heart disease, there would be national outrage.

Because people on these courses talk to each other, and wind each other up. Because, as those doctors and psychologists well know – after all, this is the principle behind the CBT they teach – negative thoughts make the pain more prominent, and there can be no thought more negative than 'this is never going to get better'. Because telling someone their life is essentially finished is going to screw them over.

In short, a pain management course may well end up making John Smith worse.

There were 10 of us on my course. When we started, six were in full-time work, two were students, one person was working part-time from home, and I was signed off temporarily. By the time we had our six-month reunion, only four of us had any kind of employment, and both students had dropped out. One of us was using a stick, one was on crutches, and one of us had progressed to a wheelchair.

I was the one with the stick.

Our course took place over two months during summer 2012, around the London Olympics. In one way, it was an inspiring time to be ill – the Paralympians were everywhere, defying expectations and redefining disability. For the first time, they got a closing ceremony; for once, everyone was at pains to give them equal billing. Pistorius, back then, was as feted as Bolt.

But in another, it was the most depressing time to be ill. If Ellie Simmonds could set a new world record; if a 40-year-old who lost her legs in the London bombings could represent her country at volleyball from her wheelchair, I would harangue myself, why could I not even type an email, or sit for more than two minutes, without my body erupting in pain? And anyway, those of us who couldn't sprint or play boccia were still invisible. I spent a day at the Paralympic stadium with tens of thousands cheering on equality, but when it was time to go home, nobody wanted to give me a seat on the Central Line. I was, I swiftly realised, the wrong kind of disabled.

'Disabled' was a loaded word, of course, but disabled was what we were, according to the psychologist running the pain management course. It wasn't what I wanted to hear. My biggest dread, when the pain had first crippled me, had been that my life was over; I was thrilled to be accepted onto the COPE course because I believed it would fast-track my recovery. Instead, it was an eight-week reinforcement of my darkest fears. There would be no quick fix, they told us on day one; indeed, there would be no fix at all. They weren't here to cure, because there was no cure. They would teach us coping strategies – ways to live despite the pain.

That wasn't what I'd signed up for.

They introduced us to the concept of pacing, which helped. They led group stretches, as if they were imparting some kind of divine revelation that stretching a sore muscle made it feel better. They made us live our lives by the stopwatch, calculating our tolerance for every activity: walking, sitting, reading, washing up, lying in the bath, 'sensate touch' (the chronic pain patient's gruesome alternative to sex). They set an alarm to sound every 15 minutes, so that every 15 minutes we would get up, move about, stretch, roll around on the floor, or do whatever might gift us some minute comfort in that moment.

They did guided meditation and taught us CBT, which was outrageously, offensively obvious. They made us set 'goals', even if the goal for the next week was, as mine once was, to ring up a friend and ask whether she had somewhere for me to sit at her wedding (planning for pain means freedom from it, they said). When, at the next session, I confirmed I had done this, I was congratulated as if I'd got married myself.

The premise of the COPE course was that chronic pain doesn't get better, but by accepting it, it can bother us less, and we will suffer fewer flare-ups. Flare-ups, they said, were when, for reasons known or unknowable, everything suddenly gets worse. They generally last a few days. My arm was a flare-up of my underlying chronic pain, they told me.

But it's lasted eight weeks and counting, I said.

Sometimes flare-ups take longer, they said.

To me – and to my GP, who was as frustrated and baffled as I was – it seemed obvious that there'd been some kind of injury that day at my computer, writing about wine cruises. Yes, as it happened, I'd had aching joints for so long that I'd always assumed it was normal (in fact, shortly before my injury, I'd been diagnosed with a genetic condition that causes chronic pain). But the arm pain was an entirely different kind of pain, we argued. It had exploded from one second to the next. It was an injury, and if it was an injury, that meant it could recover.

Oh no, said the pain team; it's a flare-up of an incurable underlying problem. Acceptance, they impressed upon me, was the first step towards pain management. The physio suggested I'd come on the course too early, while I was still in the initial, denial stage of grief. The psychologist took me to one side when she caught me rolling my eyes at an especially patronising cameo from a rheumatologist, and told me to stop being so *angry*. I wasn't helping myself, or the others, she hissed. When I wrote, one day, that my six-month goal was to have a firm diagnosis for my arm and a way forward for my life, they told me it was unrealistic. 'You have to accept that you already have a diagnosis, and that the pain might never go away,' said the physio. 'So the next question, Julia, is how are you going to progress *with things as they are?*'

'He says no one but myself can help me out of it,' writes the *Yellow Wallpaper* protagonist. 'That I must use my will and self-control.' She ends up beaten down by the professionals. So did I.

By the time I finished the course, I was walking with a stick and describing myself as disabled. 'My condition is incurable,' I'd tell people, parroting the phrases the psychologist had taught us for dealing with questions about our health. 'But there are coping strategies to live with it.' I'd try to look bright – the Great British Public prefers its cripples plucky after all – but inside I felt hollow, in mourning for the life that had been stripped from me, the life which the medical profession insisted I'd never get back. If it was never going to get better, what was the point of trying to cope? I wasn't the only one to feel this way, either. On day one of the course, the room had crackled with anticipation and we had hovered on the edge of our chairs, craning for a revelation. By the last session, we mostly lay on the floor between the ghosts of our ambitions, the air heavy with grief.

Hopelessness is contagious. Is it any wonder I turned to God?

THE ODD ONE OUT

*Ironshod horses rage back and forth
against every nerve.*

Audre Lorde (1934-1992: cancer patient, writer)

Around half of all chronic pain patients are indulging in some kind of alternative therapy at any one time.

It doesn't sound a lot, 50 per cent. For every supine body on the massage table, that means another on the sofa, splitting open the foil blisters on a new pack of painkillers, wondering whether this will be the one to work. It probably won't, because the '30 rule' means drugs typically reduce pain by only 30 per cent in just 30 per cent of patients – and anyway, chronic pain patients are more resistant to both painkillers and placebos. But if you compare that 50 per cent to the general population – only one in five of whom have tried complementary medicine, ever – it's a pretty striking figure. Every other one of us hopes that we will be the odd one out. The one who defies the doctors. The miracle.

The scientific community laughs at us, of course. Its members talk of 'quacks' and 'placebos' and proselytise about 'evidence-based medicine'. They deride talk of 'cures' in favour of 'management'. They do, of course, have a point. Real, medical-grade proof that any complementary therapy works is close to non-existent.

But if we listened only to our doctors, all we'd hear is 'side effects' and 'no real cure'; 'Sorry, I can't help,' or, 'Have we talked about counselling?' Chronic pain patients are 14 times more likely to kill themselves than the general population. When the medical profession deals with our illness by confiscating our future, the only wonder is that it isn't more.

Luckily, human beings are born to hope: for a better job, the partner of our dreams, a healthier bank account or an epiphany revealing the meaning of the universe. Think of the ebola survivors who, once they've made it through, say that in the deepest troughs of their illness, the fear of the disease seemed deadlier than the virus itself. Hope can mean the difference between life and death.

Human beings hope – and always have hoped – that, against all odds, it will get better. We don't have to believe it will; just in the possibility that it might. Hope is what keeps us alive – and hope is why so many of us in pain are so willing to sweep aside our scepticism, mute our doubts, and give the people who say they can heal us a chance.

Some rush into alternative therapy the minute the pain begins; others wait until conventional medicine has written them off. Some commit to their first practitioner, while others play the field. It took me seven months, and I started at the top.

In those first seven months, I'd tried everything the medical profession had suggested. I had bounced from hospital to hospital and from specialist to specialist. On the NHS, I'd seen one rheumatologist, two physiotherapists and two psychologists. Privately, I'd added a neurologist and an expensive physio who specialised in my underlying condition. I'd even been sent to a cardiologist and a gastroenterologist, in case my problem could be linked to an abnormality of the nervous system. All had drawn a blank.

I'd tried medication: anti-inflammatories, opioids, anticonvulsants (epilepsy drugs are sometimes used for nerve pain) and old-school antidepressants (now used as muscle relaxants). I filled two bathroom cabinets with drugs: ibuprofen, diclofenac, naproxen, gabapentin, tramadol, amitriptyline, pregabalin, co-codamol, Vicodin, celecoxib, dexketoprofen. Some of them did nothing; others took the edge off, but shut down my brain at the same time. Nausea, dizziness, brain fog, dry mouth, memory loss, vivid dreams, halitosis, headaches, suicidal ideation, faecal impaction and overflow diarrhoea. The better the pills worked, the worse their side effects. My life disintegrated.

I did physio exercises four times a day, but they aggravated the pain. I practised pacing until I could sit and walk for five-minute stretches, both major achievements. At the recommendation of the rheumatologist, I fixated on remedial pilates – but although my body felt slightly less susceptible to the background aches and pains that had scored my whole life, none of it helped my arm. The fire ants were still doing their circuits, the carving knife was still wedged in my armpit, and my neck still felt like I was balancing a lorry on it. In fact, more often than not, the exercises made the pain worse.

It was beginning to spread, too – creeping up my skull and across my back, millimetre by millimetre. There was talk of my developing Complex Regional Pain Syndrome, or CRPS – dubbed 'the suicide disease' by doctors, because its progression, starting with nerve pain in one limb and leaching inexorably through the body, is unbearable for many patients. I was also showing signs of allodynia – when nerve endings on the skin which report touch and pressure morph into pain receptors, meaning the gentlest touch can be agony. Brushing my arm against someone on the bus would spark a neural explosion. Off came the jewellery – the slimmest necklace felt like an anchor round my neck. The only clothes with sleeves I could tolerate were soft cottons and fluffy hoodies: patient-wear. Of all the tiny attacks on my identity, the one on my wardrobe was the most overt.

There were only two things that helped the pain. Half a bottle of wine would tone it down nicely, as would a hit of some medical marijuana mouthspray, which I'd tried in California. But, long-term, I didn't want to go down either of those roads.

The doctors gave up on me. Not my GP, Dr Good, who was steadfast in his support, writing off a new referral or prescription every couple of weeks; but the specialists he was sending me to. The more desperate I got, the more indifferent they became. Thinking it might help to make my invisible illness visible, I did away with shampoo, makeup, dress sense and my English reserve. If I weep at them, I reasoned – if I show them my desperation and beg for their help – they'll take me more seriously. But the more I cried, the more they smiled politely, proffered tissues and sent me on my way. Months later, I learned about Yentl Syndrome: a modern version of the Victorian preoccupation with female 'hysteria', in which male doctors are less likely to prescribe adequate painkillers for women than men, and more likely to dismiss female pain as psychological. *I am a doctor, dear, and I know.* Perkins Gilman wrote *The Yellow Wallpaper* in 1892, yet 120 years on, it felt like little had changed.

They treated me not as a patient, but as a statistic; they wanted to diagnose but not to cure. While I was wholly under the care of western medicine, living with its insistence that I would never get better, not a day went by when I didn't think about killing myself. Coming out of every miserable appointment, a part of me would long to be hit by a bus. After seven months of relentless negativity, I realised I needed something more. I would continue with the doctors, but I wouldn't pin my hopes on them. Those I would pin to a miracle.

It was in Georgia that I first turned to God. An editor friend had flown me to New York (officially to dictate a 600-word article, but actually to cheer me up), but, knowing I couldn't cope with the city in my state, I had carried on south to Savannah, where I found a quiet B&B run by an elderly couple. I'd chosen it because it was cheap, but I began to wonder whether it had chosen me when, over breakfast on my first morning, Robin – an eightysomething Anglophile sporting a velvet burgundy dressing gown and Gandalf beard – started talking, apropos of nothing, about healing.

He spoke of a woman he'd known, decades earlier, who could cure any ailment instantly. He told me how, 20 years before, his dog had 'taken on' his heart defect and died in Robin's place. Everyone has the power to heal, he told me. Once, cutting logs high up in the mountains, he had fallen and broken his tibia clean in two; he would have died had he not knitted it back together through the power of thought, enabling him to drive to hospital.

'You should come to my church,' he said, when I told him about my pain. 'We have a healing service on Tuesday; it's very powerful.' I was meant to be leaving that morning, but he urged me to stay, so I did. Could fate really have brought me my miracle so quickly? I'd always believed in God – or, at least, a god – at my core, and I believed in an afterlife, too. But I disliked the idea of the church and, somehow, found the concept of an individual endowed with miraculous powers easier to believe in than a congregation of mere mortals praying to a system I wasn't sure I didn't despise.

'I think it worked,' said Robin as we came out. It didn't, but it had sparked something in me. Robin, I decided, was the first step on my journey, an Ariadne figure handing me a spool of thread. It would be up to me to navigate my way out of the darkness.

It turned out soon enough that the thread led somewhere, too. Robin's church was affiliated to one in London which, in turn, was an offshoot from a shrine in Norfolk: Walsingham, one of the best known pilgrimage sites in medieval Christendom. I couldn't afford to fly round the world in search of a miracle, but here was a miracle-giving spring a day away from London. I had never been one for signs (at least, not then – soon I would be noticing signs with every gasp of hope), but Robin had flipped a switch. It was too neat to be a coincidence.

At the London branch I collared a priest and told him everything. I looked as unhinged as I had for all my hospital appointments, and I cried at him, too. But unlike all those other figures of authority, instead of fobbing me off, he sat me down and asked how I was coping. Instead of acting like he had worthier people to serve, he told me to pop by whenever I wanted. He gave me his phone number and asked whether I was surviving financially. 'Don't worry,' he said.

'We *will* get you to Walsingham. Keep in touch and I'll let you know when our next trip is.' He said he believed in miracles and thought the shrine could help me, asked my permission to pray for me, and urged me to stay in touch.

But I was scared he'd let me down, so I never contacted him again.

I did get to Walsingham, though. Two months later, I was in Norfolk for a wedding, staying with friends who happened to live eight miles from the spring. Still in the optimistic, early months of my quest, I was sure it was another sign, so I went up a day early to fit in my healing before the ceremony.

The vicar in London had told me that there was a well in the church, whose water you could use to anoint yourself. I could do this quietly, privately, I had thought. I wouldn't have to get embarrassed or tearful at anyone; whether it did or didn't work, nobody would ever know.

The well was down some steps, a brick semicircle dug in at crypt level. There was a pitcher of water with a giant ladle beside it, but a barricade in front.

'Can I help you?' said a voice from the gloaming. A tiny priest was eyeing me accusatorily. 'The church is closing now,' he snapped. It was December, dark at 4pm.

I told him I'd been sent by his colleagues in London and Savannah, that I just wanted some water. He softened instantly. 'Is the water for you?' he asked. 'What do you want it for?'

'A miracle,' I sniffed. 'I know it's stupid but they told me I could get a miracle here.'

He moved the barricade aside. 'What do you think a miracle is?' he asked, and I silently screamed, *like I came here for theological discussion.*

'I don't know,' I said, sourly. 'It's a cure, isn't it? Like Jesus waving his magic wand.' Suddenly I was desperate to leave, to run to my happy, pain-free friends and wedding champagne in a warm pub two villages away.

He nodded, and led me down the steps. He swilled the ladle around in the water, took a scoop and held it out to me like a goblet of communion wine. Tactfully, he looked away as I dribbled it over my neck and rubbed it into my armpit. Just do it already, I told the universe, because I can't live like this any more.

'I do believe in miracles,' he said thoughtfully. 'I've seen several here. But a miracle isn't always what you think it is.'

'In what way?' I muttered, but I wasn't sure I wanted to hear.

'I've never seen someone be instantly healed,' he said. 'There are no biblical miracles here. But I have seen times when God has given people the strength to cope with their burden. That's what I think a miracle is – gaining the strength to cope.'

That word again: 'cope'. It wasn't what I'd come for.

'Maybe,' I said. 'Thanks.' I slouched out, wanting, needing more, and he locked the door behind me. As I walked to my car, I prayed again. Screw strength, I told God, and screw this acceptance that the doctors are smothering me with. What I need is a cure – I need my arm back. And the second I said it – and I swear this really happened – every single street light in Walsingham was suddenly snuffed out. A sign?

I would think back to that priest again and again over the following years, threading through his words like worry beads. Should I have listened and saved myself the heartbreak? Or was it fear of his words that kept me alive? I don't know. I don't know I ever will.

But that night, I drove to the pub with terrifying confidence. I knew I would prove him wrong.

A STARTER MIRACLE

*When the doctors did no good she had climbed
stairs all over town to rooms where incense burned
and where men or women in traffic with the devil
gave her white powders, or herbs to make tea, and
cast spells upon her to take the sickness away.*
James Baldwin, *Go Tell It on the Mountain* (1953)

The person who eventually gave me my life back was an angel therapist called Kevin, who I met exactly two years and two weeks after my injury.

The odds were inauspicious. He charged twice the local going rate, and worked out of a darkened booth at the back of a Los Angeles nail salon. But I was desperate for a cure, and willing to pay anyone who claimed they might be able to help me.

After two years shuffling from consultation to consultation, my conventional options were by now all but exhausted. I had seen a pain management consultant – an anaesthetist who sedated me three times to give me epidural nerve blocks, two with anaesthetic, and one with pulsed light. We cancelled the fourth, because the first three had made no difference and there was a small chance each could end in paralysis.

I had seen another, very eminent rheumatologist, who had taken more interest in the Italian book I was reading than my body, and, once we had discussed 'il bel paese', as he insisted on calling it, asked me, 'What can we do to get you back to work?'

'Well, I'd really like a referral to a neurologist to see where this nerve pain is coming from,' I said. 'And some physio on my neck and arm.'

'Oh, but you already had six sessions of physio this year,' he said.

'That was on my bum,' I said. (I had been prescribed lower-limb physio to see if that would help my aching legs, and it had turned into six miserable weeks of glute exercises.)

'Yeeees,' he hummed. 'Perhaps that was a mistake? Come back in a year's time, and if you're still off work we'll consider more then.' I waited 51 weeks for that second appointment and then, right before we were due to meet, I discovered he'd retired some months earlier and I'd been erased from the clinic. A re-referral to his replacement took another four months.

I had seen a second gastroenterologist, who'd run more tests and declared there to be absolutely nothing wrong with me. I had seen an endocrinologist, who'd suspected Addison's disease after routine tests showed dangerously low levels of cortisol. Soon after, I was rushed to A&E with suspected adrenal failure and pumped full of steroids, but after three months my levels bounced back to normal and he declared himself mystified. At the time, I attributed it to the healing power of reiki; later, I realised I'd come off some pain pills around the time of my miraculous recovery. Since each consultant had been interested only in his niche diagnosis, nobody had been monitoring the bigger picture.

I had seen one dentist who'd declared my neck pain to be coming from tooth-grinding, and charged me £600 for a mouth splint. Another thought my misaligned jaw might be the culprit, and referred me for an operation, but the surgical team said that even if they sliced off part of my face, realigned it and sewed it back up, however functional my bite would become, there was no guarantee it would solve the pain.

I had seen two hand therapists who'd diagnosed previously unnoticed issues with my wrists and fingers – 'deformed', one called my curly left pinky – and given me strengthening exercises for them, which made the arm pain worse.

I'd seen another expensive physio who thought perhaps

the problem was coming from weak eyes, and an ophthalmologist who said my eyes were fine. I'd been put on a daily arm exercise programme by a ruthless 'rehabilitation consultant' appointed by my work insurance, which was getting tired of paying out half my salary every month. The exercises aggravated everything, but she wouldn't let me stop. The flare-ups came weekly.

I'd tried NHS acupuncture, which did absolutely nothing. I'd had 'adjustment counselling' from a fierce lady in my GP's basement, and therapy (or what was supposed to be therapy) from a psychologist paid for by my employer's insurance. His name was Dr Jannie Van Der Merwe, and he was the only one I liked.

Jannie was a chronic pain specialist and, unlike his colleagues, he believed me. From the first appointment, he made it clear that he had no doubt that my pain was real, and that it was having a debilitating effect on my life. Even though he was paid by the insurance company and worked in tandem with their rehabilitation consultant, I trusted him.

After the priest I'd run away from, Jannie was the first person to treat me as an equal. Although he was being paid to teach me CBT, he accepted that I loathed it, so instead he gave me six months of science lessons. Where the pain management team had issued the edict that we'd never get better, Jannie taught me the neurology of pain to explain why that was the accepted view. Where other doctors had declared me unhelpable, Jannie showed that this wasn't a reflection on me, but a reminder that science didn't understand everything. Jannie, though, worked with chronic pain patients every day, he reassured me. And his experience indicated that it was possible to get better.

It wasn't a given, he levelled with me – 'better' didn't mean 'well', and the attempt would be the hardest thing I'd ever done. I would have to keep it up every day for the rest of my life, and there was no guarantee that I would ever make a complete recovery. But Jannie believed that if I worked at it, physically and mentally – tried to flip my old neural pathways back into action – I could eventually live a relatively normal life again.

I spent six months with Jannie reading books about pain and neurology, bombarding him with questions and testing theories that I would come up with. As well as giving me a grasp on what was wrong with me, our studies were also a much needed confidence boost. After 18 months of being treated like a child by the medical profession, here was someone who allowed me some authority. For the first time, I realised that even if the pain did turn out to be in my head – and neither of us knew whether it was – it wasn't anything to be ashamed of, it wasn't my fault, and it wasn't any less real.

Those last six months before I met Kevin were hellish. My employers, having long since given my job away, were scrambling to find me another position. The insurers, presumably sick of paying out, were trying to rule me fit for work. The rehabilitation consultant was drawing up start dates for a week's time even though I was still signed off indefinitely. Jannie was my rock through all of it. He gave me back my self-belief and crushed my underlying fear – planted by all those doctors over all those months – that I was making it up. I'm still not sure I'd have made it without him.

In the March of my second year of pain, I saw a third rheumatologist. He took me more seriously than his predecessors, admitted that my care so far had been less than ideal, listened from scratch to my symptoms, and suggested I might have something called thoracic outlet syndrome, where the main nerve to your arm is compressed at a crucial channel, resulting in constant pain. I was ecstatic – finally, a breakthrough – and sobbed my way triumphantly through another stifling MRI.

He'd promised to call and talk me through the results the following week, but in the end I heard nothing from him for four months. His letter was waiting for me on my return from LA: there was nothing abnormal about this pleasant lady's thoracic outlet, it read (though she did, by the way,

have a thyroid tumour which should probably be investigated); he was therefore discharging her from his clinic.
Luckily, by that time I'd already met Kevin, and didn't care
about doctors any more.

I'd also, by then, met Stella – my fifth physiotherapist since
my pain had started, and the only person in the medical
profession who, during those two years, provided a diagnosis
that made any kind of sense. She was in Cornwall, which
meant that although she'd been recommended to me several
times previously, I had dismissed her. Everyone knew the
care was best in London, I scoffed; for months, despite living
with my mum, I'd insisted on travelling to the capital for
treatment.

But one day, during a vet's appointment to get my cat's
claws cut (at 20, Miffy could no longer sharpen her own),
I got talking to Victoria, a nurse I'd known for years. I told
her about my pain, and she insisted I call Stella. 'All the girls
here go to her,' she said. 'The surgery couldn't run without
her!' Her colleague even paid me a house call to evangelise
about her. Katie was back at work after two months off with
chronic jaw pain, she told me; it was Stella who had made
it go away.

I saw Stella a couple of weeks before I went to LA. She
assessed me and immediately suggested I had thoracic outlet
syndrome, as the third rheumatologist had done. I told her I
was still waiting for the results of the MRI, but warned her
that my posh London physio had dismissed the idea. She
had already 'tested' for thoracic outlet syndrome by holding
my arm in the air and seeing if the pulse in my wrist disappeared, and it hadn't.

Stella pushed back. Neither test nor MRI was conclusive –
they were looking for bone spurs constricting the nerve, but
tight muscles could have the same effect. She showed me that
my shoulders craned skywards when I lay on my back, and
that the muscles were so tight they'd heaved my second rib
out of place. Finally, a physical clue to my pain – one that in
two years, nobody else had noticed. After Charmayne, Stella

was my second wise woman. I went to California with her words ringing in my ears.

Ostensibly, I was going to LA to cat-sit for a friend: free accommodation, flights slapped on my bulging credit card. I would relax in the sun for three weeks before returning to London, at which point we would start drawing up a plan for a return to work. I had discussed the trip with my rehabilitation consultant, and she had ruled it an excellent idea. Jannie, too, thought it was the best thing I could do. I had already confided in him that there was no way I could return to my old job after the way I'd been treated, even if I did make a miraculous recovery. The past few months had turned me into a nervous wreck, and I had developed an unfortunate Pavlovian response: a panic attack every time a job-related email dropped into my inbox. I was desperate to work again, Jannie understood, but I couldn't do *that* work. He thought going away would buy me some clarity.

I arrived in LA crippled by the 11-hour flight, and awoke the next day feeling like I'd been in a car accident. The cat jumped on top of me and it felt like a cannonball against my ribcage. I wondered how I would ever make it back.

A massage might help, I decided – Stella had said it was all about the muscles. 'Best massage North Hollywood', I googled. Across all the review sites, there was one name that kept popping up.

I nearly didn't call. His website was sickeningly New Age – as well as massage and reiki, he offered angel card-reading and 'loving guidance'. But I was in too much pain to find an alternative, and I figured an angel therapist was unlikely to damage me with an unnecessarily deep tissue massage. Three hours later, I was at the salon, filling in his medical history form.

I had seen dozens of these over the past few years. Are you claustrophobic, they would ask. Do you have allergies? Please list any medical conditions you have. Could you be pregnant? Have you been drinking?

Kevin's form was different. It had the normal health questions, but then it went on.

'Do you believe in angels?' it asked. 'Yes', 'No' and 'Unsure' sat beside it, waiting to be circled. I ticked 'Unsure'.

'Have you ever received energy treatment?' it continued. That was easy – I was a reiki fiend. I circled 'Yes'.

'List three things/people you are grateful for,' it finished. There were three blank lines below. I wrote:

1: My mum
2: My cat (20 yrs old!!)
3: My work skills (now I just want to be able to work again)

I was chortling at his specialities – angels, meditation, auras, chakras, self-healing, law of attraction, crystals – when he bounded up.

He didn't look like a Kevin; even less like a healer. He was early thirties, a meathead extra from *Jersey Shore*: head shaved and over-inflated biceps ballooning out of his sleeves, making his arms as stumpy as a T-rex and blocking them from resting by his sides. He wore the unprepossessing uniform of the young American male: tight white T-shirt, beige cargo shorts. I could better imagine him ogling himself in gym mirrors than channelling angels. I would die, I decided, if, during the next hour, he saw me naked.

He led me to his cupboard at the back of the salon, a tiny room with dimmed lights trying to disguise a plywood ceiling. There was a cod ethnic curtain draped across the glass door, a lamp masquerading as a translucent crystal, a framed print-out of his aura reading next to his massage credentials on the wall, and a pencil sketch of a long-haired, slightly wild-eyed man on the counter.

'Who's that?' I asked. He looked confused.

'It's Jesus,' he said, and rolled up his sleeve to show me a doppelganger tattooed across his right arm and shoulder. He had a black panther on the other side, too, he said. It was his 'totem animal'.

I told him I just wanted something gentle to unstick me from the flight. I asked him to go easy on my right arm, as there was a trapped nerve there. I had been off work for two years because of the pain, I said, and even the doctors couldn't help, so please don't try anything weird. He asked what the diagnosis was, and I said nobody really knew but the latest suggestion was thoracic outlet syndrome. He had no idea what that was. Why would he?

It probably wouldn't feel like a normal massage, he warned, because, unlike most therapists, he didn't have set moves. Instead, the angels told him what to do. I scoffed inwardly. And then he started.

Massage, deconstructed, was how I described it later. There was no smearing of oil or butterfly shapes traced on my spine. Instead, he flipped me onto my back and homed straight in on my right collarbone: one of the 'trigger points' which Stella had identified as a problem area, but which nobody else – no massage therapist, physio, chiropractor, doctor or consultant – had ever looked at twice. He turned me back over to work into the shoulder blade, not crunching the knots with his elbow, as most people did, but smoothing things out, firm yet pain-free. At some points he stroked a crystal across my skin; at others, he just dug his thumb in and yawned theatrically. Sometimes he would wiggle his finger into my flesh, as if he were practising vibrato. Every now and then he'd exhale fast, like he was blowing out a candle.

At the end of it, I felt transformed: not healed, but better than I could ever have imagined feeling after a single treatment. Although the pain wasn't gone, it was as if Kevin had implanted me with the memory of feeling well again, and somehow I knew without a doubt that a corner had been turned. I didn't believe in his guiding angels, but it didn't matter that I didn't, because whatever he'd done had worked.

I was ravenously hopeful for what he could do next. But it took a while to get him to allow me another appointment.

'I think you need to wait and see how it goes,' he told me on the way out, as I quizzed him on his availability for the rest of the week.

'But I feel amazing,' I pleaded. 'I feel so much better!'

'But I want to check whether that's temporary before I take any more money from you,' he said firmly, and told me to call him in three days.

The following morning, I woke up to an email. It was a link to a YouTube video, discussing constriction of the C7 nerve – the one I had damaged, according to the nerve conduction studies from two years earlier.

'This is the exact spot where the muscles I was working on were inflamed,' he had written. 'I think this is what you are dealing with. The guy also goes on to say that massage will only give temporary relief.' And Kevin, of course, wasn't interested in that.

'I just don't think it's ethical to take your money if I don't believe I can really help you,' he said when I called, the second I had read the email. 'What would you gain from another massage if it'll go back to what it was in a couple of days?'

'Kevin,' I said sternly – for I had found The One, and wasn't going to let him go without a fight. 'Who's the person who believes in miracles?' And I heard him smile.

It was so good, his angel therapy, that I came back six times in three weeks. By the end of it, I had begun to work a little. I was driving round LA, going for mini hikes in the canyons, and the pain stayed in remission through it all. I wasn't healed, of course – the fire ants would stir if I did too much, and I could sense the crushing weight looming over my neck if I didn't keep up my stretching sessions and thrice-hourly lie-downs – but, after two years of flailing blindly for it, I had taken hold of my life again. Or, rather, Kevin had handed it back to me.

The transformation wasn't confined to the physical, either; decisions were easier to take now that my brain was no longer slicked in pain. I resigned from my job, found a part-time gig I could do from home, and decided that home would be Cornwall, not London. As Jannie had predicted, with distance had come clarity. Finally, the fog was beginning to recede and I could make out the road ahead.

'It's astonishing,' said Stella as I lay on her table for my first post-Kevin appointment. 'If I hadn't assessed you last time, I honestly couldn't have believed you'd been as bad as you were. It's as if you have a completely different body.'

'Do you mind me asking what you put your recovery down to?' said a consultant, two months later. 'It's just that from your notes, I was expecting a very sick person. I had to double-check we'd called the right one in.'

'Interesting,' said Dr Good when I skipped into my monthly check-up and told him I'd signed myself back on without asking his permission. 'I reckon for about eight out of 10 of my patients without an obvious diagnosis, it's all down to stress. Do you think it was a case of you relaxing enough to let something work, and everything spiralling from there?'

It was, of course, but I was sure there was something more to it, too. Several times, I'd been relaxed enough for a therapy to work; several times, I'd been convinced that the next treatment, whether medical or alternative, was going to heal me. In fact, several times, I'd even made headway; once, deep in a meditative trance, I'd even managed to unhook myself from the pain entirely for a few blissful minutes.

But each time, sooner or later, things had fallen back into their neurologically unsound place – either the effects had worn off, or I'd started to doubt myself. How could reiki possibly be working, I'd wonder. How could mindfulness actually shut down my nociceptors? And, once I'd tasted that grain of doubt, each time I'd thudded straight back down to earth.

I vowed not to doubt Kevin, though, and the pain largely stayed in remission. There were good days and bad, of course – a flight to Singapore, one of my first new work trips, slammed me back into my original levels of pain for two terrifying weeks – and I was still far from capable of working full-time, but overall it was manageable. Sessions with Stella, who did excruciating deep needling of the muscles, kept it under control; and I continued the scientific reading that I'd started with Jannie. With the pain on a more even keel, I started to want more.

Kevin may not have cured me entirely, but he had shown me that alternative therapists could do better than doctors; that people who believed in angels could care more, change more, than the men in white coats. That it wasn't insane to think that if a guy with a Jesus tattoo could get me this far, there could be someone out there who could go a step further.

I wouldn't give up on doctors – I still believed that science was capable of achieving more than it had up to now. But Kevin was my starter miracle. And he made me hungry for a real one.

I AM A DOCTOR, DEAR

You see he does not believe I am sick!
Charlotte Perkins Gilman, *The Yellow Wallpaper* (1892)

The reason all those experts were convinced my pain was just a flare-up of my underlying condition is because of my medical history. Girthy is the word for it, though I don't think the thickness of the file is down to the severity of my illness. Actually, I put it down to those same experts and their joy of diagnosis.

Look at my medical records and they'll tell you I have Ehlers-Danlos Syndrome. EDS type three, to be precise, otherwise known as EDS hypermobility type. Joint Hyper-mobility Syndrome was another term for it in 2012 when I was diagnosed – in fact, that's what my rheumatologist's letter said at the time. She told me they were interchangeable terms, just a matter of semantics; today, they're seen as different conditions. I've never been told which I have, though. Or whether I have any of them at all.

Depending on which doctor you discuss me with, I might also have Postural Orthostatic Tachycardia Syndrome, TMJ, fibromyalgia, ME, CRPS, migraines, IBS, anxiety, Benign Paroxysmal Positional Vertigo, chronic fatigue, and a gluten intolerance (experts are divided on whether gluten intolerance actually exists, but there's no room for shades of grey in medical records).

We shouldn't forget the pain of course – but depending who you ask, my chronic pain is either a disorder in itself or merely a symptom of something else. My COPE team, after all, would tell you it's just a flare-up of my EDS – even

46

after four years, when flare-ups usually last a maximum two weeks.

So many diagnoses, or misdiagnosed so many times?

I was born bendy. My childhood party tricks included trimming my toenails with my teeth, pulling my fingers back 90 degrees at the knuckles and excavating my nose with my tongue. I could contort my body into poses yoga bitches can only dream of, but it wasn't all Cirque du Soleil stuff. I was flat-footed, knock-kneed and pigeon-toed, and bullied relentlessly because of it, even by my friends. Being 'double-jointed' – because hypermobility wasn't a thing in the nineties – was cool only as long as it wasn't freakish.

One of my earliest memories was at some doctor's surgery – I must have been about four. My mother had taken me in because she was disturbed by the way I used to sit: on the floor, semi-kneeling, calves splayed out to either side. Nowadays, that's one of the textbook flags for hypermobility – you'd put a kid like that through physio immediately – but back then, the doctor dismissed her as an over-worrier.

At 13, I fractured my left wrist and it never recovered. With hindsight, I know that putting a hypermobile limb in a cast is the worst possible treatment, weakening already unstable joints; back then, nobody could explain my phantom pain. My mother even dragged me to London to a special NHS 'musicians' clinic', because I'd been pretty good at the violin, and one of the more tangible side effects of the fracture was that I could no longer play it. I remember a team of doctors sitting round a table, making me perform my circus tricks. 'Definitely hypermobile,' said one – it was the first time I'd heard the word. Yet they discharged me with neither explanation nor diagnosis, and I never played again.

My left arm withered and became unusable; then, just before my A Levels, the right one went – throbbing to the bone with relentless cramps. Must be RSI, said the orthopaedic surgeon, because X-rays and ultrasounds showed nothing. I got through my exams thanks to a homeopath in Truro: before every paper, he'd put electrodes on my arm, immerse it in water, and turn on the current, Russian roulette by TENS machine. Inside, I got extra time and wrote with special fat pens and old-person grips. I still do.

At university I discovered the miracle of computers: typing was a hundred times less painful than handwriting. I could do all the work I wanted – which, at the time, was only a few hours per week. In my last year, when I had to do more, my arms went again. I dictated my dissertation and my finals, too, but at least that meant I got to do them in a room of my own, wearing normal clothes rather than the Harry Potter robes everyone else had to wear.

By that point, something else had happened: I'd contracted glandular fever, and it had never left. After two years, it was reclassified as ME. At the ME clinic (which, I later discovered, was part of the mental health unit), they put me on antidepressants 'because they improve the quality of sleep'. It wasn't until my COPE course that it was explained to me that, back then, ME was classed as a mental disorder.

My arm improved after university, but not completely. I worked in a shop but couldn't stack shelves or man the till, so I didn't last long. I trained as a journalist, and was given special dispensation to skip shorthand. I had flare-ups when I started work, but with weekly physio and regular massage, I kept it in check (secretly of course – what kind of journalist can't type?). The ME had shuffled off, but it had left its markers: I was permanently exhausted, needing six coffees and three chocolate bars a day to stay awake. Of course, I got fat.

My limbs ached all the time, my head and neck too. I took to having a bath every night, an old lady in my twenties. Next, I developed crippling vertigo, or BPPV. Nobody knew why, although one specialist put it down to migraines. But I don't get headaches! I protested. Oh I think you do, he said. You just aren't aware of them.

I am a doctor, dear, and I know.

I lost my job in London and moved to Vegas in search of work and rebirth. There, amongst the showgirls and go-go dancers, I resolved to lose the chocolate-induced pounds. I started walking in the desert every day; then I started running. But every time I ran, I'd injure one or the other of my knees. They'd always made strange clicking noises with every step, but this pain was new. I stopped running – but then it started happening when I wasn't running. By the time I moved back to London, 18 months later, one or the other of my knees would go after just 10 minutes on my feet.

One of my first acts on coming home was to see a doctor. 'I can't walk more than half a mile without my knee giving out,' I said. He stared at the screen. 'Hmm,' he said, prescribing ibuprofen gel. 'You've just turned 30. I'm afraid this is part of the ageing process.' In retrospect, my pain was at the early, abortable stage of gestation. But he didn't catch it.

A couple of months later, starting a new job (the website one) fired up the arm symptoms, so I went back. My knees are still hurting, I said, plus I need some physio on my arm. I had moved up a tax bracket with the new salary, and become a ball-breaker.

Maybe it was my attitude or maybe today was a good day, because this time he took me seriously. As he inspected my arm, he noted that it was long. He checked my wingspan (wide) and my palate (high), then asked if I could bend over and touch my toes. Easy, I said – I can even do that with my knees bent back the wrong way. (No one had told me that joints bending the wrong way wasn't normal.)

'Hmm,' he said this time. 'I wonder...'

Six months later, I was standing in front of a rheumatologist, who stripped me to my underwear and inspected my body. From my posture and my gait, it was obvious, she announced. I had Joint Hypermobility Syndrome, otherwise known as Ehlers-Danlos Syndrome type three.

In essence, EDS is a genetic condition that causes faulty collagen – it's too stretchy, like an elastic band that's been used one too many times and doesn't snap back into shape. Collagen forms all our connective tissue, from the blood vessels to the ligaments, which means that EDS is an all-encompassing illness.

Your ligaments exist, but they're effectively useless – too stretchy to hold your joints in place. That's why 'double-jointed' people can ply thumb to forearm and do the splits, but it's also why the most innocent action can dislocate or subluxate their joints – like the time my shoulder popped out as I wiped down the hob, or when my neck went while I was parallel parking. Of course, what slips out so easily can also slide back in before a doctor takes a look, so though the damage is done, you've no proof of it happening. The best theory anyone has for why reaching for a cup of coffee ended my life is that some anonymous joint in my neck must have fallen out of place and onto a nerve. But – EDS is unsettling – nobody actually knows.

With EDS, since your ligaments don't work, your muscles have to work overtime to hold your joints in place. They feel like they're running a marathon a day, and they get tight, knotted and swollen – that's where the all-over joint pain and exhaustion comes from.

The other place EDS has taken its toll on me is my ability to stand. I have a heart condition, I tell people when I ask for a seat on a bus, because that's the easy thing to say when they're glaring at you. Technically, though, POTS – or Postural Orthostatic Tachycardia Syndrome – is just a condition that affects my heart. Since our blood vessels are made of connective tissue, EDSers' blood vessels are baggy. They don't pump the blood effectively round the body, and they let the blood pool in our feet at any opportunity (this is where my 'massive weird feet', as a school friend once thoughtfully called them, come from). So if we're standing still – in a supermarket queue, say, or in an art gallery – the blood pools, the brain starts feeling starved and tells the heart to pump faster and faster. We feel dizzy, and then we pass out. That's why I don't go to galleries any more.

That's why I needed a Kevin.

NOT YOUR AVERAGE GURU

All of us can change ... we can be made foreign
to ourselves, suddenly, by illness, accident,
misadventure or hormonal caprice.
Hilary Mantel (1952- : endometriosis patient, writer)

Nine months after I met Kevin, I was on a flight from Gatwick to Newquay, crossing the country in 50 minutes. That wasn't fast enough for me, though, as I was flying back with a mission: to heal my ailing Miffy with the skills I'd just been taught by a man called Patrick San Francesco. To take my mind off the task ahead, I was leafing through a list of Balinese healers that a hippy friend had sent me – in six weeks, I would be in Ubud, ready for my miracle – and my eyes were cramping with the stress. Who would cure me, was I capable of saving Miffy? I switched to the book I was reading: *The Death of Ivan Ilyich*, a novella by Tolstoy about a man who succumbs to inexplicable illness after a risibly minor accident. Nobody – not doctors, friends nor family – can understand what's happened to him or why he's wasting away and, eventually, he dies. Obviously, I thought Tolstoy had written it for me.

I had got to the part where Ivan Ilyich, having run through various doctors without success, turns to alternative medicine. A homeopath delivers yet another hypothesis about his illness, and gives him sugar pills that don't work. Next, he overhears someone talking about the healing power of religious icons.

'Ivan found himself listening carefully and believing the reality of this,' wrote Tolstoy. 'This incident frightened him. "Have I really become so feeble-minded?" he said to himself.

"What rubbish! It's all nonsense. I mustn't give in to hypochondria."'

I set the book down, pretended to study Exmoor 20,000 feet below, and wept silently. Then I remembered I hadn't sent my daily email to Patrick. I grabbed my phone and quickly drafted it, so it would send the minute we landed.

Everyone knows that mysticism begins with India. 'Miracles? They happen every day there,' Ajay, the owner of a holistic resort in Cyprus, had told me. Ajay had introduced me to mindfulness when I'd stayed at Zening during an early low ebb – it was under his instruction that I'd unhooked myself from the pain for a few heavenly minutes. A year later I returned, informed him he was now my guru, and asked where to find a miracle. I'd got the contract for this book, you see, and was convinced it was my ticket back to health. Not only was I sure that every doctor and healer in the world would clamour to speak to me (as it turned out, they mostly ignored me), but I had money for the first time since the coffee incident – not a lot, but enough to cover flights. Suddenly, the entire globe was open to me, and it was as obvious to me as to Ajay where I had to start. Then it got even easier. I didn't have to go to India, it turned out. India would come to me.

Patrick San Francesco is not your average guru. Half Dutch, half Goan-Rajasthani, he was raised Catholic and started talking to God at the age of four. Even more unusually, God talked back. Patrick Jr healed his family, his friends, his neighbours. His fame began to spread throughout India – even by the standards of the land of miracles, he was extraordinary – then beyond. People started flocking to him from all over the world.

Today, Patrick San Francesco is the most modern of gurus. He flies round the globe giving masterclasses; he's abroad as often as at his base in Goa. He has a non-profit organisation and a YouTube channel. He runs live webchats and streams full moon meditation sessions. He's spoken at the United Nations and done reconciliation work in the Congo. His followers have their own groups and mailing lists in their different cities, states and countries. For reasons I don't really remember, I ended up on the Austrian mailing list, and suddenly one day I received an email announcing that Patrick would be in Vienna the following month.

It was fitting for Patrick to be the first person on my quest for a miracle that Kevin had sparked, because I was absolutely certain – at least, almost absolutely certain – that he had to be a fake.

On the face of it, of course, it made no sense. I was on this journey in order to be cured and I wanted to find that cure as quickly as possible. But that didn't stop me being frightened of what a cure might mean.

A miracle – in the shape of a Jesus figure who pointed his arm at me and magicked me better, immediately, effortlessly, permanently – would delete my personality as well as my pain. No more questioning, no more cynicism, no more agnosticism. No more sitting at the back feeling superior to the Kevins at the front. Omnipotence demands discipleship; a real miracle would mean a radical repositioning of all the beliefs that had made me *me*. I had no interest in finding myself; I only wanted to find a way back to my old self. I was going out into the world, desperately seeking something that terrified me.

At least I wouldn't be in for that with Patrick. His claims – or, rather, those of the people around him – were preposterous. He had cured cancer, they said. He had disappeared HIV. He had made the barren fertile and a flatlining heart beat again. When I asked Magdalena, the organiser of the Vienna meeting, how she'd met Patrick, she said he'd cured her eye problem. He'd been recommended to her by a friend whose cancer he'd made vanish into thin air. He *had* to be a con artist, I decided. That made him the perfect person to start with.

By the time I met him, though, I was desperate for him to be the real deal.

I'd gone for a walk in the Stadtpark beforehand – despite

my mantra, *this is bullshit, this is bullshit, this is bullshit*, I was feverish with hope that, against all odds, Patrick might be The One. I felt mildly panicked. A wad of anxiety had lodged in my throat.

I was at lunch when my mum called. 'Nicky's just left,' she said, sounding grim. 'I thought you'd want to know—'

The bottom of my stomach lurched away, George Clooney in *Gravity* pitching into nothingness.

Miffy was nearly 21, now, and she'd been reeling from crisis to crisis. First her kidneys were failing – but with medication, they rallied. Then they found a mass on her liver – a tumour, it had to be – but I'd called a friend who did long-distance reiki, and suddenly her liver function tests were back to normal. He'd sent her some more when she snapped a ligament in her foot, and yet again she had recovered. Nicky the vet had called it inexplicable.

This time, her lymph node had swelled up. Antibiotics did nothing but I wasn't worried – I knew Johnny would deal with it. He'd sent more reiki and I'd cupped my hand around it before I left for Vienna, sure it had shrunk. Her check-up was due the day I would meet Patrick.

The lump was bigger, Mum said. Nicky had measured it with her calipers. She thought the only thing it could be was cancer.

I left the money on the table along with my food, and walked through the park on jelly legs. Back at my hotel I lay on the bed, gulping down the air but unable to breathe. Go to Patrick, my mum told me. Forget Miffy and focus on yourself. You went to Vienna to see if he can help you.

I can't, I said. My hands were shaking so hard I could barely hold the phone.

But maybe Patrick can help her too, said my mum – ever the pro at cajoling me to do what I needed to do. And I thought, yes, what if he can? So I washed my swollen face, put on a top that had cats on it – in case it would sub-consciously channel healing energy – and went.

We met in a gallery just off the Ringstrasse. It was silent

when I arrived, a heavy door barely ajar and uninviting. I wanted to run away – the road ahead was suddenly yawning in front of me, and I realised it had no destination, that it just coiled round Mount Purgatory – but I told myself: I'm here for Miffy.

From what I could gather, Patrick was used to big groups at his workshops. Believers flocked to him in California, London and, of course, in Delhi, where he was famed for conducting mass healings of thousands at a time. Luckily for me – because nothing breeds suspicion like a populist healer – there were only about seven of us.

I introduced myself to Magdalena – she knew I had come all the way from England to be healed. 'You must meet Patrick!' she cried, beaming like a schoolgirl. She led me to a side room. Here he was, my first miracle man.

Lustrous black hair flowing down towards his waist. Salt-and-pepper facial hair. Hypnotic, almost black eyes. Jesus crossed with Russell Brand.

Even at first glance, my hackles rose.

He wore a nondescript, long-sleeved top under a neat gilet, smart ink-coloured jeans and trainers. He smiled with his mouth but stared with his eyes. He was small – slight, too – but with the gravitational pull of an A-lister.

'This is Julia,' said Magdalena, proudly. 'She's come from England.'

Patrick turned his imperious gaze on me.

'Do you mind if I take notes?' I stuttered.

'Of course not.' His voice was soft.

'I'll leave you alone,' said Magdalena.

Christ.

We stared at each other. What can I do for you, he asked, gravely. I'm in pain, I said. Where, he asked – *shouldn't you know?* flashed through my mind – and I put my left hand on my right arm, running it up and down as the allodynia crackled underneath. From my neck and my shoulder all the way down, I said.

He swayed gently on his legs, and glanced at the floor.

55

When he looked up, he'd crossed his left arm over his front and tucked his right arm over left wrist, index finger cocked up and at me like a Byzantine saint giving a blessing.

'You have a slightly compressed vertebra,' he said. 'Only at certain times, though, when it moves.' I felt the fire kindle under my shoulder blade. A sign?

Several specialists had said that what I really needed was a 'functional MRI' – a scan taken standing up instead of lying down – since bodies with EDS move differently from others. Parts that fan out gracefully lying down for a traditional scan might slide onto a nerve the moment gravity hits.

Not that I was going to tell him that. I held my poker stare.

'It's because the ligament is not working,' he said. 'So in certain positions, the vertebra is compressed.'

I tried not to blink. EDS was all about faulty ligaments, but I hadn't said anything about ligaments or EDS to Patrick.

'It's between the C4 and C5,' he added helpfully. I tried to hide my shock. Was this a cold reading or witchcraft?

Then he said, lighter this time, 'But it's okay – I've taken it away. What else?'

'My cat!' I blurted, gesturing frantically at my chest, desperate for him to be real. 'I wore this top so you could try and help.'

Patrick smiled inscrutably. When I started to cry, he kept smiling. I leaned against the table, on the verge of passing out, and whimpered something about her being my baby. He stared.

'What else?'

I flicked through my mental rolodex of health issues.

'Joint pain,' I said.

'You have Marfan syndrome,' he declared.

'Don't say that!' I screeched. 'It's serious!' Marfan's *is* serious – a connective tissue disorder that's related to EDS, but worse. Instead of causing stretchy skin and chronic pain, it can collapse lungs, detach retinas, tear aortas and prolapse mitral valves. It also has a signature look – tall, thin, sunken-chested, curved spine. The GP who'd first sent me off to be diagnosed had mooted Marfan's as well as EDS because I'm six foot, so I'd asked the rheumatologist and she'd said, 'No, you don't look like an alien.'

I couldn't have Marfan's because Marfan's could kill you.

'Don't worry,' Patrick said calmly, standing there, still pointing at me. 'I will heal it.' He looked at the ground. 'It's gone.'

'Can I record this?' I asked. I knew I wouldn't believe it unless I played it back.

'Why?' he said. 'I'm nobody.'

I told him numbly that my neck still hurt, and he told me to keep reminding him about it. 'In a few days, it will be better,' he declared, leading me out of the side room. As he walked to the front to address his audience, I noticed his jeans were Armani.

The room had filled during our absence: there were now about 20 people there, mostly middle-aged and earnest. They sat ramrod straight as Patrick walked to the front and I slouched at the back, embarrassed – the fangirl who'd demanded her healing before the party had even begun.

He sprinkled us with a smile. 'What would you like me to speak about? Mango pickle recipes? Rocket fuel?' He spoke in English, his accent as light as his tone. Magdalena giggled and translated into German.

'When I was four years old, my brother fell very sick,' he told us. 'The doctor said he wouldn't live. I had always been told that God would look after everything, and I was sad he wasn't looking after my brother. So in that innocence, I went outside and shouted – "FIX MY BROTHER!" Then I went back in and said to my family, "Don't worry." And he was fine.'

It spiralled from there. He'd come home from school and find people waiting for him, proffering their selves and their pets. 'They would say, "Patrick! Heal me!", and I'd say to God, "Whatever it is, fix it, so I can go play."' And God would fix it. At 17, Patrick was paralysed from the neck down; within a month he was walking again.

He used colours to heal, these days, he said – colours from another dimension, and celestial music, too. The Austrians nodded, rapt (I'd read that one in 10 Austrian GPs also practises homeopathy). How, I tried to unscramble, could he have taken one look at me and guessed the problem was my ligaments?

This talk was free, as was the healing – there was a donations box but it was placed so discreetly on a windowsill that later I'd walk out forgetting to add anything to it. I looked at the empty seats and wondered how he made his money. The workshop the next day – in which he'd teach us how to heal people ourselves – cost €125, but even if all 20 of us turned up, it'd barely cover expenses for a trip from Goa.

I wondered that night, over a plate of spätzle, whether he could be the real deal. But my pain was still there, so he couldn't be.

It was still there the following morning, too, when I arrived for the workshop, and I could tell I was an instant annoyance. I positioned myself at the back again, so my writhing would be invisible to the other recruits. 'Does it still hurt?' he asked quietly, walking past, and I grimaced and nodded. 'Don't worry,' he said. 'It will get better.' It didn't, though. I tried not to think about it but the more I tried to disengage – to decrease my somatic focus, as the doctors would say, because the more you focus on your symptoms, supposedly, the more you feel them – the deeper the knife in my armpit dug. I was a poor ambassador for his skills.

As Patrick taught us how to heal people, I began to piece together how I reckoned he did it. It was obvious, really, I decided. It was the same reason he'd said to me, 'What can I do for you?' instead of 'What's the problem?' or 'What's wrong?'. It was the placebo effect in all its potent glory. At least, that's how it seemed to me.

'When a patient comes to me, I say: "Tell me." I ask them to tell me what they think is wrong, what they want me to heal. Today, because of the internet, they think they already know. They've gone tap-tap-tap "I'VE GOT CANCER". I smile, I listen, and then I find out myself what's really wrong.'

He could heal masses at a time, he said, but preferred to treat people individually, because 'part of the therapy is allowing the patient to speak'. Listening to them, though, was just for show. By the time they've opened their mouths, he said, they're already healed.

Words were important. Never ask someone what's wrong, or talk down to them by offering to 'help'. Instead, we should be attentive but caring, listen carefully, and extract the maximum information in the minimum number of questions. After all, even Hippocrates knew that a good bedside manner amplifies the placebo effect. 'Some patients, though conscious that their condition is perilous, recover their health simply through their contentment with the goodness of the physician,' he wrote 2,400 years ago.

It wasn't all theatrics, though. Again and again during our six-hour masterclass, Patrick insisted that the healing was real, and being done by otherworldly forces.

'I don't heal anyone,' he said categorically. 'The energy heals, I'm merely the conduit. I will awaken you to the fact that you've been healing yourselves all along.' We were part of God, he said, and as such, we had the ability to heal ourselves. I clearly hadn't made a very good job of it, though. I turned my chair around, away from Patrick, to rest my head on the wall.

'When you walk out of this room,' he was saying, 'you'll be able to make a blind person see, a lame person walk. You'll have at your disposal universal energy, and with that you can do anything for anyone.' It wasn't instantaneous – cancer generally took a month, autoimmune disorders six – but it was definitive. Unless, of course – and here came the get-out clause – the illness was there to deliver us from this world to the next.

He took us through the six emotions that, he said, caused physical issues: anger, jealousy, fear, insecurity, sadness and stress. By scanning a patient's aura – standing a metre away and bringing our hand towards them until we hit the energy – we could tell which was dominant. They all feel different, you see – jealousy makes an aura clammy, for example, while a pulsating energy means anxiety.

As healers, we would identify the dominant negative emotion. Then we'd scan the patient by sweeping our hands down in front of the body three times: first to check the bones, then the skin, and finally the organs. We would feel the same sensations, but this time they signified different things: a presence, absence, infection, toxin or oxygen deficiency. Once we identified the health problem, all we had to do was pick an appropriate celestial colour and spin it at the other person's solar plexus. There were eight colours to choose from, each doing something different, from dilating to inhibiting, disintegrating or isolating (aura-healing, it seemed, was reasonably scientific). Then we'd seal up their solar plexus and they'd be done.

It was our turn. We practised groping each other's auras, scanning organs, diagnosing negative emotions and disease and then spinning them away. After lunch, Patrick physically manifested various illnesses in himself – cancer, arthritis, HIV, depression – and made us heal him, one by one.

'You are healers now,' he said at the end of the workshop. 'I have given you all the tools.'

He hung back at the end to finish some individual healings, and the rest of us milled around, attempting to feel each other's auras. I was flying home in a few hours, but I wanted to press him about Miffy – he hadn't responded the night before when I'd talked about her, but during his speech he'd looked at me darkly while explaining that every illness is curable other than the one that's destined to kill us.

It was almost as if he knew my plan, I thought half an hour later, as the clock hands inched towards my flight time. Somewhere in the Innere Stadt, my coach to Bratislava airport ('Vienna Bratislava' in Ryanair parlance) was pulling out of the central bus station; here in the gallery, Patrick was studiously avoiding my gaze as he attended to those who had nowhere to go. 'It's embarrassing,' he'd said the night before. 'I can read people's minds.'

As I attempted unsuccessfully to penetrate my neighbour's aura, I remembered my foot.

Five months earlier, in Burma (an add-on to my post-Kevin work trip to Singapore), something inexplicable had happened to my right foot. There'd been a short, sharp pain – a bite or a sting, it felt like, though when I'd looked there'd been nothing there. But the pain had stayed with me ever since, shooting me an electric shock every time I bent it, even to walk, almost as if there was a sting left inside. After four months, I'd gone to the doctor. I was waiting on the referral to a specialist when I went to Vienna.

'Oh! I should ask Patrick about my foot,' I thought out loud as Magdalena assessed my aura.

'What's wrong with it?' she asked.

'Guess,' I said, trying to eyeball Patrick.

She scanned my body: bones, skin, organs. 'There's definitely something there,' she said. 'In your right foot. It feels so swollen!' She called over another woman who scanned me tentatively and decided my ankle was giving off negative energy. 'Oh!', they squealed in unison as I rolled the leg of my jeans up for them. 'So swollen!' I toyed with explaining that fluid retention was part of my Condition (I had named it by now, now that I was stuck with it) – the other side was just as elephantine – but it felt like telling a child Father Christmas didn't exist.

I'd missed two buses by now, and even a taxi to Bratislava was pushing it, but Patrick was locked in another intense conversation. As I drilled my eyes into the back of his head, I prayed he was everything he said he was. I don't even care about myself, I said silently. You don't even have to heal me. Just. Heal. Miffy.

He looked up, and Magdalena rushed me over. 'You have to check out her foot!' she squeaked, excited.

'What's happened?' he said.

I don't need the therapy of vocalising it, I thought to him. I'd be far more impressed if you just told me what had happened.

'I think I was stung five months ago,' I said meekly. 'It still hurts when I flex the foot, like there's a sting still inside it.'

Patrick glanced down. 'A spider bite,' he said. 'It'll be healed within six months.'

'Six *months*?'

'Yes, or a month if I work on it,' he said.

The gauntlet had been thrown.

'Yes please,' I murmured.

'You must email me every day asking for healing,' he said. (He'd told us during the workshop that we must involve the patient in their own healing, that they must be as invested as we were. The easiest way to do that, he said, was by having them email us daily. 'On any given day I heal 18,000-20,000 people,' he'd said. 'I am healing them as I sleep and drive.')

Magdalena wrote his email address on a Post-it note and passed it to me slyly, so no one else would read it. I handled it like it was the Holy Grail.

'What about my arm, can I email you about that too?' I said.

'Yes,' he said. 'With emailing, that should get better within a week.'

I chanced it. 'How about my cat?' He smiled, repeated the line I didn't want to hear about everything being curable apart from the illness that's fated to kill us.

I thought hard about Patrick in the taxi. The stuff about the foot had convinced me, for some reason. His finances, too – he didn't seem to be charging enough to be a fraud. Yes, my arm and neck still hurt, but he'd said it would take a week. I should give him that.

And imagine if he was genuine! My foot would be healed. My pain would be gone. I could heal my cousin's rheumatoid arthritis, my mum's lung condition, my friend Marc's MS. I could heal Miffy's lymph node and keep her well until it was time for her to go. Nobody I loved would ever have to suffer again.

Suddenly the idea of a miracle wasn't so frightening. I would do anything to make Patrick real.

On my return to England, I brought forward my flight to Cornwall so I could get going immediately. I swirled colours at my solar plexus in the mirror, at my mum's, at Miffy's, which I felt pulsating with anxiety. I emailed Patrick every day for a month, asking him to heal my foot, my pain and my cat, even though he'd said my pain would go in a week and he hadn't mentioned Miffy. Although I doubted myself all the time, I tried to have faith. I trust him, I told myself as I sent my chirpy emails every day – *Hi Patrick! As requested, please keep healing my pain, my foot and my cat. Thanks so much* – I have complete faith in him.

Eight weeks later, Miffy died.

PEELING OFF THE LABELS

*I do not suppose that women invent their ... pains
out of anger or jealousy ... But the It, the unconscious,
drives them into illness against their conscious will.*
Georg Groddeck, *The Book of the It* (1923)

Pain is like gastroenteritis: once it's out of your system, it's impossible to recall just how brutal things got back there.

You may remember the image of a broken bone poking through your skin, but you forget the physical sensation the minute it's out of plaster. You forget how fearsome a hangover can be until the next time familiar mallets are pounding your brain. Apparently, you even forget the agony of childbirth once you're wreathed in oxytocin, clasping a baby. You know that it hurt, and it hurt a lot, but try to summon up the exact way it felt and you can't. That's because while we store emotional memories, we don't lodge immediate perceptual ones. Every dose of pain is served with a chaser from the river Lethe.

I remember things about pain: that when I fractured my arm at 13, it didn't hurt as much as I expected, that when I fractured my ankle the pain was so minimal that I didn't go to the doctor for six weeks. I know the worst pain I've ever been in was in 2011, when, out of the blue, a knife fight seemed to kick off in my belly. I remember the joy of being filled with morphine and wondering, as the drugs wore off, whether I could knock myself unconscious if I hurled myself out of the hospital bed. That's how I know it was the worst pain of my life; but if I try to remember exactly how it felt, I don't have a clue.

So if you aren't in pain at this precise moment, it's unlikely you'll be able to conjure up exactly – to feel, viscerally – what pain feels like. I, too, have this amnesia, but of a different kind: I can't remember what it feels like to *not* be in pain.

There was probably a time during childhood when I wasn't hurting – at primary school I was a fast runner, and I couldn't have managed that if I was in pain. But all I can remember, looking back now, is a life scored by a quiet soundtrack of hurt: an aching joint, a stiff neck, a back that won't bend, a shoulder that creaks, a knee that pops with every step.

And because it's all I've ever known, I thought it was normal. Because nobody else I knew complained about body parts hurting (least of all my family, who've borne everything from autoimmune disease and cancer to heart and lung disorders with textbook stoicism), I assumed that what I felt as pain – the constant aches, the low-to-mid-level soreness, the twinges as my joints slipped in and out, the dizziness that seeped through my skull if I spent too much time on my feet – was normal, and I was just lazy, spoilt, unfit and self-centred. I spent two decades despising my lack of stamina and moral weakness. Ultimately, although my EDS diagnosis sounded a death knell for my future, it also relieved me of a weight that had spent the previous 20 years suturing itself onto my self-esteem.

Getting a diagnosis for something that's plagued your whole life should, of course, be a breakthrough moment. 'Yes,' said the rheumatologist, looking me up and down as I stood there awkwardly in bra and pants. 'It's absolutely clear.' She showed me how my pelvis was twisted the wrong way and my legs emerged at odd angles; how my knees folded back on themselves and my fingers were as flexible as a Balinese dancer's. She congratulated me for holding down a full-time job, was surprised when I said I walked to work (the two-mile commute was my concession to a healthy lifestyle; I'd walk in the morning and collapse in a bus on the way home, assuming the fact I couldn't manage both ways was testament to my fatness). This was a debilitating condition, she said; I was doing surprisingly well.

Well fuck you, I thought to the GP who'd told me I was just getting older. Fuck you, I thought to the colleagues who'd looked quietly disgusted three months earlier when my limp had slowed us down on a group bonding walk. Fuck you to my friends who acted disappointed when I bailed on a night out in favour of a bath. Fuck you to the commuters who shot disapproving looks if I sat down when a fiftysomething woman was standing up, the people who made me feel I had to swell my belly out to mildly pregnant to justify my need for a seat, the ones on the Tube who looked aghast if ever there were no seats but a black curtain was sweeping across my vision and I had to sit on the floor with my head between my knees.

Fuck all of you, I thought, suddenly standing tall in my pants. I was never lazy; I was ill. And then, as I pulled my clothes back on, I thought: now I know I'm ill, I can get better.

She discharged me with a referral for those six physio sessions on my bum, an unofficial prescription for vitamin D, and a stern warning to stop walking to work because I could do myself untold damage. 'Wait until you have the physio,' she said. 'You need to be taught how to stand and walk from scratch.' Except, she added, I could walk for pleasure, just not to work. When I asked her to explain the difference, she got angry and kicked me out. Women can have Yentl Syndrome, too.

I came to realise that a diagnosis isn't always a step forward.

You have a name, at least, that proves it isn't all in your head. You have a name you can spout at non-believers, sympathisers and HR. You have a name you can google and join support groups for. You have a name that gives you access to hundreds, even thousands of fellow sufferers – the key to a community you never knew existed. But what's in a name if it stops there?

I was discharged from that rheumatology clinic the same

day I was admitted. Months later, six ineffectual physio sessions were followed by a six-week gym programme which turfed us out into the real world at the end. Condition diagnosed, budget dried up, hands dusted. During the COPE course, as I tried to suggest that my arm pain was separate to the underlying EDS and they assured me it wasn't, I realised that sometimes a diagnosis can be a millstone round the neck. A domino, too, teetering on the edge. And the first consultant flicked it, and that first diagnosis spawned another and another, and before too long my whole structure came crashing down.

I was sent to a gastroenterologist because I was always exhausted after eating and EDS often goes hand in hand with digestive issues. He asked after my bowel movements, and, wanting to be helpful, I told him that since renouncing vegetarianism, my poos were more solid and less frequent. Suddenly it was on my medical file that I had IBS. I was tested for food intolerances and passed with flying colours, but nevertheless I was probably gluten-intolerant, they said, and urged me to start a diet which was similar to Atkins yet even less pleasurable. I was dismissed from the clinic when I failed to attend two initiation sessions.

Next in their crosshairs: my heart. I was diagnosed with POTS – those baggy blood vessels, they said, were making my blood pool and my heart pump faster, sending it up and down like a rollercoaster. There was talk of putting me on heart medication – for life – until I asked whether I couldn't just carry on as I had for the past three decades, sitting down where possible and holding onto walls when standing up. How bad was the POTS, really? Technically, said the cardiologist, you don't have it – your tests came out fractionally below the marker. But since you have the symptoms, I diagnosed you anyway.

I am a doctor, dear, and I know.

It was a rollercoaster that, once strapped in, I couldn't get off. They were asking leading questions and taking the answers they wanted to hear, slapping labels on me that helped their research (and research funds) but did nothing for me, crossing me off one waiting list and adding me to a colleague's to-do list without asking what *I*, who'd lived 30 years with this body, made of it all. And once they'd applied those labels, they would read only those labels, instead of listening to what I was trying to tell them.

Eventually, diagnosis became a straitjacket. I could refuse medication or skive diet classes, but I couldn't force a doctor to take my arm pain seriously when my notes insisted it was just an EDS flare-up. And as the weeks ticked by and I waited – for second opinions, tests, courses and discharges – the chance of curing the pain ebbed further and further away. The longer it stayed with me, the harder it would be to get rid of. I knew that, and Dr Good knew that, but no matter how many letters he wrote, no expert was prepared to peel off the labels their colleagues had already attached to me. All those diagnoses actually worsened my health.

When we finally jumped through the hoops to earn a third opinion about the pain, the rheumatologist did the same tests everyone else had, and announced that I wasn't even hypermobile. Maybe the pain had made me stiffen up, he said – it had been two years since my original diagnosis and 23 months since my arm had short-circuited – but if he were seeing me for the first time today, he'd say I didn't have EDS.

'Can I get that in writing?' I asked. 'Because I think having the EDS label has stopped me getting a diagnosis for my arm. If I don't have EDS, I want it to be officially recognised.'

'That should be the least of your worries,' he said. 'We won't bother with that right now.' And the note to Dr Good falling through the letterbox the following week said that there was nothing more he could do for this pleasant EDS patient, therefore she was discharged from his clinic.

———

If overzealous diagnosis plagued my first two years of pain, later I would be reminded of the flip side. It happened at my fifth appointment with an endocrinologist to find out what, if anything, was going on with my thyroid.

My history with Mr Bloggs (as we'll call him) was long, drawn-out and frustrating – the NHS seen through a tabloid filter.

It had started when a neck MRI uncovered a rogue lesion on my thyroid, but it had taken almost 18 months to establish that I didn't have cancer. First, an ultrasound revealed more lesions, one of them deserving of a biopsy. I returned for my biopsy, except they did a second ultrasound. Next, I saw the consultant – he was lovely, Mr Bloggs was, that first time round. It was probably okay, he said, but since the wait between having the ultrasound and my appointment with him had been so long, I should have another scan, just in case. So I had another scan.

I saw his deputy at the follow-up. It looked benign, she said, locking eyes with my notes instead of with me; but since the waiting time between the third ultrasound and follow-up had been a couple of months, the team wanted to re-scan it to be sure.

Groundhog Day.

Another ultrasound, another follow-up, and finally they confirmed I didn't have cancer. It wasn't over yet, though. This doctor noticed I had thyroidy symptoms – things like tiredness and dizziness, which had previously been put down to my EDS, though now, of course, I was no longer hypermobile. She dispatched me for blood tests but at the follow-up, six months later, Mr Bloggs said the results were out of date and needed to be repeated.

Five consultations, multiple scans. Hours wasted waiting in late-running surgeries, thousands wasted on tests that were out of date by the time they were evaluated, appointments wasted because all that happened in them was that the doctors looked at my notes and realised they needed up-to-date results. Hell it was not, but it was certainly third-tier purgatory. So I was longing for this clinic to be the last.

I got the top man himself this time, Mr Bloggs again. The last time we'd met, he'd treated me as an equal. This time, running an hour late, something had changed.

'So, you were last here in April, and your ultrasound was fine,' he started.

'Actually,' I ventured, channelling the invested, self-aware patient that the COPE course had trained us to be around doctors – a substantial part of the eight-day course spent teaching us psychological tips to get the NHS care we needed – 'since then I've seen *you*, just a couple of months ago.' He looked back at the notes.

'Ah, so you did,' he said. 'And your bloods were fine. I'll write to your GP.' He clicked a window on his screen shut and whirled round in his chair, going in for the goodbye handshake.

There was no way two years of purgatory were going to end like this.

'That's great,' I said, in my most engaged and alert voice – there's a fine line between knowledgeable and hypochondriac, the psychologist had taught us – 'I'm so pleased. But I'm still having symptoms.'

'The blood tests were normal,' he said. 'That means there's nothing wrong with your thyroid.'

You really are better, dear, whether you can see it or not.

I leaned forward, casually slipping my prop – a Ben Goldacre book – onto his desk. Doctors are more impressed by people who show an active interest in their health, we'd been taught. I smiled back. 'Any chance you could run through the results with me here?'

He sighed, and turned back to his screen. My bloods may have been normal, but they were at the very highest end of normal. Infinitesimally higher, and they would be abnormal.

Don't be demanding. Don't be emotional. Don't be annoyed.

'The reason you wanted to rerun the tests,' I said, innocently – never dictate to a doctor! – 'was because of symptoms that had been ascribed to my EDS but didn't quite make sense. I don't *want* a thyroid problem, obviously, but I'd like an answer, because the last rheumatologist I saw said he wouldn't even diagnose me with EDS right now. So it'd be wonderful if we could get to the bottom of this once and for all.'

'What made you think you had EDS in the first place?' His smile had turned from professional to avuncular. 'Joint pain?'

'That, exhaustion, dizziness, feeling faint all the time, being unable to stand up for more than a few minutes,' I said. 'I was hypermobile when I was diagnosed but I'm not any more, so the rheumatologist was unsure whether I've just stiffened up since my diagnosis or whether I was mis-diagnosed in the first place.'

He looked me up and down – I had put on my go-getting patient uniform of a dress, leggings and big cardigan, signify-ing professional yet comfortable, the kind of thing one can wear to a meeting but also do stretches in.

'If you have joint pain, the best thing you can do is lose weight,' he said. 'If you lose weight, you'll feel fine.'

I stared at him. All that effort – the clothes, the makeup, the book, the carefully controlled facial expressions and studied words – and he thought I was just fat? His team had been calling me in, again and again, for the past two years and he was dismissing me as lazy?

'If you have joint pain,' and he spoke more slowly this time, 'the best thing to do is to lose weight.'

I should have pointed out that my pain was centred in my neck and I was pretty sure my skull wasn't overweight, that my arm pain came from a malfunctioning brain not my bingo wings. But I didn't.

I said, 'I know better than anyone else I should lose weight' (this was true – I had glimpsed my whale-like body only that morning as I rolled around pulling on my leggings, my back so stiff I could no longer curl over). 'But it's hard to build an exercise programme when your doctors have forbidden you from doing more than a couple of minutes' exercise at a time.'

'Here's a secret,' he said. 'Burning calories is always hard. What's easier is not taking them in in the first place.'

I blinked back tears, tried to crack a pointed joke about

cake being the only pleasure left to those who have no life left, but he'd already stood up, opened the door and was standing there, hand extended.

'There's absolutely nothing wrong with you,' he said, as I walked out. 'You'll be absolutely fine if you only stop worrying.'

If you only stop worrying.

'If a physician of high standing... assures friends and relatives that there is really nothing the matter with one but... a slight hysterical tendency – what is one to do?' asks the *Yellow Wallpaper*'s protagonist, before she goes mad.

It had taken me over three decades to be told I wasn't lazy, I wasn't fat, I wasn't a slob. That the reason I couldn't walk as far as others, had to sit down more than others, couldn't sit at my computer for as long as others was because there was something wrong with me – not something I'd brought on myself, but something genetic. Over the past four years, I'd slowly dismantled the barricades of self-hatred and shame I'd built up around me, and replaced them with a thin buffer of understanding. And, just like that, this man had sent in the wrecking ball.

Women with chronic pain have to go through 12 doctors before they find one who provides them with adequate medical treatment, writes Paula Kamen in *All In My Head*, her memoir about migraines. 'There is a great deal of evidence showing that women's complaints of pain are taken less seriously by physicians than men's,' says Joanna Bourke in *The Story of Pain*. 'Female patients routinely get treated differently than male ones, in part because of deeply entrenched ideas about the female body (as more capricious, emotional and prone to "women's problems"),' she told me via email. The term 'Yentl Syndrome' was coined in 1991 by Dr Bernadine Healy, named after the protagonist of a short story by Isaac Bashevis Singer who masquerades as a man in order to receive the education she wants. The story was set in the 19th century, yet a 2011 study in *Cardiology Today* showed that women suffering coronary heart disease receive better treatment if they present with symptoms that are more common to men.[2] If they present more naturally, they're undertreated and are more likely to die. Yentl Syndrome crosses cultures, too – the same mortality gap was noted in Korea in 2016.[3]

If I saw Mr Bloggs now – secure in myself, boiling with rage like Lilith, first woman and first monster in Hebrew mythology, literally demonised when she revolted against Adam's domination – I'd ask why he'd thought it appropriate to say what he did. How much he knew about EDS, or POTS, or neurology, or thoracic outlet syndrome, or chronic pain. I'd ask whether it had been professional to contradict colleagues who specialised in my condition, and debunk rheumatology diagnoses when he wasn't a rheumatologist. I'd ask how he thought losing weight would help my neck pain – was my skull swaddled in rolls of flab? Was my brain made up of fat tissue? Were my nerves misfiring because they had to reroute around extra lipoid cells?

Had he read the studies that show male doctors are more likely to dismiss female pain as psychological, that younger women delay seeking treatment for heart attacks out of fear of being labelled hypochondriacs? Had it occurred to him that it wasn't me referring myself to his clinic over and over again, but rather he and his colleagues who'd kept summoning me back? Had he been tested for Yentl Syndrome? I'd heard it was rather contagious amongst hospital staff.

But back then, I said nothing, of course. I handed in my discharge paperwork and snivelled my way out of the hospital. Then, inspired by Mr Bloggs, I went for a walk. I walked to an amazing French bakery and bought a croissant, butter oozing from its every pore. I took it home, and I ate it. I didn't leave the house for the rest of the day, and when the pain got worse, because I too had Yentl Syndrome, I told myself it was all my fault.

BAD BALIANS

It is in your mind to pretend she is mad.
Jean Rhys, *Wide Sargasso Sea* (1966)

There was a lot of Yentl Syndrome in Bali.

'Hahaha, you so fat!' said the first guru I saw in Ubud. I had expected so much from this town, the epicentre of today's New Age healing culture since Elizabeth Gilbert outed it in *Eat Pray Love*. After India, it was the obvious place to go. I had found a villa with a pool, in the middle of rice fields, for the princely sum of £32 a night on Airbnb. At check-in, I asked the owners for the nearest healer and their eyes widened.

'Why you want balian? You ill, Julia?' said Made Reni, the mother (balian is what they call healers in Bali). 'If you are ill, we take you to doctor, not balian.' Luckily Agung, their agent, had dealt with enough tourists to know that white people don't want doctors. For a fiver, he could take me to a famous balian who'd healed some former guests, he said – though of what, he couldn't say. He picked me up on his motorbike the following afternoon, Made Reni and the family looking on in bemusement, and drove me to a compound (the Balinese live in walled compounds with their extended families) half an hour away. The balian was asleep when we arrived, passed out in the May heat on a sheet printed with that iconic symbol of clean living, the Welcome To Las Vegas sign. Agung cleared his throat as we walked towards him and he sprung up, switching on a smile. He was topless, breasts bigger than mine over a magnificent bronze beer gut. He sat, legs crossed, like a chubby Buddha.

'You so fat!' he said in Balinese, as Agung translated solemnly. 'Hahaha!' He was giving me an 'electric massage', which consisted of him squatting on a threadbare mat wired up to the mains, and running his hands up and down my body. It was to stimulate my muscles, he explained as they convulsed under his electrified touch. Except, once he got to my legs, there wasn't so much as a twitch.

'He has never seen such fat legs before,' said Agung, gravely, as the balian laughed. 'He says they are so fat, the electric cannot penetrate.' The balian caressed my buttocks, which twitched obligingly, and then swept his hand down to my calves – nothing.

'You must exercise,' said Agung. I thought of Patrick, who'd at least had the decency to diagnose me as mortally ill. Of Charmayne, for whom my lipoid cells had had no bearing on my wellness. I had crossed eight time zones in search of sympathy, and ended up with a man no different from Mr Bloggs.

'Actually,' I said firmly, 'I do exercise.'

The balian hauled himself over to a rattan mat, squatted between two empty litre-bottles of Bintang beer, lit a cigarette and blew smoke in my face.

'This is not possible,' translated Agung. 'Because you are still fat. You must do running to make your legs thinner.'

'I have a problem with my health,' I tried again. 'This is why I have come to Bali. I know I am fat but I am not allowed to run. My doctors say it is not possible with my disability.' Usually the D-word shut people up.

The balian spoke, and took another drag of his cigarette.

'He knows this,' said Agung. 'You are fat. If you run, you feel better.' Then he suggested a traditional Balinese massage.

I'd already had one of these at a hotel on the coast, and it had felt more like an assault than a massage as the balian had positioned himself between my legs and groped me all the way up to my knickers. Still, it was better than being lectured or electrocuted.

I sat on the floor as the balian instructed, between his legs as he squatted behind me, sweat trickling down his cleavage.

'Please be gentle,' I said through Agung. 'I look strong, but

I am in a lot of pain. And do not crack my neck at all, this is very dangerous for me.'

Cracking necks can be dangerous for anyone – it can injure a major artery running to the brain, as happened to Katie May, a *Playboy* model who died in 2016 after a chiropractic session – but manipulating the neck of an EDS patient is asking for trouble. It can put something out of place, as I did reaching for that coffee, or it can kill you. It is an absolute no-no.

'No, no,' translated Agung. 'Very gentle, no cracking.' I gasped as the balian dug nicotine-stained fingers into my shoulders. 'Oww!' I said. 'Too much!' The balian pounded my shoulders as if they were concrete, my back like it was unbreakable, then started on my arms, taking them in a vice-like grip and squeezing, inch by inch, down the over-sensitised nerves. 'It hurts,' I whimpered, wondering if I'd pass out from the pain. 'It's good for you,' said Agung, reassuringly.

The balian went back up my arms, across my collarbone and started kneading my neck. I felt his breath hot on my skin. 'Gentle,' I begged. And then there was a noise like a thunderclap as the balian cracked my neck.

There was a scream – mine, I realised – and a searing pain, as if he'd torched me with a branding iron. The yard seesawed in front of me, the balian's grinning face spinning gently round. Was it the adrenaline, I wondered at one remove, or a haemorrhage? How far were we from Denpasar? Why had I not memorised the number for the Indonesian emergency services?

'I told you not to crack my neck!!' I bellowed. The noise – the thunderclap – was burrowing into my skull. It didn't come out until I'd put several time zones between us and I can still hear the echo now.

'It will not be good if he has only cracked one side,' Agung was saying. 'You must sit down and he will do the other. If not, it will not be equal.'

'No,' I shouted. Then I had an idea. I had heard that the Balinese can never be seen to lose face.

'Maybe the next time I come, he can do the other side,'

I said. My neck was slightly anaesthetised, as I imagined a stroke would feel.

'Okay,' said Agung. 'Balian says he teaches many western people meditation. Maybe he can teach you meditation too.' The balian handed me a business card, and I clasped it to my heart and shot him my doctor's smile. On the way out, we bought some spicy fish sticks from a relative of the balian. I was sure Agung handed over a fifth of what I did, but he swore I was mistaken. 'Suddenly I'm beginning not to trust my memory at all,' says Ingrid Bergman in *Gaslight*, the 1944 film in which her husband tries to slowly drive her insane.

Made Reni and the family were waiting for me at the villa, but I put myself to bed and cried myself to sleep.

It took about two weeks to recover from the neck-cracking – the fire mellowed quickly but left pain and ominous creaking in its wake. Ketut, Made Reni's husband, took me to a real doctor who concealed a laugh as I told him what had happened, and told me the balian had probably sprained my neck. Never one to let a sprained neck interfere when there were miracles at stake, I combed the island for The One, aided and abetted by Iluh, Made Reni's daughter. Unfortunately, there seemed to be an epidemic of Yentl Syndrome in the balian community.

Iluh took me to Cokorda Rai, a medicine man so famous that he treated only foreigners. In thickly accented English, he diagnosed a lack of boyfriend and an over-used brain, almost the exact definition of 19th-century hysteria. When I protested my physical ailments, he told me they were all in my head, and suggested prayer and a diet.

Ketut Liyer, the seer from *Eat Pray Love*, was too old to read palms by the time I went; instead, he sat mutely beside his son, a schoolteacher who'd suddenly, miraculously, developed his father's gift. I was healthy, Ketut Jr told us, glancing at my left hand, and would soon find a husband who'd bring me three children and plenty of money – but first I should go on a diet. That night, Iluh asked me to excise her from a photo we'd taken of the four of us together. If people saw her with Ketut Liyer, she confided, they would assume she'd sought help because she was a few grams overweight and unmarried at 21. Yentl Syndrome, it was clear, crossed all cultural boundaries.

Yet that was the wonder of Bali, I realised long after I'd left, as I yearned to go back to a place which hadn't only not cured me but had dented my health and my ego, too. Bali taught me that there was more to the journey than the cure. I spoke no Indonesian and their English was poor, but Iluh and Made Reni understood what I was doing and why I needed to do it. They came over twice a day to ask how I was feeling – not just physically, but emotionally, too.

Made Reni did kerokan on me, a traditional Balinese treatment to let out toxins from the body by scraping the skin, leaving red welts across the back. She didn't think it would work for my pain, she said, but she would try. Iluh took me to her boyfriend's grandmother for boreh, a treatment for aches and pains in which she chewed through a bowl of what looked like thin porridge and spat it out over my arms, reading my health and my future in the shapes she had sprayed. She was less interested in my health than in the dead grandmother who she said was with me – a strong woman, she nodded, like the one I would eventually become.

When I returned, broken, from each bad balian (not that they liked me calling them bad balians – superstitious, they were terrified of what my heresy could unleash on us all), they comforted me. And they prayed. One day Made Reni announced that she'd made an offering at their family shrine for my good health. 'I pray for you, Julia,' said Iluh, rubbing my arm another morning when she came in unexpectedly and found me weeping. Made Reni commiserated with me about the patriarchy – 'He fat too!' she said, outraged, about Agung's bad balian. 'If I there, I tell him: "Do not call me fat, when you so fat yourself!"' It was an issue close to her heart, you see, because she, too, had chubby legs. 'Don't listen him, Julia, he wrong,' she told me. Made Reni didn't need me to explain what Yentl Syndrome was – she already knew. And she gave me the confidence to trust myself when it came to my pain and what caused it, and not to override that trust if a professional told me it was all in my head. If I hadn't grasped that on the first leg of the journey, I'm not sure I would have seen it through to the end.

I left Bali with the knowledge that I wasn't alone. But before I left, there was Jero Pura.

———

It would be a lie to say that every balian I met on Bali was a disappointment before Jero Pura. Only four out of five were – the fifth was a 78-year-old called Ketut Suwitra in Munduk, part of Bali's unspoiled north. He had a wonderful bedside manner, but told me openly that he specialised in internal problems, not bad arms or misfiring brains. Don't hurry back, he told me at the end of a gentle massage. If your symptoms aren't better in a week, I am not the balian for you.

To be healed by a balian you need jodoh, explained Nyoman, a friend of Agung's, as he drove me to Bangli, three hours away but home to a balian I needed to see. Nobody could tell me anything about the balian – his name, what he specialised in, why I had to see him. But every person I'd asked – everyone I'd told about the bad balians – had said the same thing. *I hear there is a very powerful one in Bangli.*

'You must not say Corkorda Rai is no good,' Nyoman admonished me. 'He did not help you because you had no jodoh with him, not because he is bad.'

'What's jodoh?' I asked.

'Jodoh,' he said, and shrugged. 'Jodoh is jodoh! With Agung, I have jodoh. With my wife, I have jodoh. Some-times one healer can't make you better but another one can. Because of jodoh.'

It reminded me of a conversation I'd had with my London acupuncturist, Dr Cuong. How come the acupuncture I'd had on the NHS had been useless, I'd asked, but when he did it, I felt different every time? He'd talked about qi and train-ing and targeting the whole system rather than an individual point, and then he'd said, 'It's chemistry, too. You can't

79

help someone if you don't have chemistry.' He was right. A supportive doctor can increase relief from IBS symptoms by 18 per cent, according to a 2010 review.[4] Patients of a surgeon who is rude to operating room staff, a 2011 study[5] showed, are more likely to die than those of a polite one. Jodoh can mean the difference between life and death.

I hoped I would have jodoh with the man in Bangli.

We pulled up on a potholed track on the outskirts of town, and Nyoman handed me the offering I must give the balian: a rattan basket filled with rice, boiled eggs, cake, fruit and bread, prepared by his wife for less than a fiver. Iluh, meanwhile, had dressed me in her favourite traditional sash and sarong.

We walked between lion-topped pillars into a grandiose compound and joined a small line of patients. The woman beside me clasped a limp little girl covered in blisters to her chest. Opposite, a family chatted to a woman in a green sarong and red shell-suit jacket. She was middle-aged with hair tied back in a neat ponytail and an authoritative stance. I wondered if she was the balian's wife.

She smiled as she came over and talked to Nyoman, a gentle tone with an iron lining. 'Hello,' she said to me in English. 'What's your name? Where are you from? You want tea?'

'She asked from where I know this place and how much I was charging you,' said Nyoman as the woman strode off. 'She wanted to be sure I wasn't making big profit.' He sipped his tea. 'She said I must not remember this place and I cannot bring more tourists. Not unless they come for the right reasons.'

We waited for about half an hour – the balian takes as long as he needs, Nyoman said. The little girl slept heavily on her mother's lap. A dog dozed in the sun, its flank twitching with fleas or dreams. Who was the woman, I asked aimlessly. A nosy patient or part of the family? Did balians have secretaries?

'I don't know,' said Nyoman. 'Maybe she's the balian.'
She?

I looked around. Frilly pink curtains over the shrine in the waiting area. A pink towel hanging up to dry. Pink flowers in a pink jar. It was all so obvious, now I knew. Behind us, there was even a display case filled with handbags. Next to it hung a photo of the shell-suited woman with an elderly lady. 'Mamma Loren,' said Nyoman. 'She was a very good paranormal healer.' *Mamma Loren and Jero Pura*, said the caption. At last we had a name.

My shoulder burned. A sign?

'What is your problem?' asked Jero Pura inside her consulting room, a shrine to her Hindu gods. I told her. 'What do the doctors say?' They can't help, I said.

She took my hand in hers. Her face shone like a born-again Christian, but instead of shying away, I bathed in its warmth. Nobody had looked at me with this kind of empathy since Charmayne.

'Do you believe in karma?'

'Karma? I think so.'

She raised an eyebrow, but lovingly.

'Yes, I think I do,' I stuttered.

She smiled as she gripped my palm. She spoke to Nyoman, quiet but authoritative.

'Your problem is from a past life. You had bad problem in this arm in your other life,' he translated.

The only thing I knew about past lives was that the only people who'd had them always had to be famous in their past lives. A king, a saint or a celebrity. My old violin teacher had been Joan of Arc as well as a Knight of the Round Table. What were the chances?

I had been paralysed in my previous life, she said; my bad arm was a karmic debt. 'Luckily you have a strong spirit,' Nyoman translated. 'It protects you from bad things, it is very strong. But you will always have this problem in your right arm. It is very serious. Maybe you will have a stroke. But she will try to stop it.'

She crouched behind me, hands on my shoulders. The hundreds of feet that had visited Jero Pura before me came wafting up from the plastic mat.

'No cracking,' I said. 'No massage.' She laughed gently, stroked my neck. 'No massage,' she said in English. 'But you must believe. I hope the god will heal you.'

She rested her hands on my head and we sat in silence. Do you feel anything, she asked. No, I said. Not hot? Only where your hands are. But I wanted it to be hot, and suddenly I wondered if it was – a deep heat, warming my skull and seeping down my spine. Was it placebo, or something more? She moved to my neck, my collarbone, caressed my right shoulder blade, exactly where the fire always sparked. She patted me on the back.

'I hope the god has healed you,' she said. 'Now we pray. Do you have a religion?'

Brought up Protestant but really I think all religions are the same, I mumbled.

'That's good.' We prayed silently, the three of us. She flicked water on my head and cupped my hands: 'Drink.' She daubed my forehead with dry rice, then my throat, and gave us each a handful of rice: 'Eat.'

She shrank from me as I held out a wad of money. Nyoman gasped – no good balian receives it directly! – and I thought of the bad balians who'd held out their paws and grabbed my cash.

'Is it bad karma?' I said on the way out.

'No,' she said. 'It's because you had this problem in a past life.'

'But is it punishment? Was I a bad person?'

'No.' She shook her head gently, warmed me with another smile. 'Not a bad person.' And then she said, 'You are lucky. Your spirit is very strong. You don't need to do yoga.'

People with EDS should avoid yoga, as they're already too flexible. We look good at it, but it can push us over the edge, hypermobilising our hypermobility and popping our joints out of place.

'If you do it, you can do it easily. Not like the others.'

How did this woman in Bangli know about a condition that had floored my doctors for three decades?

She wrote me a recipe for a potion to rub on my neck and arm, gave me a little vial of holy oil and scented water. Twice a day I should anoint myself, pray, and rub the potion on my arm. If I was feeling better, I should come back before I left Bali.

'But you have to believe,' she said. 'How do you feel?' My shoulder wasn't burning any more, but then I had changed position.

'Do this,' she said, making like a bird. I hadn't been able to move my right arm properly since Agung's balian. Only that morning I'd tried to stretch it and it had stuck fast at shoulder height.

I swept my arms out and above my head, squealed with delight and she smiled at me. 'You must believe,' she repeated. 'Pray. I hope the god will help you.'

In three days, I would know whether or not He had. In four, I would leave Bali.

There was just one problem. My medicine – 'obat lepek', it was called, or stroke medicine – had to be made fresh twice a day, and making it was too much for my arm. But the women – my amazing women – stepped in. Made Reni donated pestle and mortar; Iluh came over morning and night to grind the tough leaves and pepper kernels into a paste. They mixed it with vinegar, rubbed it into my neck and arm with maternal tenderness, and I wore the stained skin proudly. Afterwards, I would smuggle the ingredients back home to England: I found the bag of herbs mouldering away in my freezer months later.

Four days left, three to clinch the miracle. Every morning and night, I knelt in the garden, anointed myself and prayed to the god. I don't know if I believe in past lives, I pleaded, but I will if you make me better.

And I did feel better – or so I thought. Not a lot, but definitely a little. Enough, at least, to ride around with Iluh on her scooter and to watch a public cremation of the queen of Ubud. I felt strong enough to venture into the hippy part of town – for the westerners had ghettoed themselves away from the Balinese, frequenting yoga centres where healing from a white person cost six times as much as a balian, and restaurants that served raw vegan food and listed '12 interesting facts about breastfeeding' on the menu. I even managed an hour-long motorbike lesson with Ketut in the rice fields, something I couldn't have imagined before. Did this mean the god was helping me?

I knew that my pain had been much worse because of the bad balian, and I wanted to be sure that the improvement with Jero Pura was something more than a natural regression to the mean. What about before the neck-cracking, I wondered. Just how bad had it been? On the third morning, kneeling before Made Reni's frangipani tree, I counted back.

It had been terrible since the bad balian, but on arrival in Bali it had been okay – I'd been able to work, at least. I counted further – normally a plane journey would flare it up for a week or so, but it had been unremarkable from Singapore to Bali, and Hong Kong to Singapore before that, and even during the 11 hours from London to Hong Kong. In fact, I had done my normal routine – 'Please may I have an extra pillow, I have a trapped nerve in my arm' – but, for the first time since my pain had arrived, I hadn't used that extra pillow. I'd ended up putting it by my feet.

I spooled further back. Before Hong Kong I'd gone to Croatia on one of those cheapo deals you can't say no to. I'd felt pretty good there, too – the hotel had been a two-mile walk from the centre of Rovinj, and I'd walked it twice, something Old Julia would have done, the Julia I missed. It had been a good weekend – we had laughed a lot, my friend and I, at people we knew, people we used to know, and my fetish of sending daily emails to a man who never responded and who I didn't even like called Patrick.

Patrick.

I leapt up, ran as fast as my fat legs could carry me to Iluh and Made Reni.

I hadn't had a flare-up since the day after I met Patrick.

FOURTEEN TIMES MORE LIKELY TO

The somatic body won't be denied, it's like a freeway.
Open up an extra lane of traffic and it'll fill up too.
Chris Kraus, *I Love Dick* (1997)

Depressed. Fat. Working class. That's the kind of person who gets chronic pain.

At least, according to one of the world's leading pain experts, it is.

'Janet Williams' is such a renowned pain doctor that the pain management centre at one of the top hospitals in Boston is named after her. She was one of the first pain specialists in modern medicine, starting in 1979 when pregnancy meant a hiatus from her work as an anaesthetist in the operating room. She ran the pain clinic at Harvard for 20 years, helped with the start-up of several US pain organisations, and was chair of anaesthesiology at a major US hospital. In short, she's the queen of pain management.

And in June 2016 we sat next to each other on a sofa overlooking the Boston River and Dr Williams told me – a chronic pain patient – that there are two types of chronic pain patients: one, very rare, where there's a specific injury that has caused the pain, and the other – a 'pain syndrome person', where you can't put your finger on the root cause.

'I would say the personality of the other kind of patient is, you know, typically someone who is overweight, who is depressed—'

'*Already?* Before the pain?' I hadn't meant to interrupt, but I was so horrified by her words that I must on some level have thought that shutting her up would make it not true.

'You never know if the chicken came before the egg,

because people who are depressed certainly feel pain worse, and people who have chronic pain become depressed, so I think it's a personality of people who are overweight, unhappy with their jobs, unhappy with their lives, depressed, have poor self-esteem – those are the people who are kind of set up for chronic pain syndromes.'

If a physician of high standing . . . assures friends and relatives that there is really nothing the matter with one but . . . a slight hysterical tendency – what is one to do?

There wasn't a gender split, she said, but there was a class one.

'The lower you are on the socio-economic ladder, the more likely you are to become disabled from your pain, whereas people who are in very high-paid jobs tend to be able to live with their pain and work through their pain,' she said.

'Is it not a question of them having more money and time to throw at it?' I asked, tossing her a lifeline.

'No,' she said breezily. 'I think it's more that the lower socio-economic folks are less happy with their lives and less happy with their jobs, and maybe there are a lot of other people who work with them who are on disability. So I think some of it is a social thing where they have lots of friends who are disabled, and they tell them, "Here's how you get disability," whereas I don't know any physicians who are disabled. I think that people who are more educated and in well-paid jobs are much less likely to go on disability than someone in a lower-paying job who's unhappy and hasn't invested a lot in their career.'

Janet Williams isn't her real name, by the way. I changed it – even though she was happy for me to quote her – because I felt uncomfortable naming the only pain doctor who'd been decent enough to give me an interview when I'm not naming those who'd treated me so badly as their patient. That they were men, and she wasn't, made me even more reluctant to make her the figurehead for a certain kind of doctor. It didn't feel right.

I reminded her that I was a chronic pain person and she

said that my pain had arisen from a specific injury, even if it had been misdiagnosed, so I wasn't a chronic pain personality type. I had only told her about my arm – not the decades of pain preceding it.

Now, Janet Williams is a formidable expert. She opened her first clinic in 1980. She's been on countless pain-related boards. She's headed up pain departments at one of the most renowned medical establishments in the world. She's been dealing with patients for longer than I've been alive.

I, on the other hand, don't have a science degree. I can only speak from my own experience, and from that of the pain patients I know. My knowledge of pain management centres is limited to the UK; we don't tend to be as fat as Americans and our opioid abuse levels are insignificant compared to the epidemic across the pond.[6] So I wouldn't dream of saying she's wrong. All I would say is that I was horrified by her words, because, for the last four years, people had been saying the same about me.

I haven't always looked like this, I wanted to tell her: reasonably put together, hair straightened, face made up, flab belted in, brandishing a fancy notebook and a dictaphone. I didn't, of course – it would have been mortifying for us both. But listening to her words and thinking back to my appointments, I flushed with embarrassment and her every adjective was a cigarette burn to my self-esteem, because I knew that all those things were things they had thought about me.

I had gone to appointments with hair unwashed because I couldn't reach my arm above shoulder level. I'd gone without makeup because I was in pain and at a doctor's appointment not a modelling audition. I'd gone in shapeless clothes that made me look fatter than I was, because allodynia meant I could only tolerate certain fabrics next to my skin and creating a sexy silhouette wasn't top of my outpatient priorities. I had loathed my job when I became ill, and of course I was depressed – I was off work, had no money, was living with my mum in my thirties, was slipping down the professional ladder and I had unremitting, searing pain that felt like I was being barbecued like St Lawrence, pain that nobody was doing anything about. But that wasn't clinical depression, or a depressive personality, or a pain personality; it was an understandable human reaction.

Plenty of illnesses carry a stigma, of course. You're diabetic because you're fat, you got cervical cancer because you're a slag, your heart disease is down to your explosive temper. What's possibly different with chronic pain is that its stigmas are myriad and bound together. It's invisible, so they think you're exaggerating. It revolves around something every-one's experienced, so they think you're laying it on thick. It deals with symptoms that bear the same names as things people say every day: I'm tired, my neck hurts, I stood up too quickly and gave myself a head rush. And it leads to things like weight gain, depression, anxiety and a personality change, so they think, yes, she really is just a lazy, neurotic, explosive cow. It's not so much a double-edged sword as a revolving chainsaw. A knife-grinder, as sufferer Alphonse Daudet called it.

People in chronic pain have to deal with it – the pain, the stigma, the worry – by themselves. There are no drop-in centres, no coffee mornings in aid of us. There's no narrative in which to cloak ourselves, no brave warrior identity to assume – in the sympathy-garnering hierarchy, chronic pain would slide in right around gonorrhoea. Sometimes, depend-ing on who I was talking to and what I wanted from them (a seat on the bus, a cripple's discount, a kindly smile), I would tinker with my description of what was wrong, playing up some ailment that existed but wasn't ruining my life. I have a heart condition, I'd say. A genetic disorder. A malfunctioning nervous system. A trapped nerve. My arm really hurts. Guess which netted the least sympathy.

Just as many men as women have chronic pain (though EDS is more common in women), but if I had to go out on a limb, I'd say it's more obviously destructive in women. Not just in terms of how doctors react and prescribe, as demonstrated by Yentl Syndrome – you can bet Jane Smith would be taken less seriously than our friend John, for example – but also in terms of how they're affected by it.

'Men are much more concerned about their performance vis-à-vis their job – can they lift things and all that,' Dr Williams told me. 'They'll worry, "I might not be able to play basketball, and I'm going to look like a wimp." Whereas women are more concerned with, "I can't do this, I'm not going to be attractive, I'm going to gain weight." I think women are more concerned about that because society expects them to look good, whereas society expects the men to perform.'

I'd go as far as to say that women have their female identity erased by pain, because so much of female identity is bound up in what we look like, no matter how much we try to say it isn't. I was agog at the bravery of Sasha Grey, erstwhile hipster porn star and now actress-musician-feminist polymath, in a 2016 interview with *LA Weekly*. The story was accompanied by a portrait of her with a tissue clamped to her nose, and the first paragraph noted her 'cold-like symptoms'. In the interview, she revealed that she'd had chronic sinus inflammation for two years, with symptoms including pain and fatigue. It had affected both her work and her appearance. It hurt even to laugh.

I'd love to know how Sasha Grey has juggled being a sex symbol with chronic pain, but in the end she didn't speak to me for this book. I don't blame her, either – were I a tumescent male fan, I'd find few images less alluring than Sasha in an oversized cardigan, blowing her nose, as *LA Weekly* showed her. Maybe talking about it once was enough. Maybe it taught her a lesson.

It's not all about gender, of course. There are patients worse off than Jane Smith; ethnic minorities for starters. Pain should be a social equaliser – a broken leg feels much the same no matter the class or race of the person to whom it's attached – and yet, your skin colour largely determines how well your pain is controlled. Studies in America have shown that ethnic minorities waiting for joint replacements have more pain, presumably because it isn't being treated adequately. Were John Smith black and complaining of stomach pain, he'd be half as likely to receive opioids as his white counterpart,[7] even though addiction and overdose rates are twice as high in whites. Were he Latino, he might be culture-bound to hold doctors in such high regard that he daren't admit they're not managing his pain, suffering more as a consequence. Look at class and wealth and it's equally terrifying. People with an annual income of $25,000 are twice as likely to suffer disabling pain as those who earn $75,000. Unemployed households spend more on painkillers than employed ones. The figures imply that Dr Williams is correct – that there is a 'pain syndrome' person who's lower skilled, who knows other people on disability. But the figures also clearly show that the system is failing that type of person. I think of how I was treated – white, middle class, university-educated, going private when the NHS failed – and I shudder to think of what lies in wait for patients without my privilege.

I had a safety net, of course: an astonishing mother who was willing and able to take me in. She helped me practically and financially, digging into her savings deeper than any parent ever should, in the effort to give me my life back. She took out a payment plan on a disgustingly expensive bed that we were conned into believing would get me back to work, paid off two loans and took out a credit card for me in her name to get the balance transfer that, without an income, no company would give me. She paid for my pilates classes at £10 a pop, for a £40-a-month gym membership when I was only able to use the machines for two minutes at a time, for the massages and reiki that kept me alive. She paid for extra physio when my six NHS sessions ran out, and for herbal supplements that I tried for a couple of months before realising I was literally pissing her money away.

I told myself it was okay, that a parent's instinct is to help if they can, that perhaps this was money she'd saved for a wedding that was clearly now off the cards (not least because my boyfriend had dumped me seven months into my pain). And though she blanched as the bills rolled in, she never complained. But whenever we were out and I saw other people my age treating their parents – Sunday roasts, cream teas, a lone coffee that I couldn't even afford – another chunk of my self-esteem would crumble off. Saying thank you every day was humiliating, calling her the saviour that she was, impossible, so I took to calling her a witch instead.

But imagine, for a moment, if she hadn't been in a position to help. Statutory sick pay – all £86 a week of it, back in 2012 – stops after six months. After that, I could have applied for disability benefits: a demeaning, exhausting process that for people like me, who 'don't look ill', often ends in rejection. I decided not to apply because I had the promise of my half-salary coming in from my work's insurance plan (little did I know it would take 18 months to get the first payment), and because I knew the probable rejection – yet another person telling me I wasn't really ill – would crush me.

More importantly, I decided not to apply because at that stage, every assessment I had – whether for a new physio who needed to know my body or the disability tests commissioned by my insurers – gave me a flare-up of the pain, and set me back at least a month. It was a Kafkaesque process – they would injure me in the assessment of me, then recall me for another assessment the moment I had built back up to where I'd been in the first place. And I would explain the situation, point out the madness of it, and they would say yes, sorry about that, but this is how it works. Would you like your money or not?

So forget my fancy bed, my expensive alternative therapies and my round-the-world plane tickets, because they're not normal. I may have found a Kevin, but most don't. If you don't have money, the fight against chronic pain looks very different:

You take the drugs they offer you: the addictive opioids,

the antidepressants you don't need because mourning your life isn't clinical depression, the anticonvulsants that seal your bowels for weeks at a time. You're turfed out of physio after six sessions, whether or not you need any more. After your pain management course, perhaps you're funnelled onto a gym programme – half an hour's stretching, half an hour on the equipment, once a week, is what I got. Perhaps, like me, you'll go dutifully along because you have nowhere else to hoist your hope, but it will never change you physically, because for every day you've spent lying down at the start of your pain, you've lost up to three per cent of your muscle strength, and it takes two weeks of activity to undo a day in bed. Half an hour per week won't cut it, ever.

So perhaps you'll cut your losses. Perhaps, like me, you'll realise that the hour-long journey is detrimental to your health and you'll stop going. Perhaps, depending on where you live, you might be able to ask your GP for a limited-time gym prescription. Perhaps you'll try to do your own thing.

You have your £86 a week for food and rent, and if there's nothing left over for pilates or massage, better say yes to that fentanyl – it may have killed Prince, another chronic pain patient, but at least it's free. Or, at least, it's free in the UK. In May 2016, 86-year-old Florida resident William Hager shot his wife of 50 years in her sleep because they couldn't afford her pain medication any more.

I already told you that chronic pain patients are 14 times more likely to kill themselves than the average person. Perhaps you read that statistic and thought *how terrible, those poor people, crippled by pain, no other option.* I didn't. I read it and wondered if it's really the pain that does it, or the situation into which the pain tips them. Because the road to oblivion is steep.

Depressed. Fat. Poor. Uninvested in life and career. Are we really talking about a personality type, or the side effects of modern medicine's pain management programme?

Up to a third of patients visit GPs with medically un-explained symptoms, writes Dr Suzanne O'Sullivan in *It's All In Your Head* – 'medically unexplained' being longhand for psychosomatic. Saying it's all in your head doesn't mean it's not in your body – it just means your brain and body are inextricably linked, and upset in one can transfer to the other. The two most common psychosomatic symptoms, she writes, are fatigue and pain.

I've thought about this a lot since that May morning. Did they think my pain was psychological? When they taught me CBT for pain management, was it because they thought I was mad? When the neurologist said the nerve conduction studies showed some damage but not enough to explain what I was feeling, was he trying to say I was inventing it?

I don't think so, at least not all of them – even though they banged on and on about depression and anxiety. I can thank my EDS diagnosis for that – it may have smothered any chance of my pain being looked at separately, but at least it provided an organic reason for so many of my symptoms. Without the EDS, I was fat and lazy, as Mr Bloggs made plain; but with it, I was allowed to hurt. Not that this stopped me beating myself up – with every failure to help me, I heard, *it's your fault, it's all in your head*. Those who didn't believe in EDS – family and friends as well as the professionals – certainly thought it was.

But I've always wondered whether there was some kind of psychological link. Before my EDS diagnosis I was working full-time – barely coping, sure, but hanging on. 'This is a debilitating condition, I'm impressed,' said the rheumatolo-gist who diagnosed me, and eight weeks later I was written off. By the end of the COPE course, I was using a stick. Was it a more sinister version of the placebo effect?

Everyone knows about the placebo effect, of course, but most dismiss it as something faintly embarrassing – the foul smell in the room from which we're all at pains to distance ourselves. We're cleverer than that, we think; the placebo effect is for dummies. Or, rather, 'unintelligent and inadequate patients', as a 1954 essay in *The Lancet* so humanely put it. Except we're not: the placebo effect works on everyone.

If your doctor tells you this will hurt, it'll hurt more than if he reassures you it won't. If she warns you that the medication she's prescribing may make you dizzy, you're more likely to feel dizzy. An antidepressant works better if it's blue than if it's yellow, and a stimulant is more powerful if it's red rather than green. A capsule is more potent than a regular tablet, and Nurofen (£2 per packet) is a more effective painkiller than Boots' Value Health ibuprofen (35p per packet) – even though the active ingredients are identical.

It's a reaction that stems from the brain, of course, but it's not just a mental reaction. As well as ramping up the potency of a medication, it can release endorphins and dopamine all by itself. And it's not just 'wishy-washy' things like pain that the placebo effect can, well, affect; Parkinson's, angina, asthma and high blood pressure all react to placebo treatment. Sham operations for knees, backs and angioplasty can be as effective as real ones.

('Wishy-washy', by the way, is the term Dr Ben Goldacre uses in his anti-quack bible, *Bad Science*, when talking about placebos in pain relief – even though, as it happens, chronic pain patients are less receptive to placebo than others. And the medical establishment wonders why all these chronic pain nutters step away from their lidocaine patches and methadone shots and turn towards Patricks instead.)

The obvious explanation for why I'd felt better post-Patrick, of course, was the placebo effect. There was only one problem: I hadn't liked him, and I hadn't believed it would work. I had given up spinning at solar plexi after a few days. I'd felt briefly guilty – was I blocking a potential cure for Miffy? – but the hunch that I'd been taken advantage of had felt stronger.

But although I'd abandoned my own innate healing powers, what I had done was act as if I believed in his. I had emailed him every day, and my emails were always the same, kind of.

'Hi Patrick,' I wrote once. 'Would be great if you can keep going with my arm and neck, my foot and my cat's lymph node – thank you.'

'Hi Patrick,' I went on the next day. 'Would love you to keep sending healing! To me and my cat. Thanks so much.'

'Hi Patrick,' read another. 'If you could keep sending healing that would be great. My arm/shoulder/neck is doing okay (not totally better but not as bad as normal), my foot is a lot worse and my cat was much worse but now seems to have turned a corner. Thank you!'

Did I really believe that, I wonder now, looking back at that email – eyes watering, stomach tying itself into a Gordian knot – or was I writing it to encourage him in case he was real? I'm not sure. One of the things I was to learn over the coming months was that my hopes and beliefs – my entire life philosophy – could change by the day, even the hour. I could go from absolute certainty that This Was It to soul-crushing defeat in an instant. Equally, I could be snorting derisively at a so-called healer as I went to bed, and wondering whether – holy shit – their angelic army had actually cured me when my alarm went off the next morning.

In general, I remember, I was sceptical about Patrick. I didn't believe his finger-pointing had changed my aura – not least because I didn't really believe I had an aura. But there were moments when I questioned my scepticism:

When my referral to an orthopaedic surgeon about my foot came through a few days after Patrick, and he diagnosed an inflammation of the sural nerve that was so rare, he said, that he couldn't be sure what caused it, but limited evidence suggested that sometimes it occurred after being bitten by an insect.

When, a week later, the same orthopaedic surgeon was baffled that the pain had vanished entirely (could the local anaesthetic you'd injected it with to diagnose it have reset my nerve pathways, I hinted, and he said yesssss, that would technically be possible but unexpected).

When I remembered how much Patrick had charged for

the healing ('I hope you're not paying him too much,' the surgeon had said when I'd mooted Patrick as an alternative explanation, and I'd said, au contraire my friend, I walked out that first night without ponying up so much as a euro).

When I'd spent half an hour in Croatia telling my friend about Patrick's 21st-century guru setup – an autoreply saying 'I will take care' the first time you email him and nothing after that – and turned on my mobile to find an email from Patrick that read, 'How are you doing? *Sent from my iPhone*'.

When I dispatched my cousin to Patrick's next workshop in London and she wasn't charged either. When, after a month, my cousin said that her arthritis had never felt better, although she had also changed her diet so couldn't be sure it was Patrick.

Did all that make me believe without realising? Did I sub-consciously programme myself with the faith that he would help? Did the placebo effect kick in and the endorphins start flowing despite my best efforts? I don't know.

But I do know he didn't save Miffy.

That moment in Bali when I realised that, sprained neck aside, I hadn't had a flare-up since Patrick, was a turning point. It was the point I wondered whether it could all be true – whether one human being really did have the ability to change another's body by pointing their finger at their solar plexus. But it was also the point I realised I wasn't strong enough or happy enough to wrestle with the heavy questions that came in its wake. If – and that was a big if – Patrick had helped me, why hadn't he helped Miffy? If he had cured my sural neuritis, why couldn't he have cleared my cousin's rheumatoid arthritis? If he could put pain into remission, why was he not doing the same for everyone with cancer? What about war? Famine? They were the questions that theologians had tussled with for thousands of years, and still nobody had come up with a satisfying answer.

I decided that I couldn't handle the fact that Patrick had helped me, let alone healed me.

I decided to take a step back from the miracles.

Two days after Miffy died, I flew to America and took back-to-back jobs that required 18-hour days, accompanied each day by a different PR person and the same mind-numbing first-date conversation. Detroit, LA, Buffalo, NYC, New York State in its entirety. I flew to London for two days, then back to New York for another job, then South Carolina. Staying busy meant I was doing alright, I reminded myself. I was crying myself to sleep every night and throwing tantrums at strangers over the slightest things, but at least I was functioning, and I was doing so in the right place, the land where god is not God, but mammon.

It was in New York one day, when I was in a taxi stuck in traffic on the Queensboro Bridge and I'd run out of emails to send because we'd been sitting there for nearly an hour and my Bad Hand had reached its typing tolerance, that all of a sudden I was confronted with time to think, and my eyes pricked and the tears came and I missed Miffy so desperately and I wondered is this what a breakdown feels like because it felt like my mind was disintegrating and I wanted so much to get better and to find the person who would cure me but I couldn't handle any more disappointment but then I couldn't give up not yet it still wasn't time there was still time to find Him.

I wasn't ready for another faith healer, yet. So I went to Denver to get stoned instead.

JUST ANOTHER MEDICINE

Pain has an element of blank.
It cannot recollect when it begun – or if
there were a day when it was not.
It has no future but itself
Emily Dickinson (1830-1886: chronic illness patient, poet)

Between 1999 and 2014, over 165,000 people died from opioid overdoses in the United States – more than those who died in traffic accidents. Forty-four per cent of Americans know someone who's been addicted to prescription pain-killers – enough of which were prescribed in 2010 to medic-ate every single American adult, 24/7, for a month. Prince, Heath Ledger, even Elvis – painkillers killed them all. They also kill thousands of less famous patients – not only directly, but also when they turn to heroin because well-meaning doc-tors dial down their opioids.

We like to think we're better than that in Britain, but probably only by a decade or so. The NHS already writes 65 million painkiller prescriptions each year. Ten per cent of adults over 35 take analgesics almost daily, and one in seven of them risks an overdose. In 2017, Ant McPartlin of Ant and Dec fame checked into rehab after getting hooked on tramadol. 'Addiction doesn't always start in some dark alley,' said Barack Obama in 2016, as part of his war on prescription drugs. 'It often starts in a medicine cabinet.'

That I was one of the lucky ones was in no small part due to my upbringing in 1980s Cornwall, home to hippies and horse whisperers. I never avoided doctors (quite the opposite, since undiagnosed 'growing pains' are a marker of EDS), but I was never the patient pleading for drugs. That's why I didn't press the GP for painkillers after the coffee incident. And though there's a good chance that the failure to treat it swiftly is why the pain didn't go away, there's an equally good chance it's also why I'm not a statistic. Writing this book, I asked fellow EDSers what they'd taken and heard of others taking. Tramadol, some said, morphine and oxycodone. Ketamine the horse tranquilliser and methadone the heroin replacement (though if you think that's bad, Eva Peron reportedly had a lobotomy for her pain[8]). Reading their list, I realised I got off lightly with pills that made me merely suicidal when they could have made me an addict.

But while I'm not a big fan of medication, there's one pain-relieving drug I'll champion to the hilt.

In 2016, at a stalemate with her doctors and their drugs that didn't work, Izzy Armstrong turned to cannabis for relief from her chronic pain. Six months later, she was sentenced to two years in prison for drug possession; and a nation which had barely blinked when Richard Branson, Miley Cyrus and Nick Clegg had all called for legalisation began to ponder Izzy Armstrong's situation. Her case swayed public opinion: a judge at Leeds Crown Court even let a medical marijuana-growing perp walk free – because, he said, he'd seen what Izzy had gone through.

Izzy isn't real. She's a character in *Coronation Street* played by Cherylee Houston, who has EDS and uses a wheelchair in real life. But Izzy – and Cherylee for that matter – is chronic pain's Everyman.

When Cherylee dared to get out of her wheelchair and walk a few feet into her own home, a stranger knocked on her door, threatening to report her as a benefits cheat. When Izzy asked her doctor for Sativex – a cannabis-based mouth-spray made by GW Pharmaceuticals which has been proven to combat pain – she was told it was only available for MS sufferers. And when Izzy lashed out at her doctor – 'It's not every day I wish I had MS,' she said, in desperation – both *Corrie* and Cherylee herself were hauled over the coals for their heinous insensitivity. Me, I sympathised, because three years earlier I'd said exactly the same thing.

Remember my medical marijuana mouthspray? I'd discovered it in Los Angeles, soon after the coffee incident, and realised that, apart from half a bottle of wine, it was the only thing that worked where legal drugs did not. But it wasn't medically calibrated (the California weed scene in 2012 was vaguely Wild West) and back home it was also illegal, so I'd asked everyone – GP, pain specialists, anaesthetist, neurologist – for Sativex, and all had said that, without MS, it was impossible to get.

Like Izzy, I briefly lamented the fact that I had pain instead of spasticity. Then, one of my consultants had a bright idea. The next time I went to California, he suggested, I should buy another spray and pop it in my suitcase. Here was a specialist saying that smuggling an illegal drug was preferable to applying for a prescription for a researched, calibrated and regulated medication that he agreed could work for me. I was dumbstruck.

Cannabis has been used for pain management for at least 5,000 years, and was acceptable for almost as many – Queen Victoria even used it for period pain. But while we've long known about its analgesic and anti-emetic qualities, it's only recently that we've begun to understand how it works. In 1994, researchers discovered the endocannabinoid system in the human body: a network of receptors that not only process THC, CBD and the other components of cannabis, but also manufacture these chemicals themselves. They're intrinsic to our wellbeing, it turns out. Endocannabinoids have anti-inflammatory and analgesic properties, and boost our mood, energy levels and immune systems. THC not only moderates pain, but also ramps up the effects of narcotics, meaning you need a lower dose of, say, fentanyl – the drug which killed Prince and contributed to Michael Jackson's death – than you'd normally need to get the same effect. Essentially, it can make them safer.

But cannabis was outlawed in the UK in 1920, and today

the only way to get hold of it is through a dealer.* Plenty do – one NHS apparatchik who shall remain nameless once suggested I get hold of some, as many of their patients did. But there's one big problem with scoring weed in the UK, quite apart from its legality. Eighty per cent of street-bought cannabis is actually skunk, up to 20 times stronger than regular cannabis, bred to ramp up the THC (which makes you high) and wipe out the CBD (the anti-inflammatory part). Skunk is said to cause everything from paranoia to schizophrenia; it's why one consultant refused to prescribe me Sativex on the grounds that studies show that long-term cannabis use causes brain damage. I had to explain to him that his precious studies had more likely than not been done on long-term users of skunk. Skunk is to cannabis what heroin is to codeine.

Ever since trying that mouthspray in California, I'd been intrigued by cannabis. I was fascinated by the hope-giving stories coming out of the US and Israel, where they were doing pioneering research. So when Patrick gave me an inkling that there might be something to this faith healing business – something that shook my cynicism and threatened my world order – I flailed for a more worldly miracle. And there was only one place I could go.

Drawing up in the car park to score my drugs, the nerves hit. Colorado may be the cannabis centre of the United States, but Colorado Springs is a different kind of town. This is a military city, a staunchly conservative place where you can't drive to a mega-church without passing a National Guard Readiness Center, Christian University or 'Focus on the Family Visitors Center'. Strip malls house shops called Bibles for the Road (though also Hooters restaurants); 12 weeks after my visit, a 'warrior for the babies' would shoot three people dead at a Planned Parenthood clinic. Colorado Springs residents have consistently voted against cannabis retailers. And here I was, in Colorado Springs, buying cannabis. It was, I'd already been warned, a risky business.

I parked close to the door. Rang the bell, looked into the camera and explained over the intercom that I'd ordered online. I was buzzed in – to what looked like a spa reception, all comfy sofas, plush cushions and a Helen Keller quote framed on the wall. The impossibly good-looking man behind the desk asked what I needed.

'The MCT,' I said.

'The 500, 1500 or 5000mg?' he asked. 'Mint chocolate or unflavoured?'

'5000mg, mint chocolate,' I answered greedily. He went backstage to score my order and I sat down underneath a collage of cutesy child photos and counted out my money: $274.99 plus tax. Drugs never did come cheap.

He returned brandishing a paper bag. 'Are you one of the brothers?' I asked shyly.

'Yes,' he said, with an American smile. 'Well, I'm a brother. But I'm not one of *the* brothers.'

'I'm meeting them tomorrow,' I said. 'What are they like?'

'They're lovely,' he grinned as he buzzed me out. I hurried back to the car – workers here received regular death threats, it was better not to hang around – and obeyed the speed limit all the way to Denver. 'Marijuana use/possession is prohibited anywhere on property,' said a sign at my B&B, as I rammed the magic little bottle to the bottom of my bag. That night, I furtively measured out my drugs –17.5ml of concentrated cannabis oil – and swallowed it down. Not that I felt a thing, because it had close to no THC. Because here in Colorado, concentrated cannabis oil was just another medicine. Just another medicine, that is, that happens to perform miracles.

Epileptic children having their last fit. Tumours shrinking. Arthritic joints de-swelling. Pain disappearing. You name the medical problem; in Colorado, cannabis, apparently, is the pharmaceutical answer. And at the forefront of it all is a little girl called Charlotte.

––––––––

Charlotte Figi was five years old when her mother brought her home to die.

She was having over 50 grand mal seizures a day, and the

doctors had tried every medicine they knew. Then, one day, Charlotte was in the throes of a seizure when they told her mum that enough was enough.

'They said we couldn't come into the hospital, there's nothing to give her,' Paige Figi told me, matter-of-fact, over a cup of coffee in Colorado Springs. I'd gone to Colorado almost entirely to meet Paige. Charlotte's story had filled me with so much hope that I thought by meeting her – or, at least, her mother – some of her miracle might rub off on me.

'They said, there's no drug. So I brought her home, signed a Do Not Resuscitate, and put her on a hospice programme. She was on oxygen, on a feeding tube, just seizing at home. Her organs were shutting down and we were just waiting. It could be a week, a day, three months – we didn't know.'

Then Paige tried one last thing – 'one last Hail Mary', as she put it. She distilled some oil from a cannabis plant given to her by a local grower, Joel Stanley, and gave it to Charlotte.

'She couldn't swallow, so I put the oil in her tube and just waited to see,' said Paige. 'I was trying, you know, not to think about it, but there was nothing left to try. And I waited, and she didn't have a seizure for an hour. And then another hour went past, and two more hours, and then a whole day went past.'

Charlotte didn't have a seizure for seven days.

'It's hard to have perspective, because at the time it's happening you're just not believing it,' said Paige. 'And you're protecting yourself, because if it's a fluke and it comes back, you'll be absolutely heartbroken. You're like, "What if it works for a week and then…?"'

I thought of Patrick and blinked back tears.

The good news was, it didn't just last for a week. Charlotte was eight and a half by the time I met Paige. She was walking, talking, riding a bike. She has permanent brain damage from the benzodiazepines the doctors had filled her with; but she was *Charlotte* again.

'I keep her wheelchair,' said Paige. 'It's hanging on a hook in the garage, collecting dust.'

There was more to Charlotte's story, of course. Paige hadn't just been a desperate mother flinging drugs at her dying child; she'd trained as a pre-med, and had read Israeli research from the 1970s suggesting CBD was a powerful anticonvulsant. Joel Stanley, who grew the plant, was neither a dealer nor a get-rich-quick schemer. He and his six brothers – Jesse, Jon, Jordan, Jared, Josh and J Austin, all tall, square-jawed and clean-cut, Platonic ideals of the all-American male – were the Robin Hoods of the cannabis industry, using the profits they made from selling weed to make cannabis oil and distribute it free to cancer patients. They'd started their cooperative along Christian guidelines, Joel and Jesse would later tell me. It had even been endorsed by their grandmother.

When Paige had her coup de foudre, the Colorado drug laws were relaxing, but truly medicinal cannabis was a nascent industry and CBD had largely been bred out of the plants. If you're taking cannabis to get stoned, you'll be using strains with a ratio of up to 20 parts THC to one part CBD. Sativex has a 1:1 ratio. But to treat Charlotte, Paige wanted a plant that was 30 parts CBD to one part THC. A plant that everyone told her didn't exist. One that *didn't* exist, in fact, except at Joel's house, where he had a little pot with a plant that was 33:1. Paige demanded his lab reports, he handed them over, and the rest is history.

Charlotte's story went global, and families whose children had Dravet Syndrome, like her, started migrating to Colorado to be treated by the Stanleys (the brothers had given away nearly $750,000 worth of oil by the time I met them). Then people who didn't have Dravet Syndrome started migrating, too. One of America's most revered TV doctors, Sanjay Gupta, issued a public apology in the form of an hour-long, primetime documentary, renouncing his former anti-cannabis position and saying he now believed the plant to have untold health benefits.

Public opinion began to change. Texas and Utah, two of

the most conservative states in the lower 48, passed laws to allow medicinal CBD. Christians went from calling it the devil's weed to God's plant. On my arrival in Colorado Springs, I'd called in at New Life, a mega-church with a congregation of 10,000, and asked the pastor what he made of my plans. He didn't approve of recreational cannabis, he said, but for medical issues? 'I'm totally okay with it.' I stared at him in disbelief, asked whether he might not like to suggest a healing service instead. 'We'll do both,' he said. 'But I want you to be pain-free, and I am absolutely okay with you trying.' That's our work, Jesse would tell me later. The gospel of the Stanley brothers was spreading.

Refugees, they call them, the thousands uprooting their lives and coming to Colorado for the cannabis, the 21st century's Dust Bowl migration. In my first week, I met several people who'd moved for all kinds of medical reasons: Samantha, a worker at my motel ('Bud & Breakfast', as it was catchily named), who'd slashed her mental health medications from 11 to zero. Ezra, a three-year-old who'd gone from having up to 500 seizures a week to five a day, and come off morphine and methadone, halved his phenobarbital dose and tapered his valium right down. Jake, who'd come off medication for MS and fibromyalgia, and was spending time out of his wheelchair for the first time in years.

Nobody tried to convince me that cannabis was a panacea, and Joel and Jesse Stanley were clear that they wouldn't make miraculous claims. They had anecdotes, they insisted, rather than hard evidence; and yet, during the two hours we spent together, they had anecdote after anecdote after anecdote. The fact that the US government had patented various properties of cannabis – anti-convulsant, anti-inflammatory, anti-oxidant, neuro-protectant – told me that these weren't snake oil salesmen. Neither were the people working for the Realm of Caring, the Stanleys' non-profit side organisation which deals with research and advocacy. Every member of staff was a refugee with a story to tell. And they were dealing with daily death threats to distribute what they believed in.

I had bought the oil, of course, but I was aware that it was a long-term project, and after Patrick I was desperate for a quick fix. Not living in Colorado, I could only buy recreational cannabis – higher in THC, for people wanting to get stoned, not better. Not that I had anything against getting stoned, but I'd renounced the doctors' pills because they made it snow in my head, and I needed clarity of mind whatever I was using. I would find a space in the middle, I thought – and so I chose carefully. I started with the most innocent thing I could find: an orange lolly glazed with CBD.

———

It hit me right after the cappuccino. During the cappuccino, to be precise.

I was about two-thirds of the way through, sitting quietly in a cafe, wondering whether to push myself to walk the half-mile back to my hotel or get the bus. I'd arrived in Denver with back pain that felt like someone was trying to lever my pelvis from my spine with a palette knife, rocking it back and forth. It was a new pain and I, with full-blown Yentl Syndrome, no longer trusted my body – should I try and gently exercise it, as you're supposed to with back pain, or was this different, something seismic like the coffee incident? I thought of the wheelchairs I already used at airports, the swift progression into mobility aids of our COPE group, and wondered whether destiny was closing in.

A wave of vertigo suddenly barrelled over me.

I'd had vertigo in the past – they'd wondered, briefly, about Ménière's or a brain tumour before settling on those migraines I didn't know I had – but this didn't feel the same. It was softer – a tumble, say, rather than a tumble dryer. It felt like someone was pouring liquid in my head, filling it from top to bottom as I tried to imagine the golden light of universal healing doing every time I had a reiki treatment.

Whoosh, went another wave. Shit, I thought, I'm half a mile from safety and I'm stoned. I made for the door, walking through sand.

I staggered outside into the rain – wait, I could walk! My

back felt gloriously, miraculously numb! I told myself fresh air would help, but the storm was brewing. When my legs started slipping through treacle, I staggered onto a bus, but two stops later, I was lit, and halfway across a pedestrian crossing I forgot how to walk. I dragged myself towards the hotel, holding onto walls, but stumbled into a nail salon on the way. I needed a pedicure, I decided – the most significant of my life, it turned out. Because as I watched the woman sawing away at my second toenail, then watched it start to bleed as she went beyond the quick, I realised that it didn't much bother me – or, rather, it did, but at several degrees of separation. It was my first real experience of weed as a painkiller. Back at the hotel, my back felt completely anaesthetised. I've found my miracle, I thought, before passing out fully clothed at 5pm.

When I woke the next morning, my back was hurting again, but not nearly as much as it had been. It was an odd feeling – I could tell there was still a problem, but it felt as if either some nerve had been severed or I was having an out-of-body experience, witnessing it at one remove. It was a breakthrough, that much was conclusive. Now I just had to find a way of getting the pain relief without the attendant 16-hour loss of consciousness.

I tried smoking CBD-rich strains, but they did nothing for me (my limited past inhalations had taught me that I'd been born with the natural tolerance of Snoop Dogg – possibly part of my Condition, since EDS patients have a higher anaesthetic threshold than normal people).

I bought lotions – $30 for a 100ml bottle – one of which made a minor difference, but since it wasn't transdermal, it was probably either placebo or the numbing menthol in it. I had a 'Mile High Massage' using 'extra-strength cannabis crème' instead of oil – I floated out on a cloud, but not an unmistakably higher one than massage usually put me on.

I tried marijuana patches, both CBD and THC – supposedly transdermal, to push the drug into my bloodstream – but they were as useless as anti-inflammatories. I tried cannabis lip balm and a 'heavenly hash bath' of herbs, Epsom salts and weed, lying back and thinking of England in a filthy motel tub as an anonymous pubic hair swam towards me. Nothing happened.

I returned to edibles, carefully slicing cannabis-infused brownie bites into four (it turned out the lolly had contained five doses of drug, but because of my slow metabolism – finally, I yelled with delight, proof – I had failed to process it in the normal 20 minutes and therefore overdosed). They helped the pain – like ibuprofen, but minus ibuprofen's increased risk of stroke, heart attack and kidney disease – but were full of THC and made me high, and I couldn't seem to find the sweet spot between pain relief and intoxication. It didn't help, of course, that I was down as a recreational, not medicinal user. With the red card of the medical cannabis patient, I'd have had access to a completely different arsenal of CBD-rich strains to smoke, eat or rub on myself. But to do that, I'd have had to migrate 4,683 miles west.

Then, on my last day, came the breakthrough. 'I have something for you!' said my trusty concierge at a dispensary as posh as a Selfridges cosmetics counter. He'd been suggesting new products every day, determined to vanquish my pain. 'We got the delivery, like, an hour after you left,' he said, leading me to a display of e-cigarettes. 'I was like, *dude!* This would have been perfect for her.'

It was, so the label said, an e-cigarette of pure CBD. I took it back to my hotel, had a drag, then another, and another. It dug deep into the pain and took a chunk away – not completely, but as effectively as amitriptyline (the only medication that had made a real difference for me) only without the dry mouth, constipation, fatigue, dizziness, blurred vision and passing out after every meal that had followed in the amitriptyline's wake.

I was already down to drive, not fly, out of Colorado. When I realised that the e-cigarette was the Holy Grail, I bought two more. If I was caught – because although CBD was legal in Colorado, California and the UK at that time, flying it home through federal airspace was a grey area – there might be trouble. An e-cigarette could separate me from a country I loved, a place that provided me with much of my work, and Kevin and Charmayne.

But, as my consultant had suggested, it was worth the risk. In the US alone, there hasn't been a death due to cannabis overdose since records began, in contrast to the 42,000 who died from an opioid OD in 2016. Even harmless NSAIDs like ibuprofen kill up to 10,000 annually. Yes, I could find a dealer at home, but they'd probably give me skunk or, if not skunk, THC-rich cannabis, grown god knows where and with what fertiliser. I wanted Colorado weed: regulated, tested for ingredients and ratios, and often organic. Getting safe pain relief these days often means breaking the law.

At 6am the following morning – pain ramped up from staying sober to drive – I made a break for Utah. I took the e-cigarettes across five state lines and one ocean, checking over my shoulder at every stop. It was worth it – they were heaven-sent. I smoked my way through them at my desk, in bed, in meetings, with friends, at a wedding. They provided almost entirely effective pain relief – enough to help me function normally, even on a bad day – without a whiff of feeling funny. CBD is, at the time of writing, legal in the UK – if you can get hold of it, that is. In late 2016 the MHRA (the UK medicines regulatory body) ruled that it does have medicinal value, meaning that anyone selling CBD needs a licence. Supplies were quickly whipped off the shelves, and when I wrote this, it was unclear how things would pan out.*

As for the $275 oil, when I got home I did something that I couldn't process until some time later. I stashed it away in the kitchen cupboard, between some unopened spices from Marrakech and oolong from Shanghai, and shut the door on it. Every now and then I would take it out, look at it, and put it back, and for months I couldn't understand why. Eventually, I realised that I'd been so convinced that the oil was a panacea, that the Stanley brothers had the answer – that they were doing God's work, as Jesse even said – that I'd preferred not to take it at all than risk being let down. I'm not so bad today, I would tell myself, even though they'd told me – all their clients screaming 'miracle' had told me – that it was a long-term neuroprotectant rather than a quick fix. Let's wait till I really need it. And I would reseal it in its sandwich bag and pop it back in the cupboard, like some kind of amulet against worsening health.

Charlotte's Web (for the oil was named after little Charlotte Figi, who'd brought it to the world's attention) was the proof that my doctors had been wrong – hell, that the medical establishment was wrong. That if they could ignore the health benefits of cannabis when the overwhelming evidence pointed towards them, maybe they could be wrong about me. That maybe I could conquer the pain, that maybe I would be normal again, that maybe the life goals that kept breezing past me – promotion, pension, mortgage, even a man – could do a u-turn and come back for me. The oil was my talisman of wellness, and I dared not test it lest it shatter my faith. So having veered from Patrick to Paige and ended up equally scared of both, I swung the pendulum back again. It was time to see a witch doctor.

* In October 2018, after this book had been published, Home Secretary Sajid Javid announced that medical cannabis would be available on prescription in England, Scotland and Wales from 1 November.

EAU DE VIE

I am not sick. I am broken.

Frida Kahlo (1907-1954: chronic pain patient, artist)

Max Beauvoir could bring people back from the dead.

At least, that's how I read it.

Beauvoir was the protagonist – hero or anti-hero, depending on your reading – of *The Serpent and the Rainbow*, a non-fiction book from 1985 about zombies in Haiti. The author, ethnobotanist Wade Davis, concluded that zombies do exist, although not quite as popular culture has them; their 'death' and subsequent raising from the grave, he reckoned, was a combination of potent herbal concoctions and cultural beliefs. In other words, the nocebo effect.

I'd learned about the nocebo effect at the same time as I'd read about its more palatable sibling, the placebo. It's what makes you more likely to feel the side effects of your medication if you diligently read through them, or start experiencing symptoms of something dreadful if you read about it online. In extremis, it means that someone who truly believes they've been hexed will respond to that hex – right down to them dying. Such is the power of the brain.

Davis didn't say outright that he believed Beauvoir – who later became the official-unofficial high priest of Haitian vodou – was omnipotent, but there were hints, and they were good enough for me. Someone who could produce zombies could surely rewire my false-firing brain, I told myself. So when a friend planned a birthday trip to Curaçao, instead of saying I couldn't afford it, I said I'd love to come. It would be my first real holiday since the pain had arrived, plus I could fly via Port-au-Prince. I emailed Max Beauvoir that night.

He didn't reply, either to that email or the next. Ten days before I was due to arrive, I sent a chaser. The next day, Max Beauvoir died.

Nobody, it seemed, wanted to talk to me about vodou. Not Max Beauvoir's colleagues, not another media-friendly houngan (male priests are houngans, women are mambos), not someone who a cousin of a friend knew. I made sure to write 'vodou', not the westernised, racist 'voodoo' in all my emails. I tried local fixers – someone who'd work on commission would surely come up with something – but nobody did. The whole of Haiti, it seemed, was living by Sicilian rules.

What if they think I killed Max Beauvoir, I thought on the flight to Port-au-Prince, the American aid worker to my left busily predicting my rape and murder because I'd dared dress in normal clothes instead of her warzone uniform of T-shirt and khaki shorts. Beauvoir was the father of Haitian vodou, after all. What if they don't just ignore me, I began to panic, but do something worse? What if I come for the placebo effect but they kill me with the nocebo?

'First time?' said the man stamping my passport. 'Welcome to my country.'

I shouldn't have come, I decided, climbing into my hotel van as the aid worker forced her Haitian boyfriend to threaten the bemused-looking driver in Creole, just in case he'd been planning to kill me.

'Welcome to Haiti!' chorused two more hotel workers in the back, handing me a bottle of water, and I wondered who'd die first if we were kidnapped (kidnapping was one of many dire warnings on the Foreign Office website). What if Max Beauvoir's people were waiting for me?

It was a bad time to be coming here. A couple of weeks earlier, I'd been diagnosed with anxiety by yet another man who'd failed to help my pain. I had told him that, yes, I'd always been neurotic – wasn't every Brit? – but surely anxiety related to the pain that had ripped away my life and confounded my doctors was not so abnormal. It's not just anxiety but severe social anxiety, he had countered, you might be a risk to yourself – and I didn't trust myself any more to know that wasn't the case. *Suddenly I'm beginning not to trust my memory at all.*

In the end, like Ingrid Bergman in *Gaslight*, like the *Yellow Wallpaper* protagonist, I'd collapsed – physically, if not mentally – one morning on the bank of the blue Danube. It was the week before Haiti and I'd been straining to research an article on Budapest despite legs soaked in concrete and a brain packed with cotton wool. An inner ear infection, the doctor said. You're okay to fly home, but to Haiti? No.

Haiti?, said a GP I consulted back home. Christ. Don't worry, we'll get you out of that one.

But I want to go, I said, and he shivered. 'You know about the AIDS there, right?' he said. 'You know to be careful? Don't. Share. Anything. Not a drink. Not food. Nothing.'

'I can't work out whether you're very brave or very stupid,' said the doctor at the travel clinic which was inoculating me against Haiti for £300. 'You know about the HIV rates, right? Don't. Share. Anything. Don't do any ceremonies. Don't eat or drink anything you don't know where it's come from. Did you know you can contract HIV from sharing a drink?' She handed me a soluble cholera vaccine with the caveat that it wouldn't protect me from AIDS.

'Isn't that where they do that black magic?' shuddered the woman in the Post Office when I tried to order the Haitian gourdes that Royal Mail didn't stock. 'Why are you going?'

Yes, why was I going? Why was I here, having ignored them all, flown halfway across the world while my world was still spinning and my anxiety was apparently a risk to myself, when I might end up as dead as an extra in *Live and Let Die*? Why?

'Eau de Vie,' I murmured, reading the side of a water truck in the lane beside us to stop my mind spiralling into doom.

'Yes, everything here has a Christian name,' said one of the men. 'Look.' And I looked up, beyond his outstretched finger and my panic, to a lotto shop called 'La Confiance' and a tap-tap – a Haitian bus – with 'Merci Jesus' painted over it. Another called 'Grâce de Dieu' was rolling towards us. I didn't understand. This was supposed to be a nation of devil worshippers, not a Colorado mega-church-on-sea. Everyone had said so.

I thought about the extra kidnapping insurance I'd taken out to come here, my rebellion against the Foreign Office guidelines which stipulated one must never travel alone to Haiti, and tried to reconcile their words with my eyes. A thought flickered on and quickly off again, that I was too used to trusting authority figures, that I'd believed Haiti was an earthly hell, that when a doctor or healer blamed me for my illness, I blamed myself too.

The hotel men were fascinated by my mission. Two of them, Cubans, pointed out a sacred site en route to the hotel and suggested the driver could take me. But the driver was Haitian and knew better. He was sorry, he said, but he didn't feel safe taking me to places like that. Safe in what way, I asked. Because of hygiene, he said, and other stuff.

We reached the hotel – a beautiful collection of beachside bungalows – and breathed. Ten steps from my bed was a glassy-watered, tree-fronded, hammock-hung beach. Was this really Haiti? I waded in as the sun set behind the island across the bay, just me and the water, as still as a fish bowl. No wonder the sea is sacred here, I thought (Agwe, the loa of the sea, is one of vodou's more popular spirits). I gripped the pontoon and hovered in the water, the current so soft that it felt like the sea was breathing. It was the first time I'd felt the pulse of nature. What if this is it, I thought. What if Haiti holds the answers behind its omertà? What if, as an outsider, I'll never know? And I salted the sea with my tears.

I stayed two more nights on the beach, drinking cocktails under a framed picture of a *Thriller*-era Michael Jackson, waiting for a houngan or a mambo who would never materialise. In a way – a way that I was trying to force down, beneath my bowels – I was relieved. I had watched *Live and Let Die* far too young and it had lodged in my brain: voodoo as the ultimate horror, Baron Samedi rising from the grave in top hat and tails. This is racism, I told myself, and I knew it was. But that didn't stop the fear.

On day four, I got over myself and booked a car to Saut-d'Eau, a waterfall and one of vodou's most sacred sites. It was 37 miles and three hours away: a driver appeared and drove me wordlessly up the side of an unpaved mountain. At the waterfall was a guide and a handful of young men who crowded round, volunteering to translate, as curious about the fat white woman as they were keen for her tips. Two of them escorted me like an 18th-century plantation mistress into the rushing water to inspect religious symbols engraved on the rocks during the annual July pilgrimage. They knotted my skirt and pushed me up the cliff face, in search of a god-in-the-shape-of-a-serpent who lived in a cave at the top. But even the snake was hiding from me.

We went – en masse now, because I'd attracted a Pied Piper-like following – to a grotto, where I was instructed to light a candle, pray to the spirit Erzulie, and then sacrifice the rum I'd bought from the only other woman within screaming distance, who manned a stall beside the water.

I lit the candle, filtering out the male gaze around me. I already liked Erzulie, or rather, the Erzulies: Erzulie Freda, a capricious, Aphrodite-like minx who smelled of roses and demanded fancy presents from her followers, and her flip side – vengeful Erzulie Dantour, a Lilith figure, the patron saint of wronged women who wept and wailed for the things that had been done to her people. *I cry at nothing, and cry most of the time* writes the *Yellow Wallpaper* protagonist. When I'd first read about the loa, I'd decided Erzulie Dantour was my favourite.

I prayed to them both and poured half the rum into the dirt round the candle.

'Now drink,' said the guide. 'And give it to me.'

I looked down. The bottle had been refilled so many times that the label had half disintegrated and there was a sticky residue around the screwtop. It smelled of moonshine; not, as the label suggested, Barbancourt, the costliest rum in Haiti and supposedly the best in the Caribbean. I thought of the doctors in London.

'Drink it,' he said again.

I flattened my lips and took a swig.

'Now give it to me.' He drank, and handed it to his neighbour. It went round the circle, about eight of them swigging with gusto, and the next thing I knew it was being handed back to me to finish.

Unlike most people who say they have OCD when they just like a tidy desk, I have real OCD about saliva. Even the thought of my own backwash gives me anxiety and I never finish drinks for fear of swallowing my own spit.

'Drink,' said the guide.

'Drink,' said one of the nice young men who'd helped me up the waterfall.

'Don't. Share. Anything,' screamed the doctor in my head.

The men had formed a circle around me. This was their sacred place. How could I expect a miracle if I wouldn't even finish the ceremony? I looked for the driver, but he was standing a few feet away, pretending not to know me.

I downed the rest of the bottle.

The men cheered, sternly forbade me from having sex for eight days. I must tell my husband, they insisted, and I thought, how much kinder they were than the balians to assume I even had one. I paid up and gave $10 to a boy selling paintings that belonged in a gallery – 'Thank you baby, thank you,' he called after me, as if I'd descended from heaven. We took the main road, winding down the hillsides, to Port-au-Prince and the Marriott hotel, where $10 was the price of a cocktail not an unfathomable sum, where first-world bodies swam in a floodlit pool surrounded by a barbed-wire-topped wall and Secret Servicemen buzzed round the lobby. Tomorrow would be a busy day in Port-au-Prince. John Kerry would be arriving for talks with the government, and I would be meeting a houngan.

———

Barbancourt was best, said Serge. Samba El wasn't charging us to attend the ceremony, but it would be polite to make an offering. We stood there in the supermarket, looking at the shelf of rums. I couldn't help but notice that real Barbancourt looked nothing like the stuff I'd drunk the day before.

We'd started with the touristy stuff – a quick ride to the Marché en Fer, the only Port-au-Prince landmark to be rebuilt after the 2010 earthquake. We'd pulled up under the minarets (the French had originally planned it for Cairo), and walked round the touristy vodou section: iron babies with rusting nails drilled into their skulls, powders for drawing sacred vévés, pennants of what appeared to be Catholic icons but were actually stand-ins for the loa, each spirit twinned with a Christian saint under slavery, when worshipping the ancestral spirits was punishable by death.

We had crossed to the Haitian side of the market for herbs used by 'leaf doctors' and houngans to cure physical disease. Haitians were good at herbal medicine, the guys at Kaliko, the beach hotel, had told me, not because their endemic plants were more miraculous, but because it was all they had. At the only stall open to a white customer, I'd bought leaves to make a flu-busting tea, oil for my joints, and a Barbancourt bottle filled with twigs that I should add rum to, leave for two weeks and then imbibe twice a day. It was imperative to respect the timing, said the woman who sold it to me. Otherwise there would be repercussions.

We picked up the Barbancourt en route to Pétionville, driving up and up around hairpin bends at angles that almost defeated the automatic car. This was the posh part of town – there were more intact buildings, no tent cities of those who'd been made homeless in 2010, our donations for their recovery siphoned off by those we'd donated to. And yet Pétionville wasn't as comforting as I'd hoped. The poverty that had drawn Serge back – now a guide, he'd lived in the States before returning to his country out of filial duty, believing tourism the only way forward – was all-pervasive, cloying in the air.

We stopped in a rare space where, before the earthquake, a house had probably stood, Geffrard the driver shrugging as a group of boys yelled at him for parking on their football pitch. We walked up steps and along a narrow pavement winding through a mass of concrete houses – the proportions of a Greek village with none of the charm. The only sign of life was a dog twitching in the sun, a faint gust of stale urine as we rounded a corner, and then the chanting, drifting up to meet us on approach to the peristyle. The heat smothered me as we crept in – at least a hundred bodies pressed into a classroom-sized hall. People sitting in lines, like at church, round a central pillar wreathed in leaves. Samba El and his mambo wife sitting behind a desk on a raised dais at the front, and men and women – the initiates, Serge whispered, beads of sweat running into his dreads – clad in pure white in front of him, facing the congregation, heads down as they sang.

Samba El saw us, smiled, and beckoned us to the front. He wants people to see, said Serge, that vodou is not what outsiders think it is. And it wasn't. There had been no need to psych myself up for this.

Max Beauvoir had gone for spectacle. His ceremonies, I'd read – because he popped up in every book about Haiti – involved much noise and even more blood. When Bill and Hillary Clinton had gone to one of his ceremonies on their honeymoon (because, unlike Samba El, he laid on ceremonies for tourists), a man had walked on hot coals and a woman had bitten the head off a chicken.

But Samba El's ceremony was like a church service: the hymn-like songs, heads-down prayers, the solemnity and sanctity of the occasion. We took communion – cassava bread and coffee, to symbolise the body and blood of the Haitians killed under slavery. His sermon spoke of how vodou underpinned the community, giving the poor the strength to carry on in the most miserable of situations. It reminded me a little of *The Periodic Table*, Primo Levi's book about his time in Auschwitz, and I realised there was more to faith than mere placebo effect; sometimes, belief made life bearable. I thought back to the priest at Walsingham. The miracle here, he'd say, was that these people were still standing, still together.

The possessions, when they came, were different from what I'd expected. An initiate started swaying to the chant, further forward and further back until he was lurching through the crowd, crashing into elderly ladies with his eyes rolled back in his head. A girl in skinny jeans and a red T-shirt who'd shot me a shy grin earlier started screaming, her face a mask of terror. Another snatched my Barbancourt from Samba El and downed it, nearly a litre, grasping the bottle with both hands as if at any second it might turn tail and run away. Afterwards, as she sat, head in hands, soaked through with sweat, I handed her my bottle of water and she thanked me sweetly. 'From England? Welcome,' she said, wiping away her smudged mascara, suddenly completely sober.

As Samba El's congregation prepared a food run to take to the provinces, he told me he wanted to help my pain.

He took me into his sacred room while Serge stayed outside – he absolutely believed in vodou, he'd told me on the way, and was a practising atheist because of that belief. He showed me boxes of herbs, clay pots filled with the spirits of the dead, and dwarf-like humanoid figures with full-sized heads, clad in black material. 'This is my grandfather,' he said, patting one on the head, by which he meant his grandfather's skull. Another skull sat purposefully on the floor, a candle burning on top of the cranium. He wanted to help me, said Samba El, but he couldn't today – a diagnosis by the loa could take hours, and he was needed in the provinces that afternoon. 'Come!' he said. 'You'd be welcome.'

I wanted to. I wanted to go with this calm man, his slow smile and love for his people. I wanted his diagnosis and his cure. I felt grateful that he wanted to show me what his vodou was like, to send me back across the Atlantic with the news that Bond films weren't documentaries, that his collection of ancestral skulls was no different, really, from the box of Miffy's ashes sitting on my bookshelf.

But I couldn't – they weren't returning till the following afternoon and I left at midday. Plus, I'd already prepaid a hotel for my last night: the famous Oloffson, the Miss Havisham of the Port-au-Prince hotel scene, an old gingerbread mansion that, if the photos were anything to go by, had already seen better days in 1966 when Graham Greene set *The Comedians* there.

I'd already spent too much money and so much time to get to Haiti. No more wild goose chases: I had to learn when to quit while I was ahead.

'I can't,' I said. 'My flight's tomorrow at noon.'

'When you come back,' said Samba El, 'we will try to help.' He sounded as if he knew I would return, and the knowledge that I would helped sweeten the bile of disappointment that I hadn't found my cure. I'd been so close – I had almost felt it sizzling in the air that first night in the water – but it was time to admit defeat.

We left for the Oloffson. Vodou omertà or not, I told myself, nothing would stop me staying in a literary landmark.

SOMETHING PRETTY

And so I should be glad to die...
And cease from all this world of pain,
And be at peace among the dead.

Christina Rossetti (1830-1894: chronic illness patient, poet)

'The owner is a houngan,' I said to Serge as we pulled up at the Oloffson to be confronted by a lifesize Baron Samedi in the stairwell leading to the gingerbread house.

'I know,' said Serge. 'I know him slightly.' Serge agreed to introduce me, but he was nowhere to be found.

Richard Morse was his name. He was half Haitian, half American, and having stalked him online, I'd decided he would fascinate me. He'd grown up in New England but moved to Port-au-Prince in 1987 to run his mother's family's hotel. He was a houngan, according to the *Economist*, and had a vodou rock band, RAM, that played every Thursday night. Of course, the Thursday I was in town, it was cancelled.

I was at the check-in desk, asking (as the doom-laden TripAdvisor reviews had exhorted) whether I might be able to see a couple of rooms, when an American voice behind me said, 'Put her in the Graham Greene.' I turned round to find him studying me with an ironic smirk. At six foot, I was used to bending down to talk to people, but with Richard Morse, I came up to the bottom of his ponytail.

'You're a writer, right? Gotta put you in the Graham Greene,' he said. I had tweeted him, asking for an interview (I hadn't mentioned what about, lest, like everyone else, he stopped replying to me). He was in America till Saturday, he'd said, and I'd written back, great, I'll come Saturday. And he had not replied.

'Is it really where he stayed?' I asked with the ingratiating smile I usually reserved for doctors.

'I dunno,' said Richard Morse. 'Probably not.' He swallowed a laugh. 'You wanted to talk to me, right?'

'Yes!' I squeaked.

'I'll be around,' he said, and loped off. An unimpressed-looking woman showed me to my room – in an annexe which, by the looks of it, might not have been updated since Greene's stay – and brought a pitcher of non-choleric water. In the time it took to climb the stairs, the mosquitos drained approximately one third of my blood. I showered in case they were attracted to ingrained sweat, and put on the sundress that the aid worker on the plane had prophesised would get me killed. I took out my diary to circle my next antimalarial dose. Then I smothered myself in citronella and walked over to the main building.

There was reggae playing in the bar, where two busts of Jean-Jacques Dessalines monitored a taciturn barman. I walked through onto the patio and ordered a G&T, as I imagined the war correspondents did when they stayed here – for those reporting on elections, coups or everyday violence, the Oloffson was the only place to be. Suddenly, Richard Morse was sitting opposite me.

I made small talk about the hotel – how wonderful! How historic! What a place to be sitting, here where Jackie O, Mick Jagger and Gielgud had all sat! – and he looked disgusted. Richard Morse clearly didn't do small talk. I took a swig of my G&T.

'So I hear you're a houngan,' I said, boldly.

'Who told you that?' he asked.

'Read it in the *Economist*,' I said. 'Serge said you were, too.'

He shook his head: 'I thought you wanted to talk politics.' Richard Morse's outspoken Twitter feed – anti-government, anti-American government – made him the first port of call for lazy journalists.

'Oh! No,' I said, trying my best to look fearless. 'I want to talk vodou.'

He'd been brought up atheist – 'as a white man', as he put it – in America. His father had been an atheist, his mother a mambo. Richard had gone to Haiti for the first time at 16, and fallen for it. And the feeling had been mutual: on a subsequent visit, he'd heard the loa knocking on the window, calling him all night. He'd gone on to study anthropology at Princeton, but when his father died, he'd returned to Haiti and become a houngan.

Talking about his training was the first time Richard Morse really smiled. 'It was unbelievable,' he said, with the bliss of a man who'd seen God. 'It made me realise that it's all connected, yeah? Vodou, Protestants, Catholics, the Pope ... Princeton, Haiti ... it's all connected.' I remembered Jero Pura telling me to pray to my own god. What if it *was* all connected? What if vodou wouldn't just shock my pain away, but might actually heal me?

He didn't do it as a vocation, he was at pains to point out. He only did it to 'take care of stuff'.

I swallowed. It was becoming clear that I was the Oloffson's only guest tonight, but I couldn't leave Haiti without some kind of closure. I reminded myself that the scene which had played in two decades of nightmares – Roger Moore and Jane Seymour in the graveyard, Baron Samedi erupting from the earth and laughing them to hell – was a film, voodoo not vodou, and that the nocebo effect might reset my brain.

'What kind of stuff?' I asked.

'I mean, someone might come along,' said Richard Morse, and he paused. 'And I might think, you know, maybe I can do something for that person. I don't – I mean, you know – I don't have a sign outside saying "I do readings", or whatever.'

'And if someone comes along,' I said, casually, 'and you think you can do something for them, do you tell them?'

'I've helped a few people,' he said, cryptically. And then he told me.

He'd helped one woman's cancer, though he didn't want to take official credit for that. Been called to another who'd just come back from the dead to 'get her going'. Healed the paralysed arm of a woman selling art by the roadside at Saut-d'Eau, just like that. My ears pricked up.

'Could she immediately lift it?'

He paused. 'It's a miracle,' he said, jazz hands in his voice. Then he said, more quietly: 'Frightening.' He had stopped after that, because he didn't want to feel obliged to go around healing people.

The nape of my neck was prickling, and for once it wasn't a mosquito bite.

We circled each other in small talk, and then I tried again. Do you think you could heal anyone, I asked. He said he didn't know. I said: you should try. Once in a while, he said, I come across someone and – he paused, stared into the distance – give it a shot. Ask God to help this person.

'Will you help me?' I said.

I told him about the coffee, and the diagnosis, and the COPE course, and the drugs, and Kevin and Bali and everyone who'd tried to be my Jesus but hadn't been. I said: maybe you're it.

'So this is what you're doing,' he sighed. 'Looking for someone to fix you.'

'I just want someone to make me not in pain,' I said. And then, in a small voice, I added: 'And maybe you're that person.'

'Wouldn't that be funny,' said Richard Morse.

So would you help me, I asked.

Would I try, he said.

Would you try, I said.

Would you like that, he said, a hint of anger in his voice.

'I would love you to,' I said. 'Yeah.'

We both studied our drinks. *I'm still in love with you, girl*, Alton Ellis sang from the bar.

Richard Morse dragged the air into his nostrils. Once. Twice. I kept my eyes on my drink.

'Don't touch the ice,' he said. 'I have to go get the keys.'

It's a funny thing, trauma. I thought I had a perfect memory of what happened that night, even though it comes as flashes: instant followed by instant instead of the normal spool of film. Thinking about them now, they pop up, one by one, moving slowly like a turgid PowerPoint presentation, only these are slides that knot my stomach, constrict my throat and swell the blood vessels in my eyeballs as I sit through them, powerless to hit the off switch, knowing I must let them run their course.

I remember the punch of fear as he jumped up to get the keys. Realising it was on and wishing it wasn't. Offering to do it in the morning, saying 'I don't want to pressure you,' and him saying darkly, 'That's not what it is,' as he strode off.

I remember walking through the garden, breath shallow with anticipation as it always was before a treatment I prayed could be The One, stealing a glance at the dark pool, thinking, 'That's where the suicide was in *The Comedians*.'

I remember being in a building round the back of the pool – lights off, silence except for his jangling keys – walking past silhouettes of gym equipment barely lit by a feeble moon.

I remember my stomach tightening as we stopped at a padlocked door, and trying to make eye contact with Richard Morse as he rapped three times, then took a key to the padlock.

The flood of cortisol as I followed him in, to a hotel room lit by a naked oil lamp burning on the floor: clusters of religious symbols, figurines, bottles plugged with candles and strips of cloth set around the room at regular intervals.

The catch in my throat and the blood vacuuming from my legs as I took in the black top hat of Baron Samedi, cocked at a jaunty angle and hung from the headboard, his stick propped up beside the double bed, and a rush of regret as Richard Morse gently closed the door behind me and I realised I was going to die.

My pores opening like floodgates and haemorrhaging sweat, trying to make me slippery as an eel, as he started a strange, jerking shuffle – to the bed, back to me, then around me, then standing silently behind me.

His hands slipping along my soaked skin as he grappled with my neck, rubbing the skin and pulling things off – dress strap, bra strap, the pink elastic in my hair – as he yanked his fingers down the top of my spine, across my shoulder and down my arm, each time more violent than the last, each time my dress dragged a little lower. I remember saying in a tiny voice, 'Please don't crack my neck,' and him lumbering round, face towards mine, breath hot on my cheekbone and eyes rolled back in his head, possessed. 'Hmm?' I remember him saying.

I remember trying to zone out as he pawed at me, wondering whether, if I screamed, he might come out of his trance or someone in the hotel might come running. And I remember realising that not only would nobody in the hotel hear me, three buildings away with the reggae turned up, but that there *was* nobody in the hotel to hear a scream that night, other than the staff.

I wondered if he'd rape me first or just break my neck.

I remember praying: to God, Jesus, Miffy and my grandmother, to Charmayne's celestial beings and Patrick's holy colours, to whatever was in that room – because I could feel *something* in that room – to show mercy. I remember repeating silently, desperately, that I had come in good faith, that I wanted only to be healed, as he shuffled off towards a cupboard, bobbing at the knee. I remember turning for the door while he was in the cupboard, and deciding I wouldn't make it out before he caught up.

I remember a warm liquid trickling between my thighs as he shuffled back towards me, and wondering whether it was only sweat or if I'd wet myself.

I remember the relief that maybe he would only rape me

as he stood nose to nose and demanded, in a high-pitched voice, that I give him 'something pretty', and the dawning realisation, as I picked up the pink elastic band that he'd pulled from my hair and offered it to him and he pressed again, *is it pretty*, that Erzulie was in the room, now – flighty Erzulie who smelled of roses and demanded presents from her adoring male followers – and maybe she would protect me from the Baron. The flood of hope that perhaps I would survive, and the desperation to find something pretty enough to engage her sympathy. I remember telling her timidly that right now I didn't have anything, that the elastic band wasn't worthy of her, swearing to bring her something suitably pretty in the morning and adding, in my head, *if only you let me live.*

I remember feeling his heavy presence – or maybe Erzulie's, or the Baron's – behind me, as he directed me into the cupboard; then inside, gazing in horror at another flame burning, more bottles and figurines and *stuff* – stuff like necklaces and souvenir bottles of holy water and pots containing the spirits of the dead. Realising I was cornered and not knowing who I was more scared of, the possessed man behind me, or whatever was guarding the shrine in front.

I don't remember how it ended, only that it did. And that we walked back into the hotel in silence and sat down on the terrace outside, above the statue of Baron Samedi, and I realised he had let me live.

But trauma is a funny thing. Because when I look back at the transcript – I still can't listen to the recording, so I paid someone to transcribe it – there was more to it than that. It would seem I'm an unreliable narrator.

I remembered the room as deathly silent, the only sound his heavy breathing. Which is there, in the recording, but there's also a ticking noise which doubles, disappears, then starts up a rhythm – like a paradiddle, said Allie, who listened to it for me – and goes silent. There's a bottle clanking against other bottles, a car alarm honking far off in the distance. My voice near the start whispering, 'What are you going to do?' – it must have been when he touched my neck – and saying politely, after 15 minutes of silence, 'Thank you so much – do I need to do anything, like get some wine?'

And there's an exchange. One right after the long back and forth about which pretty thing I might be able to give him.

'My neck does feel much better,' I say. 'I think my back does, too.'

Tick, tick, tick, goes the sound in the background.

'There is ... you ... there was ... something,' Richard Morse – or Erzulie or Baron Samedi, because he's still possessed – says. 'I don't know how you got it.'

'What kind of thing?' I rush it out.

'Nasty,' he says.

'Really?'

'Yeah.'

'But you took it away?'

'Yeah.'

'Thank you.'

Then he says: 'Pray.'

And then it's silent for two minutes until there's a bang, a noise like sticks being slapped together four times, and he asks, 'You feel good?'

And I say, 'Yes.'

'Are you terrified?' he asks as we're walking out, and I say, 'I'm not now.' Then I order us both a stiff drink.

Whenever I would talk to professionals about my pain – doctors, psychologists, hypnotists or Kevins, because they were all the same – at some point in the conversation, every conversation, once we'd established what they thought was a rapport, they would invariably look deep into my eyes and ask me if – really, truly, honestly – I wanted to get better. Janet Williams' idea of the chronic pain personality may not be universally shared – 'It really doesn't exist,' Ronald Kulich, professor of psychology at Boston's Tufts University told me – and yet, confronted by my tear-stained face, my stomach stretched with comfort food and my gender, most doctors assumed that, on some level, I was choosing to be ill.

You can't judge someone else's pain – it's been proven that medical professionals underestimate their patients' chronic pain levels by up to 49 per cent.[9] Yet still they doubt us, and because they're the experts, we end up doubting ourselves. *Suddenly I'm beginning not to trust my memory at all.*

Whenever they'd ask me if I wanted to get better, I'd say yes as a reflex, but the scepticism in their eyes would always spark a self-interrogation afterwards. Do I really want to recover, I'd ask, or underneath all this, am I secretly happy as a victim? After that night with Richard Morse, I knew the answer.

––––––

On my first morning in Haiti, after breakfast at Kaliko Beach Club, a man I'd seen eyeing me over our plates of hard bread and bruised bananas had come over.

'I'm Jean,' he'd said.

'Julia,' I'd said.

'Julia,' he'd repeated. 'Why are you here? What are you running away from?'

'Nothing,' I'd said primly, gesturing at my Kindle. 'I'm on holiday.' He'd narrowed his eyes and handed me a business card. He was a priest.

I wasn't running away from anything, I'd wanted to scream at Jean. I wasn't a running away kind of person – if anything, I was the opposite. If something was wrong – physically, emotionally, whatever – I would unpick the situation until it was a tatty pile of string. What I should have done, what I could have done, why I'd said what I did, laughed when I shouldn't, reached for that fucking cup of coffee when I'd known it was already cold. If I had a problem, I confronted it. That's why I was in Haiti, after all. That's why I was on this whole frigging journey, building up debt that would forever cripple me, even with the book money, even if I got another job again. I was chasing down my illness.

But I hadn't been doing the journey right, it dawned on me months later, when I was going over that night at the Oloffson for the thousandth time. I'd been travelling but not engaging; in fact, I'd been turning up, acting interested, then turning tail and running away as fast as my flat feet would carry me into the next time zone.

I'd stopped swirling Patrick's colours at people's solar plexi after a few days, and packed away the CBD oil in the kitchen cupboard as if it were a rabbit's foot against a greater illness. I'd stopped my Balinese prayers the day Miffy died, used the last of the oil to anoint her dead body. I'd excised all memory of Charmayne's kindness so the hope she'd sparked in me no longer rent me apart. I'd been telling myself I was on this journey to find the truth as quickly as possible, but actually, all I was doing was legging it every time I reached the crunch.

That night at the Oloffson it all changed, though. That's why I was so shaken.

By the time I solved the puzzle, I had done far scarier things. Been cut with a razor in the AIDS capital of the world. Slaughtered a chicken and bathed in its blood. Jumped in icy mountain water and had a neck vertebra crunched out of place. And I could think back on all that stuff and process it, but every time I thought back to my night at the Oloffson I'd have the same visceral reaction: gobstopper expanding in my throat, pressure bloodshotting my eyes. Why?

Eventually I realised: that night with Richard Morse was the first time I saw the treatment through to the end. I'd always wanted to get better, but that night I realised I'd sell my soul to do it. And that ghastly desperation was more terrifying than any Bond villain or spectral murderer I could think of.

I didn't sleep well in the Graham Greene room, partly because of the trauma, partly because of the heat, mostly because I woke up at 4am with the distinct impression that someone was sharpening a razor along the line between my neck and collarbone.

Please wait till morning, I begged whatever it was. Wait for your something pretty. I won't let you down. At check-out, I walked to the lobby with a delicate, Modigliani-esque sculpture of a vodou initiate I'd bought as a souvenir the previous day, and asked for Richard Morse.

I have the thing, I said, the pretty thing. Can I go back – there?

Sure, he said, and went to get the keys.

It was different in the daylight, of course. The pool looked just tired, not sinister; the treadmill was a treadmill, not a harbinger of doom. I kept breathing as Richard Morse knocked on the door, felt perfectly calm as we walked in, past the bed and the top hat and into the cupboard. I took the elastic band that had tied up my hair the night before, and knotted it round the sculpture, just in case she'd wanted that all along. I put it down beside the little water bottles ('Holy water,' said Richard. 'People bring it to me from all over the world') and the bits and bobs perched above the flame. I thanked Erzulie for protecting me, hoped the sculpture met with her approval and begged for her help. I believe, I said, I believe in it all. Once I was back in the car, telling Geffrard what had happened, I realised I was drenched in sweat again.

It was only at the airport, once I'd been wheeled to the gate, that I realised my arm wasn't hurting.

I picked up my bag – the little carry-on case that I normally made everyone else lift in case it dislocated my shoulder – and went upstairs for a coffee. My neck didn't hurt, either.

I came back downstairs, exaggerating a limp I no longer felt to avoid questioning looks as I sat in the disabled seats. I preboarded and asked the cabin crew to lift my case into the overhead locker, asked for an extra pillow to cushion the armrest against my allodynia. But I didn't need it. I typed all the way to Miami and then to Curaçao, and it didn't hurt. My friends were at dinner by the time I got to the villa – it was Tanya's 40th birthday and I'd promised to come straight out. Instead I found some rum in the kitchen, took the bottle down to the bottom of the garden where the sea smashed against the wall, and sacrificed it to Agwe, one of Erzulie's three husbands. Then I got into bed and prayed.

I felt fine the next day. And the next. My friends stared as I went down to the sea twice a day to make the rum sacrifices, outraged at my waste of good liquor. I tried to explain it, but all they wanted to talk about was shagging, not possessions. Although they did quite like the idea of the demon cat.

Back in the bar that night, drinking rum straight up – neither food nor ice was allowed after a ceremony with the loa – I'd asked Richard what had happened back there. He didn't know, he'd said – he never knows. But there was one thing he did.

'I saw what was bothering you.' He'd lowered his voice even though we were the only people in the hotel.

'It looked like some kind of beast,' he'd said. 'Some kind of black cat shape.' Wrapped around my neck.

How? Why? I love cats. I don't believe in demons.

'I don't know,' he said. 'I don't know what you do, where you've been. It was just there. Nasty. Mad at me.'

He'd pulled it out through my fingers, he said – that's why he'd been dragging his hands down my arms. Then it had started towards him, so he'd taken it to the flame in the cupboard shrine.

I told him that I had a general phobia of people touching my neck, but that it had been worse recently, and I'd been having recurring nightmares in the lead-up to Haiti in which someone would stand behind me and quietly break my neck, and I'd wake up from them in a sweat thinking about Baron Samedi.

'That's where whatever it was, was,' said Richard. 'I would have searched more, but you were a little … you know.' He was kind, Richard Morse. Even when he was possessed, he hadn't wanted to frighten me. He'd chosen not to pull it out through my legs for the same reason, he said. I wondered if all houngans were so paternal.

I confided in him that I'd nearly wet myself. I didn't say that, actually, I might have.

'Do I have to believe for it to work?' I asked, and he didn't reply.

'How do I know it won't come back?'

'I have no idea.' My journey worried him, he said. I shouldn't be going around offering myself to people, telling them to do whatever they wanted to help my pain. 'Just don't start going round, opening yourself up,' he said, all fatherly. 'You've got to figure out a way so that when you're going around doing this stuff, you're not susceptible to ... stuff. Because everyone's not nice. And if you get a vibe, like, "get the fuck out of here", get the fuck out of there. See what I'm saying?'

'Yes,' I said meekly, but in my head I added, *I don't care what they do to me, as long as it helps the pain.*

'Did you get the vibe to get the fuck out of there today, or were you just scared?' he said.

Oh, just scared you were going to rape and murder me.

'I didn't want to get out,' I lied. 'I was just sure that Baron Samedi was going to kill me.'

But today wasn't Baron Samedi's day, he said, it was Erzulie Dantour's. Erzulie Dantour, represented as the black Madonna. Erzulie Dantour, the protectress of abused women. Erzulie Dantour, who raged and wept at the injustices she suffered – when I'd told Richard earlier about wanting to kill myself and the non-stop tears, he'd said, 'That's very Erzulie Dantour.' Erzulie Dantour, the hysterical woman, the Medea and the Lilith of the loa. I wondered what Erzulie Dantour would say about Yentl Syndrome. *I cry at nothing, and cry most of the time.*

After delivering the sculpture to Erzulie I was completely pain-free for 48 hours. It was astonishing – wonderful and horrifying in equal measure. I'd had occasional respites from the pain in the previous three years, but they'd either been brief – a matter of minutes – or incomplete (I hadn't had a bad day for over a month after seeing Patrick, but the pain had always been there, just muted). Vodou, though, had spirited it away in its entirety.

It was probably the placebo effect, I told myself – after all, houngans had mastered the nocebo effect like nobody else.

In a way, I hoped it was, because I preferred to believe in an all-forgiving God than in vengeful spirits who freaked out when they weren't given presents as pretty as they deserved.

But I knew that what I'd felt in that room hadn't just been in my head.

I took it badly when the pain sloped back on the third day. I woke up with a sore neck – maybe because I'd tried to swim four lengths the day before, maybe because I'd tossed and turned one too many times, trying to block out the sound of my friends carousing till 4am, maybe because my offering had only been pretty enough to merit two days' respite, maybe because the placebo effect is notoriously as instant in its passing as in its arrival. Either way, it hit me harder than any of the disappointments that had gone before. I got a cold. Which turned into food poisoning. The next day I woke up with a fever and crushing pain through my body. I couldn't move, only gasp for help. My friends iced and monitored me until they were scared enough to call a doctor. An ambulance was called – my symptoms were those of a heart attack, the dispatcher said. Of course, there was nothing wrong with my heart when the paramedics scanned it. It was the nocebo effect in its full, raging force.

For the first time in my life, I'd risked everything, offered up my soul as well as my body, and it still hadn't worked.

I couldn't talk about Haiti for a while. I wanted to forget I had ever been. And so I went back to the medical drawing board.

THE WORLD'S MOST FAMOUS
MEDICINE MAN

Why did the doctor inhabit another world from hers?
Why couldn't he hear what she was saying?
Zelda Fitzgerald, *Save Me the Waltz* (1932)

In the eyes of a sceptic, faced with a world of 'quacks' and 'charlatans' – even Radovan Karadžić had a thriving business masquerading as a Belgrade faith healer before he was caught and convicted of genocide – acupuncture stands out as the most acceptable, and accepted, of alternative medicines. Scientists may argue over the statistics, talk about small sample sizes, say that for every study showing acupuncture may be effective there's another that implies it's the placebo effect – but, for pain, it works. Why? Who knows? It may reduce pain by triggering the release of adenosine, a compound which stops pain by tamping down our nociceptors.[10] It seems to increase opioid receptors in pain-controlling parts of the brain.[11] Or maybe, as devotees would have it, we have an unmeasurable life force flowing through us called qi, which acupuncture revs up when it's down. Either way, the fact remains that if you have an operation and you follow it up with acupuncture, your pain levels will probably be lower and you'll need less medication.[12]

I'd tried acupuncture in the past and hadn't been convinced, but then, no alternative therapy had ever really convinced me. Not that I'd been fully sceptical – the anti-quack militants had always seemed so angry to me, so outraged by people they'd never met and things they'd never tried for issues they'd never had. But on moving to London, I'd realised my upbringing amid healers and wart charmers hadn't exactly been normal, and I burned with embarrassment. After that, on the rare occasions that I tried something, I would sit through the consultation wondering what I was doing there, and leave as furtively as from a Soho peep show. But then, in 2009, I met Dr Cuong.

A colleague had recommended him to me for my nuclear hayfever. 'He's expensive,' she had warned – and he was, but I could just about afford his Harley Street prices back in those halcyon salaried days. 'But he will change your life,' she'd added. And he did.

He was a doctor for starters, an actual GP with a surgery near Dr Good's. He split his time between there and his father's private acupuncture clinic. He came from a long line of Vietnamese acupuncturists, and he said that for many ailments, he found acupuncture worked better than western medicine. Now here was a quack I could trust.

That first session, he said my qi was low, that although he couldn't blitz my hayfever mid-season, he could work on my system as a whole. Maybe it was placebo or maybe it was my qi, but as the weeks went on, I started to feel more energised. I only needed three coffees to get through the day, instead of six and three chocolate bars. Then suddenly it was March, then April, then October, and I'd made it through the hayfever season on one Zyrtec a day. I was sold.

Of course, he was the first person I ran to when they told me my pain was never going away.

He didn't want to treat it in isolation, he said, and he didn't want to interfere with anything my doctors were trying, but he was happy to work on my qi as a whole. We did a couple of sessions – they helped my fatigue and suicidal ideation, as doctors coyly call it, but they weren't what I'd hoped for. Then one morning, when my pain was through the roof, he took pity on me and zeroed in on it. Afterwards, I raced off to COPE class, no time to think about how I was feeling until I was running up the steps so as not to be late, then realised my arm didn't hurt. It lasted the rest of the day.

I was, of course, living on £344 a month at this point,

the amount deemed by the government sufficient to live on for those of us too sick to work. Chronic pain responds particularly well to acupuncture – a 2006 study[13] showed patients like me demonstrate a greater increase in activity of the hypothalamus (which regulates the nervous system) and a larger decrease in amygdala activity (which keeps us in fight or flight mode) than healthy people – but I couldn't afford Dr Cuong's £80 fee. Instead, Dr Good dug into his budget to get me some free sessions.

Critics of complementary medicine on the NHS say acupuncture's a waste of money, and this absolutely was – a guy who'd done the requisite three years of study and had learned it by the 21st-century scientific book. Instead of working on my system, he focused exclusively on the pain, digging needles into my neck, along my collarbone and above my shoulder blade. In our 30-minute sessions (Dr Cuong's were an hour) he would start with six, say, and ask me to tell him if I felt anything. Yes, I'd say, it burns here, and here, and here ... and he'd quickly remove them. Once, I mooted that the burning might be a good thing – Dr Cuong's needles tingled as he tugged at them to stimulate the qi – but he insisted he didn't want to hurt me. So I'd lie there for the rest of the session with a single needle – two if I was lucky – lodged in the only place it didn't hurt, and I'd dutifully thank him as I was pulling on my top (the sessions were so rushed there was no time for modesty) but inside I'd be screaming you useless idiot, you waste of space. When we completed our six sessions he told me his funding was being cut and I – the girl who'd grown up on beansprouts and homeopathic toothpaste – said to myself, thank god the NHS is stamping out this nonsense.

After Kevin's intervention, I was living in Cornwall, but going up to London every month or so for treatment. I could have gone back to Dr Cuong, of course, but I subscribed to the belief that the acupuncture he was practising in London – perfected through the generations of his family – must automatically be inferior to what was being practised in the land of its birth. So when I was traumatised by what Haiti had revealed about myself, and was groping for something less scary and more of this world – yet still brandishing two fingers at western medicine – I happened to notice that flights to China were really rather affordable at this time of year, and the next thing I knew I was drifting past the mountains of Yunnan province as we commenced our final descent into Lijiang.

———

That I might be flying 6,000 miles to meet a dead man was a distinct possibility. Doctor Ho Shixiu was, depending on reports, anything from 92 to 108 years old. He lived in the mountains, they said. He had a website that appeared to be from the early 1990s: a single page which Google struggled to translate, listing an email address that bounced back and a phone number that rang and rang without ever being answered.

I asked my friend Shiwei what she thought. She consulted with a journalist friend back home in Shanghai. 'Based on her experience with old people,' Shiwei wrote, 'she would encourage you to go as early as possible. Several old people passed away right after she interviewed them.' Max Beauvoir had died. John of God, a ridiculous faith healer I planned to see in Brazil if all else failed, had just been rushed to hospital for a heart bypass. Ketut Liyer had died soon after my visit. Potential saviours were dropping like flies.

The good news, Shiwei said, was that she had phoned herself and Dr Ho had picked up. He didn't speak Mandarin, so they'd conversed in English. 'He was keen to hang up the phone,' she wrote. 'But I guess that's a typical thing for senior people. All he said was "okay" and "no problem" plus a sentence I did not understand at all.'

I tried to call again, to make sure he could help me before I took five flights totalling 19 hours to reach him. But the phone was cut off for a few days, and then it returned to ringing out again.

Go, said Shiwei, before he dies and winter comes, because

he's halfway up a mountain and you don't want to get snowed in.

Go, said a colleague – a photographer who had, several years earlier, shot Doctor Ho, the world's most famous medicine man.

Go, said a friend who worked in TV, and was used to doing stuff like flying halfway across the world on a whim (and a budget), in case there's something to it. Sometimes you just have to take a chance.

I didn't want to take a chance, of course. My whole life had turned into a merry-go-round of taking chances, round and round and round as my money spun into thin air and the end of the ride remained out of sight. But I went anyway, without speaking to him, emailing him, or having any proof that the thought alone of my visit hadn't killed him as it had Max Beauvoir.

Dr Ho Shixiu wasn't strictly a doctor. A member of the Naxi minority people, he was a self-trained herbalist. He was also, so the story went, a man who could cure anything from cancer to diabetes with concoctions of plants picked from the mountainside by the light of the full moon. Or something.

It was a story that appealed for its romance as much as its hope. This ageless old man had retreated from the Cultural Revolution to his birthplace, a tiny village on the banks of the Jade Dragon Snow Mountain in the wilds of Yunnan. There, he had stalked the foothills, gathering the local flora and turning it into medicine. The plants were organic, of course, and many of them were endemic to the mountain – no wonder he was popular with idealist westerners. The fact that he had apparently cured an American of prostate cancer was the icing on the cake.

Dr Ho had first been brought to western attention in 1986, when Bruce Chatwin had stumbled on him during a trip to the area and written about him for the *Sunday Times*. Chatwin focused on his charisma and family life rather than his medical credentials, but nevertheless a legend was born.

Dr Ho's clinic became an essential stop for any journalist travelling through Yunnan; the guidebooks caught on, and countless blogs followed. 'He's a Naxi-minority country doctor (and probably half a loon) who has become a bit of a celebrity,' Shiwei's friend, who'd first told me about him, had written. 'Apparently western cancer patients keep visiting him hopeful for treatment.'

Baisha, where Dr Ho lived, was at high altitude, and with my myriad health concerns I didn't want to fly straight there from the plains of Chengdu, so I went to a city called Kunming to acclimatise. I'd chosen it for the name, but almost immediately on arrival, things – fate, if you will – slotted into place. There was an English guy working at my hotel, and I told him why I was there. I don't know about Dr Ho, he said, but you need to meet Nick.

Nick was technically a TCM doctor, yet in reality so much more. William had met him in Lijiang, when Nick had arrived at his hotel, taken the hand of his colleague and told her: you have cancer. No I don't!, she'd yelped. Get a scan of your liver, Nick had said. And she'd gone to the doctor, and lo and behold she had early stage liver cancer. She survived.

Six years later, Nick was William's main healthcare provider. He had found cancer in William's body many times, but cured it with herbs before it could take hold.

'Wow,' I said. 'And you confirmed every time that you definitely had cancer?'

'Oh no,' said William. 'Nick spots these things before they'd show up on a scan, and he cures them himself, so a doctor would never know. Say there's a scale of one to 10, and 10 would be stage one cancer. He catches mine at a six.' I thought of Patrick, who'd said in Vienna that he could spot cancer at a molecular level. Just cure it, he'd told us. Cancer scares people, so don't tell them, just deal with it. I still didn't know what to make of Patrick – I tried not to think about him much because his possible powers scared me – but even so, I wanted to meet Nick.

He charges a lot, warned William – about £300 for a

consultation – but for that, you get a six-month supply of herbs.

Nick told me it would be £2,000 for a consultation, more if it turned out to be cancer. 'I'm very angry he would do that,' said William when I told him. 'He said he was raising his prices but...' he tailed off. As I left, the cogs were still turning in his eyes.

Lijiang had been a beautiful town once upon a time and it was still pretty, though it had somewhat lost its edge of authenticity by demolishing its Han dynasty buildings, rebuilding them to Epcot standard and charging tourists £10 to enter. At the hotel I met Lea, who spoke fluent English and immediately understood what I had come for – when they'd found a tumour in her neck five years earlier, a TCM doctor had told her it would disappear if she could only be happy, and lo and behold, it had disappeared. She called Dr Ho, established he was alive, and agreed I would come over the following day.

The guidebooks had described Baisha as an unspoiled village, an antidote to Disneyfied Lijiang, and it probably was when they'd written that. But while the Chinese tourists stuck to Lijiang, western travellers had branched out. The first faces I saw belonged to a group of hearty, Teutonic-looking pensioners; the lopsided wooden buildings – so charmingly not tarted up, as they had been in Lijiang – shilled Naxi shawls and printed fabrics. One building had been done up as a New England-style shack and advertised tea and cappuccinos.

'Doctor Ho,' said the taxi driver in English, pulling over with a flourish. He'd picked me up in Lijiang, 40 minutes away, but every taxi driver in Yunnan knew exactly where to go. 'All the white people want Dr Ho,' as my driver the next day would say with a grin.

The people who'd feted him – Michael Palin, the *Telegraph*, the *New York Times* and Sue Perkins – had described it perfectly. It was a wooden bungalow, his famous clinic, with 'Jade Dragon Snow Mountain Chinese Herbal Medicine

Clinic' painted over the doorway and newspaper clippings and internet printouts in every language stuck on boards, forming mini towers of Babel either side of the steps.

There was an ancient woman – Dr Ho's wife, I would later learn – sweeping the pavement outside. She wore traditional Naxi dress: maxiskirt, long-sleeved top, jerkin and oversized flat cap in varying shades of blue, with a white harness criss-crossed from front to back – all the better for lugging baskets around on one's osteoporosised vertebrae, because Naxi women do all the physical work for their men.

Two middle-aged couples, who I decided looked Dutch, were emerging, calling out 'Thank you!' as they came down the stairs. They smiled at me standing there, as if I was hanging back for them to pass. I wasn't.

I pretended to be engrossed in the reviews as I rehearsed what I wanted to say. With other people I'd just winged it, offering up my body to heal as they saw fit. But because Dr Ho was a doctor, or kind of a doctor, I'd prepared a list of symptoms to discuss with him, symptoms I thought he might pinpoint to one malfunctioning meridian. They ranged from 'burning shoulder' and 'carving knife' to 'heartburn' and 'eye focusing hurts'. One never knew, in Chinese medicine, what could be related to what.

I climbed the steps, four of them, into a shrine to Dr Ho. Pennants hung from the walls, scarlet with gold fringing – inscribed with thanks, I would later be told, for his achievements. Flimsies stuffed with testimonies, interviews and articles hung from the polystyrene ceiling. Frames on the walls were filled with business cards from every continent.

'Hello?' I called – it was still light outside but the room was so full of ephemera that it was hard to see. Nobody answered. 'Hello?' I tried again. A faint shuffling came from out the back.

'Doctor Ho?' I said, and the shuffling turned into unsteady footsteps and a silhouette in the back doorway.

He came towards me, a slip of a thing: barely five feet, slight, but with a broad grin that transcended his white lab coat and wisdom that filled the room. My god, he was as old as they all said: liver spots dappling his lined face, grand canyons from nostril to age-thinned lips and the wispy goatee of Confucius.

'Doctor Ho,' I said. 'My hotel called. I'm the journalist from England. I've come for a consultation.' (I had decided Dr Ho was media-friendly and would doubtless be more thorough if he thought I was going to write about him in a magazine.)

Dr Ho looked up at me from under a navy woollen hat. He beamed the gummy smile that had launched a thousand blog posts. He motioned at a bench, and wordlessly thrust a sheaf of reviews at me.

'No,' I said. 'I'm here to find out what's wrong with me.' He grinned. 'No big problem,' he said in what sounded like a deliberately exaggerated Chinese accent. 'Be happy.' And then he looked me up and down – I must have been three times his volume – and said, 'High cholesterol. Diabetes.' And he mimed an obese belly as far as his little arms would stretch.

———

'He called me fat,' I shrieked to Lea that evening when I stumbled in, so tired I was struggling to stand. 'He said, "No problem, be happy," and he kept saying I was fat.'

'Diabetes,' he had said again and again, miming an expanding belly. 'High cholesterol.' Are you trying to say I have diabetes and high cholesterol, I asked – the benefit of having been tested for everything under the sun in the past few years being the knowledge that I had neither – and he said no, not now, but I would if I got fatter. 'Don't worry, be happy,' he recited like a stuck record. 'Be optimistic,' said the slip of paper that he gave me, that he normally handed over with his magic herbs. Only the paper, mind, because for chubsters like me, there was no need for herbs.

From Mr Bloggs to the bad balians to Dr Ho: three countries, different disciplines, all transfixed by my gender, my tears and my belly. *Cheer up love, it might never happen. I am a doctor, dear, and I know.* I yearned for Charmayne and for Jero Pura.

'Dr Ho will diagnose ailments (in good English) and talk herbs, health and happiness,' the *New York Times* had written. 'He has been praised around the world for helping to solve specific medical conditions among many that western medicine had not been able to solve,' read one of the dozens of blog posts. And here he was, 'one of the leading lights of Chinese traditional medicine,' according to Michael Palin in *Himalaya*, refusing to take my pulse.

Maybe it was because of his age. Maybe everyone else had been embarrassed by the emperor's new clothes, hadn't dared point out he could barely speak English. Maybe it was because female + journalist didn't compute any more than female + genuinely ill. But when I changed tack and started asking him questions about his life, all he did was thrust a potted bio at me and said, 'Read.'

I looked down at my notebook, the careful list of symptoms and three pages of questions, and pinned on my medical smile.

He was saying things about blood tests, something normalising without having any therapy.

'Doctors come here for study so I'm very happy,' he said.

'Which doctors?' I asked. He paused.

'You have no big problem,' he said. 'Many girls have problems, so you must be happy. No stress, no depression. You have PMT.' Then he did his jolly fat mime again. 'Make people fat. Many girls have this. And men. No big problem. Be happy.'

Hot tears were pressing on the back of my eyes, of sorrow or of rage – *The Yellow Wallpaper* or Erzulie Dantour – I couldn't be sure.

'Can you take my pulse please?' I begged. He grabbed my wrist and jabbed it with his index finger.

'Be happy, no problem.' If you say that again, I thought, we're going to have a big fucking problem.

'Do you treat cancer?' I asked, remembering the mythical

American whose miraculous cure had turned Dr Ho into a pilgrimage site for sick westerners.

'Oh! Yes. Cancer, leukaemia. No side effects. I have saved many people.'

One of the central tenets of the Dr Ho myth – along with the idea that he was a doctor, and had cured cancer – was that he had been his own first patient. He'd been suffering from some deadly disease, had retreated to the countryside, boiled up some herbal concoction and cured himself. I asked him what the problem had been.

'Not being well,' he said. He handed me another photo-copy. 'All here.' It was just another article about him, fellatio in 500 words. I pushed – what was the name of your disease – and in response he knocked my dictaphone onto the floor.

When I announced, wiping away tears, that I was a journalist and that his father didn't seem to understand my questions, Dr Ho's son, Dr Ho Shulong (an equally talented doctor, according to the blogosphere) whisked me off to the family home, a huge compound a block away, surrounding a large garden full of plants – plants used in Dr Ho's surgery, his son said, although of course the family still collected all their herbs from Jade Dragon Snow Mountain. It was as big as Ketut Liyer's place in Bali, which he'd built with the proceeds of his *Eat Pray Love* fame: newly constructed but traditional in style. Wooden panels around the cloisters were being painted with tributes to Dr Ho's triumphs: quotes from guidebooks, blogs and letters carefully copied out in thin black cursive, extolling him to the skies. One was taken from a letter that Ho Shulong said had been written by the Mayo Clinic on 23 January 2002, when Dr Ho had successfully treated an American with prostate cancer. 'He has never had any chemotherapy,' it read. 'He is doing well on herbal treatment alone. His disease is dormant.' I asked Ho Shulong if I could see a copy of the letter or if he could give me the name of the person who'd written it, but however many times I asked and however I phrased it, he couldn't understand my question.

Dr Ho Shulong told me that before his father had opened his clinic in 1985, he had been a poorly man, suffering from many diseases – though which diseases he wasn't sure, other than TB, which he had cured with his herbs. He talked of Chinese medicine seeing the body as a whole rather than compartmentalising it as the west does, how it treats health problems psychologically and socially as well as biologically. He spoke of the importance of mental healthcare along with the physical.

'To cure sometimes, to relieve often, to help always,' Ho Shulong said was the duty of a doctor. Great, I said. So can you help me? Because your father didn't seem to understand that I wanted a consultation.

Not right now he couldn't because – so sorry – a neighbour had just died. But I insisted it was no trouble to return the following morning.

'I will come with you,' said Lea, that night.

Lea had gone to Dr Ho herself, some time ago, to ask about a birthmark she wanted to disappear. That he hadn't helped was her own fault, she said, because, seeing no progress, she'd eventually stopped taking the herbs. I wondered whether it was a peculiarly female trait to blame oneself when a treatment fails. 'A child cannot help believing that those who are stronger and wiser than he must have the means of giving him aid for his sufferings,' wrote Tolstoy in *War and Peace*.

'Dr Ho is very famous with you foreigners, but the Naxi people rarely go for help,' said our taxi driver on the way. 'Maybe because western people and eastern people have differences in their bodies. Maybe he's good at treating your bodies, not ours.'

'Or maybe we're gullible,' I said, and she (for she was Naxi, so worked instead of her husband) and Lea both clamped their hands to their mouths and laughed delicately. When I told her what was wrong with me, she said she feared I needed a doctor, not Dr Ho.

Dr Ho Shulong seemed reluctant when I brandished my

pulse at him, but this was China, where to say no is to lose face, and I smiled sweetly. We squatted outside on low stools as he took my pulse for a very long time, his grimy fingernails dancing over my wrist. Are you married, he said, and when I said no, he asked to see my tongue. How is your sleep, he said, and I said it's okay. How about your period, he tried; it's late? No, I said, throwing him a bone, kind of painful but regular. How are your breasts, he said, and I said I don't know, Ho Shulong, but I think they're okay.

Your body is okay but the lower jiao is a little unbalanced, he decreed, and you have weak qi. It is very common for ladies. You are not young but not old and it is not a big problem. My father says don't worry, be happy.

You'll be absolutely fine if you only stop worrying.

I glanced at Lea, but she was suddenly absorbed in the traffic along Baisha's main street.

'Can I have some herbs?' I asked.

I didn't really need them, he said, but he would give me some to regulate my liver and kidney. Normally they charged about £6 for a three-month supply, but as I was an important journalist he would give me some for free. The poor also got theirs free, but the Drs Ho always tried to charge because people don't believe that something they're given for free will cure them. It was a neat extrapolation of the placebo effect. I said I'd pay.

Ho Shulong took me outside onto a patio overlooking the garden where plastic barrels of paint were filled with various powders: herbs from the mountain, he explained. He filled a bag from a single barrel – 'What is it?' I said, and he said 'herbs' and I said 'which herbs?' and he laughed and said 'herbs' – and tied a neat little knot in it. I must take one spoonful, boiled into tea and sweetened with honey, three times a day. 'Optimism is the best medicine,' read the instructions. 'Avoid smoking or drinking. Eat simply, live simply but above all be optimistic.' Then he showed me business cards of all their visitors – pilots, diplomats, lawyers and estate agents from all over the world but especially Belgium. He reminded me that John Cleese had been, and Terry Jones. 'And Sue Perkins,' I said. 'She's very famous.' Ho Shulong shook his head, confused. 'I don't remember a lady.' He showed me how to stimulate my qi by massaging my cankles, and sent me on my way.

'I think his son is really good at the media,' Lea said diplomatically, as we brunched on 'traditional Naxi snacks' at a cafe down the road. 'I think his father's strong with his expertise – that must be why he's so famous.'

But yesterday, I said, his father didn't even take my pulse.

'And that's what's really worrying,' she said. 'I think he's lost his memory or something. The TCM doctors, they're all ageing but their sons and grandsons don't necessarily inherit the skills. They inherit the cash but not the medicine.'

I remembered when I'd gone to Shiwei's wedding in Shanghai and had asked the staff at my hostel where I could get some acupuncture. They'd looked blank, asked what the matter was. I have a bad back, I'd said, my standard response when I couldn't be bothered to get into it – everyone could sympathise with a bad back.

You don't need acupuncture, they'd said. If you have a bad back you must go to a hospital. You need real medicine! TCM patients, it seemed, were dying off as quickly as the doctors.

I drank the tea when I got home: it tasted sweet. A colleague got her Chinese parents to taste it, and they said liquorice and gingko. Gingko wouldn't grow on the Jade Dragon Snow Mountain, said a botanist I checked with, but it could grow in Baisha. Liquorice grew at altitude. Technically these could both be what they purported to be – and yet for some reason I doubted it.

I emailed several people who'd left their business cards with Dr Ho. All had fond memories of their visit, but none had been healed of anything; they'd mainly gone as tourists. One, a Foreign Office staffer who'd written an effusive letter following an official visit saying he felt better for the tea, told me that it had been a spot of diplomacy. 'The tea he gave me was very pleasant, and I certainly drank it when back in Beijing,' he wrote. 'I am not sure it actually did me any good, but it certainly did me no harm. Our letters were really to encourage someone we regarded as a decent man, whose company we had enjoyed – their fulsomeness should be seen in that context, rather than crediting Dr Ho's medical skills.'

I asked the Mayo Clinic if they had a record of the letter upon which Dr Ho had built his empire. 'No one here has any knowledge of this clinic, this provider, or the letter that he claims to have received,' they wrote back. 'It is extremely unlikely that we would send such a letter, 1) because patient privacy laws in the US would prevent us from communicating with an external party regarding our patient's protected health information, and 2) as an evidence-based organization, we would not give much credence to the "cure" of only one patient by any given means of unproven treatment. The outcome of one patient is just not enough to draw any meaningful conclusions.' They said they were forwarding details of the letter to their legal department.

Before I slunk back to Dr Cuong, I had a few days in Chengdu. There was time for one last throw of the dice.

TRUST THE BODY OF YOURSELF

If pain is a language, I have the accent on my tongue.
Sonya Huber (1971- : chronic pain patient, writer)

I was staying in the best hotel in Chengdu – partly because I was reviewing it, mainly because all I wanted was familiar, western luxury after Dr Ho – and I asked where to find a TCM doctor. Every member of staff I'd spoken to swore by their own tui na masseur, acupuncturist or TCM guy, but no one wanted to recommend them. The clinic wouldn't be up to your western standards, said one; he speaks no English, said another, and his massage is very painful. That one I was happy to renounce.

Then Steve on reception suggested a clinic affiliated to a local university. It was popular with expats, safe, and the real deal, he said – the website even mentioned treatment for chronic illness. It seemed a world away from Dr Ho – light years away when a young man in lab coat and owlish glasses took my pulse and diagnosed me, via a translation app, as deficient in yang, causing nausea, hand shakes and a numb arm. He had me at 'numb arm'. I thought of Richard Morse – *don't start going round opening yourself up* – and told him to do whatever he liked.

He wanted to do 90 minutes of excruciating tui na, it turned out, plus an hour of acupuncture, sticking me like a pig with needles thick as turkey darners as I squealed and burned and the young man told me that it was good, that pain cures pain, and Richard Morse's voice bellowed *get the fuck out of there*. When it was over I found a large red lump, two inches in diameter, had sprouted from my neck. First it was nothing, he said; then, a bone had come out

150

of place – a herniated disc, he suggested, when Steve called him later to ask why his guest had returned to the hotel in a state of hysteria. There in the cubicle he bore down on it, his whole bodyweight on the flat of his palm as black spots waltzed across my field of vision. I politely agreed to return for another session and got the fuck out of there.

I promised Steve I'd stick with western medicine from there on in, but I knew that TCM could help me, if only I could find someone with good jodoh. And what do you know, the following day, a chance encounter at a temple where I'd limped to try my *please-heal-me* mantra on yet another god, led to a Post-it note being pressed into my hand – not an email address like Patrick's, but a phone number this time. A famous clinic, I was told, and very expensive – about £30 per hour – but very good.

Steve insisted on coming with me. I think he felt guilty.

Zan TCM, said the unobtrusive sign on the street; inside, it was as smart as a Mayfair spa. We walked past the pharmacy, where masked workers bundled up piles of herbs into prescriptions, towards an open door, and Steve said: 'This is Mister Wong.'

I used to raise my eyebrows when people talked about meeting the one who became The One. 'I just knew,' they'd say piously, and I'd roll my eyes and think about reinforcement theory. But when Mr Wong stuck out his hand to shake mine, I suddenly understood: this was it. He looked younger than me, but wisdom seeped from every pore. He had the same smile as Dr Cuong: gentle but paternal, invested but reassuring. And he radiated calm and confidence, the knowledge that he could and would help, an aura that beamed endorphins and oxytocin straight into mine.

He was from Tianjin, he told me through Steve, a city with a strong TCM tradition. He specialised in sports science and bone-cracking, and worked mainly at a hospital tending to the injured sports stars of Sichuan province. Even as he sat me down, asking respectfully if he could take my pulse, I thought: here it comes, the coup de foudre.

Wordlessly, he took my right pulse for 90 seconds. Then my left for two minutes. He asked to see my tongue. Then he said something in Mandarin.

'Do you have your period?' asked Steve.

'No!' I squeaked. It was a lie – I did have my period – but there was no need to share that with Steve. Mr Wong looked at me and furrowed his brow.

'Mr Wong says your pulse says you do,' said Steve. Mr Wong shot me a knowing smile, then turned and said something to Steve.

'Is your poo okay?' asked Steve.

'My poo?' I echoed.

'Yes,' said Steve. 'Your poo.'

I'd woken up that morning with diarrhoea, my first in nearly a fortnight in China, and my desire to be healed tussled with three decades of English embarrassment.

'Yes, my poo is fine,' I said, and added, sternly, 'This is all very intimate.'

Mr Wong looked at me again, over to Steve, back to me and raised his eyebrows. And then he grinned.

'Doctor says usually is your mouth dry, bitter in the morning?'

Recently it had started to taste like I'd spent the night with a 2p coin under my tongue. I'd bought a fancy electric toothbrush and taken to cleaning my teeth for five minutes at a time, but it hadn't made any difference.

Mr Wong mumbled something else.

'The doctor says you have some pain in the shoulder and wrist,' said Steve.

'No!' said Mr Wong, springing from his chair. 'Here.' And he leaned around me and put his index finger halfway along the bottom edge of my right shoulder blade, right where the fire had been kindling for three and a half years. It flickered under his touch. The sign.

'Shoulder,' he said quietly, in English. 'Yes.'

I turned to Steve. 'Did you tell him this before?'

'No,' said Steve meekly.

'Do you swear?' I said.

'I swear.'

Mr Wong muttered something in Chinese.

'This is amazing,' I said as the tears welled up. *I cry at nothing, and cry most of the time.* But not at nothing this time, because this was it.

The problem in my shoulder was genetic, said Mr Wong (EDS is thought to be genetic), but my pain came for many reasons, including non-flowing qi and the job I had hated. By working too hard, I had caused the qi to clog and then the pain had come.

'Mr Wong says if you want to clear the pain, you must make the blood and qi flow smoothly,' said Steve. Do what you want with me, I said, switching off the Richard Morse in my head. So he needled me and did more tui na which made me cry out in pain, but pain from Mr Wong wasn't the same as pain from the others, because Mr Wong was The One. At the end, he said he was off until Thursday but he'd like to see me every other week for the next couple of months.

I leave Wednesday morning, I said, distraught.

Then Mr Wong did a Charmayne.

'He will see you tomorrow night,' said Steve. 'After he finishes his shift at the hospital. Mr Wong want to help.'

I felt better the next morning – not physically, because I still ached all over and my arm still burned, but for the first time since Kevin, something had shifted. This is my perfect day, I thought, staring at foot-long baby pandas at the Chengdu breeding centre. First this, then a cure. This is it.

That night, Mr Wong welcomed me with a paternal smile, a kind reassurance that I had only ever seen on Samba El and the vicar in London. Both of whom I'd run away from, I realised with a start. This time, I must see it through.

Did my neck still feel tight, asked the woman from reception who was on translating duty. And to my surprise, I heard myself say, *yes, but it's okay.*

It used to be assumed that pain was a process of cause and effect – you tear your ligament and it instantly hurts. But in World War II, Henry Beecher, a US army anaesthesiologist, studied 215 of the worst wounded soldiers in his field hospital, asking them, as they were stretchered in from the Italian front, whether they were in pain that very moment. Forty-eight said yes and requested morphine, but the rest – men with horrendous tissue damage, broken bones and deep wounds – ranked their pain as minor to non-existent, and needed no painkillers.

Beecher theorised in a 1946 paper that the circumstances of an injury affected pain levels and that 'strong emotion can block pain'. A soldier being removed from the battlefield is relieved that he's survived – things can only get better. For you and me, it's different. 'The civilian's accident marks the beginning of disaster for him,' wrote Beecher. He went on to become the first chair of the Department of Anaesthesia at Massachusetts General Hospital.

Did I have tenderness in the shoulders, Mr Wong was asking. Yes but I was working late last night, I found myself saying – I don't mind. And, like Beecher's soldiers, I really didn't. Western doctors would say I had decreased my somatic focus, that the pain mattered less because I was busying myself with work and panda-watching. That wasn't it, though – the reason I didn't mind the pain was because I knew it was about to come to an end.

What's the most uncomfortable thing going on right now, he asked – the first time a doctor had looked at my body as a whole instead of its parts – and I was surprised to hear myself saying it wasn't my pain but my dizziness. For several months, I'd been having trouble focusing if I was looking at a screen. Glasses and contact lenses hadn't made a difference, and I had headaches every other day. I'd mentioned it to Dr Good, had my sight tested, even flagged it to the endocrinologist in case it was thyroid eye disease, but everyone had drawn a blank.

'Yesterday the doctor feel your pulse and feel there are some problems with the neck, some things in the wrong place,' said the woman. Bonesetting would make it better. With my consent, he would adjust it today.

I remembered Samba El's gentle smile as I'd promised to see him again, the vicar in London's furrowed brow as I'd walked out saying I'd see him around, Charmayne's look of love as I'd sworn I'd call. I had run away from them all.

'You have the wrong joints in the wrong place,' said the woman. 'If we put it in the right place, you will not feel the dizzy, or the headache.'

'No pain,' said Mr Wong, in English. 'Wish you'd believe me.'

I thought back to Ubud and the thunderclap when the bad balian had crunched my neck. To Port-au-Prince, where Richard Morse had merely stroked it and I'd maybe wet myself. To a chiropractor at the end of the Metropolitan line who'd blamed me for my lack of progress when I'd shielded it from him, and the *Playboy* model who'd died after a neck adjustment like the one Mr Wong was planning for me. It could kill you, I told myself. But what if it cured me? If he could diagnose the state of my most intimate functions from my pulse, surely he could tell whether a joint was out of place. Kill. Cure. Where was the line?

He demonstrated on the woman and I felt the beginnings of a panic attack: elastic band round my throat, weight at the back of my eyes, lungs beginning to heave.

'Where did you do this last time, and why are you so afraid?' said the woman, and I told them about Bali.

Mr Wong mumbled something.

'He says it's safe,' the woman said. And I tussled with myself: to die or not to die, to risk it all for the chance of getting it back, to establish whether or not this was my Jesus by putting my neck on his altar.

Mr Wong chuckled to himself and spoke to the woman. Then he looked at me and said, in English, 'Acupuncture'.

I would wonder, afterwards – I still wonder to this day – what might have happened had I let Mr Wong reset my neck. I might have died, of course, but might he have cured me? Miracled me there and then, and saved me the purgatory that was to come? And although I've tormented myself with that thought since the day I walked away – wound it round myself like a cilice – now, when it appears, I try to remember something else he said that night.

'Maybe you don't trust the doctor, but you should trust the body of yourself,' the woman had translated. 'Don't you agree?'

Why trust the body of myself when I can trust the doctor, I had thought when she said it. Why trust the body of myself when all the doctors have told me my body is untrustworthy? *You really are better, dear, whether you can see it or not. You'll be absolutely fine if you only stop worrying.*

You didn't let Mr Wong crack your neck because it didn't feel right, I tell myself now. Because for the first time, in his little room in Chengdu, you listened to the body of yourself.

'Do you feel good?' he asked as he sank his fingers into my stomach, deeper and deeper, rootling around in my organs under the guise of tui na as I shrieked that no, I didn't.

The problem was my stomach meridian, he announced. The blocked qi there meant that the pain was worst in the neck and round the shoulder, that the arm sometimes felt numb and tight inside, that I had big clots with my periods and insomnia, an explosive temper but very little energy. He told me all this, holding up a mirror to my life with his hands in my guts, and he laughed when I said yes, yes yes yes Mr Wong, all of it, I do. It was the most painful of all my treatments – I listen back to the tape and it's full of gasps, screams and noises like a cow lowing – but I felt safe within it, like I was being burned to cinders but would re-emerge a phoenix. As Beecher could have predicted, the emotion had blocked the awareness of the pain.

It would be several days before I felt better, he said – and as it happened, it was. But before it got better, it got worse – worse than it had been in months, as bad as it had been when I first reached for the coffee, so bad that I couldn't wash my hair or even hold a fork. Mr Wong hadn't prepared me for a downturn, though, and it felt like the worst betrayal, a jilting at the altar. And, just like that, I snuffed out my faith.

Just like that, six days later, the pain switched off, and I wondered if that's what he'd been meaning all along. The problem was, I wasn't sure I believed in Mr Wong by that point. Those six days had been so bad that I'd already turned back to God.

RIDING THE ROLLERCOASTER

My steady hope turns into weeping
Isabella di Morra (1520-1545/6: honour killing victim, poet)

When Michael Phelps disrobed at the poolside in Rio for the 2016 Olympics, the focus was less on the six medals he'd go on to win than on the circular welts covering his back. There was a veritable outbreak of them amongst the American athletes – swimmers and gymnasts all looking like they were wearing blood-blistered clown suits. Team USA had started cupping.

I'd first heard about cupping in the mid 2000s, when Gwyneth Paltrow and Jennifer Aniston started appearing at film premieres with the spots all over their backs. It's a Chinese technique similar to the kerokan Made Reni had tried on me in Bali – glass cups are put on the body and heated, sucking the air out and drawing the blood to the skin. The marks last roughly as long as bruises; adherents say it removes 'toxins' (the ever-present bogeymen of today's alternative therapy industry), improves the flow of blood and qi, and soothes sore muscles.

Phelps would get cupped, he told curious reporters, before almost every event. His gymnast teammate Alex Naddour said that cupping worked better for him than massages, saunas, hot tubs and even cortisone injections. 'It's been better than any money I've spent on anything else,' he said. 'It's the best thing I've ever had. It saves me from a lot of pain.'

Of course, the American Cancer Society swiftly put out a po-faced statement mid-Olympics: 'There is no scientific rationale for expecting any health benefit from cupping.'

Over here, David Colquhoun, professor of pharmacology at UCL and a regular basher of alternative medicine, was rolled out to call it 'nonsense' and 'desperately implausible'. Tell that to the greatest Olympian of all time.

I'd had cupping twice, once during the Gwyneth period and once in Colorado, in between my attempts at getting stoned. Unlike Team USA I took no tangible benefits from it, but at least a single treatment didn't break the bank. No, it was the cumulative effect of all those treatments that did that.

The UK population spends £5bn a year on alternative therapy, wrote Simon Singh and Edzard Ernst in their 2008 book *Trick or Treatment?* A decade on, the industry is booming. A 2015 YouGov poll revealed that a significant proportion of the public think it can be effective, too.[14] And while my pain was at its worst, I was a major donor. I tried everything from the mechanical to the physical, the spiritual to the mad.

I tried chiropractic with three different practitioners, including one who told me I had scoliosis (I didn't) and declared it my fault that his battery-powered mallet wasn't making me better, because I refused to rest for 24 hours after his sessions. I tried the Alexander Technique, a single lesson in which a woman contorted me into painful-for-me positions then scoffed at my discomfort.

I tried homeopathy – not because I believed in it (it purports to take an active ingredient and dilute it hundreds of thousands of times, on the basis that water molecules will hold its 'memory'), but because I hoped it could stimulate a placebo effect. A 2005 study[15] had shown that 70 per cent of homeopathy patients with chronic conditions experienced improvements over a six-year period, and I wanted some of that. Except I didn't want it enough – when the same guy who'd got me through my A Levels by electrocuting my arm told me I'd have to give up coffee to make his sugar pills work, I walked out.

I saw two practitioners of the Bowen Technique, which

claims to work by manipulating the fascia, or connective tissue covering the muscles. According to Bowen theory, 'memory' of physical trauma can lodge in the fascia and tighten them, in turn ratcheting up pressure in the muscles and causing pain. The practitioner pinches the fascia at various points to spring them back into shape, releasing the muscles underneath. But despite the miracle stories – one of the practitioners swore it got her back to work after a car crash – it did nothing for me.

I invested in *stuff*: voice recognition software that ended up straining my neck, foam rollers and footballs to lie on that did nothing, a giant computer monitor that gave me eye strain. I ran up nearly £1,000 on supplements designed to combat inflammation and improve nerve function, but the difference was negligible and regularly they made me vomit. I overhauled my diet, swapping cheap carbs for organic meats and expensive superfoods – it made the POTS symptoms marginally better, but bit into my bank balance and didn't touch the pain.

Others tried to help. Access to Work (a government-funded programme to get disabled people back to work) bought me £3,000 worth of ergonomic equipment, but one person's comfort is another's bed of nails, and the only thing that didn't exacerbate my pain was the laptop stand. My mother took out a payment plan on that £2,000 Vispring bed that the salesman was sure would cure my pain. In a way, it was fitting that she paid for it, because once it was clear I felt worse after sleeping in it, I donated it to her.

I tried physical treatments: massage, which always gave a temporary nirvana of relief. Craniosacral therapy, which left me ready for sleep. 'No Hands' massage, done with the arms, which stretched instead of poked and was blissful, but two hours away. Cryotherapy, where I stripped down to my pants and stomped around a room chilled to -110 degrees as Robin Thicke sleazed, 'You the hottest bitch in this place' (for it was Monaco, and the room attendant piped *Blurred Lines* into the freezer).

I bought products: strong-smelling lotions and ointments filled with things like camphor and peppermint that cooled the skin, distracting it from the pain. I emptied the contents of the Dead Sea and Himalayan caves into my bathtub, because a scalding bath and a hot water bottle were the only things that allowed me to sleep.

In desperation, I said yes to every coincidence that brought me to the door of a therapist, however laughable their trade. I saw one shaman who told me I needed to connect with my womb more; another who exorcised me of a spirit attachment that, she said, was calling me a cunt. (Neither was wrong, really, because, raddled with self-hatred by now, I thought I *was* a cunt, and yearned to be a man so the doctors would see past my gender and treat my pain.) I bought a crystal, not because I thought crystals were therapeutic, but because someone who I knew really did want to help – Charmayne, as it happened, for I saw her several more times, absorbing more of her wisdom with every visit – told me I needed one. For a couple of months, I made weekly payments of $50 to a man in Las Vegas who swore he was sending me daily distance healing by banging a little clay figure on its pressure points. That was Tong Ren.

I went for healing at London's College of Psychic Studies; I went to a healing service given by a friend who'd become a priest. I prayed – to God, gods, the universe and myself. I did a past life regression, in case that held an answer. The cunt-ghost shaman told me I'd been stabbed in my armpit, centuries earlier, and just needed to clear the trauma. That seemed too easy. Of course, it didn't work.

It wasn't all terrible – massage and aromatherapy baths aside, those thousands of pounds I flung into the ether did unearth two things that made a difference. One was mindfulness meditation – not because it cured my pain (apart from that glorious moment in Cyprus), but because it calmed the anxiety around it: the panic attacks that I'd never get better, the gasping for breath as I drowned in my debts, the sobbing fits when yet another path turned into a cul-de-sac.

The other was reiki, which disturbed me because it was patently ridiculous: healing where the healer purports to be channelling universal energy, rather than claiming super-natural powers for themselves. It was as implausible as it was popular with the kind of people I despised, and yet every time my neighbour would do it to me, I'd be mortified to find that, to varying extents, the pain would recede. Maybe it was the jodoh I'd learned about in Bali, or maybe it was the relaxation, because there couldn't possibly be anything in it. At least, that's what I told myself openly; deep down, I was hoping that maybe there was something out there after all.

Thousands of pounds spent with barely any reaction – how the sceptics and quack-haters would laugh. And they'd be right to laugh at the money I spent – an obscene amount, money I didn't have. But what they'd be missing, as they sniggered at another dumb female pissing her money away – because although anyone can be a sceptic, the angriest sceptics always seem to be men – was the strength it gave me to carry on. Strength that the medical establishment had been chiselling away at.

Every time something worked enough to make me relax a bit, take my mind off the pain for five minutes or focus on a nice smell or a smooth crystal, it was worth every penny. Every time something made me feel a tiny bit better – even if that feeling of betterness barely lasted past the moment of payment – I felt a little pinch of hope. That moment when I floated away from the pain at Zening might even have saved my life – because however much I urged myself to keep going, at that point, a year in, I was flagging. Of course I felt better because I was on holiday – of course the pain shot straight back once I was home, waist-deep in bills, medical appointments and exercise programmes – but that wasn't the point. The point was that for one perfect minute I had found a place in my brain untouched by the pain, and I knew that if I'd found it once, it wasn't beyond the realm of possibility to go there again.

Of course, hope could be just as devastating as NHS

nihilism. I can't begin to count the number of times I'd have good jodoh with a practitioner, feel a little better or be sure the events which had drawn me there couldn't be mere co-incidence. When that happened, the hope would swell in my chest till I could barely breathe, and instead of catastrophising I'd start fantasising about my new life once I was back at work, bumping up the tax brackets, living in my own home, having a life. Sometimes I'd be so sure I was about to have a breakthrough that I'd tell someone. Sometimes I'd keep the fanfares in my head, scared of jinxing it if I breathed a word. Sometimes I wouldn't even tell the practitioner I felt different, hoping that if they thought it wasn't working, they'd try harder next time.

When I had one of those experiences, however much hope it gave me in the moment, the thud back down to reality was bone-shattering. And what was devastating when it happened on a local level – if I'd travelled an hour, say, or forked out £100 – was magnified a thousand times once, buoyed by my experience with Kevin, I started looking further afield.

Spending weeks researching a person and a place, taking out another balance transfer to book a trip (because the book money finished long before my travels did), enduring longhaul flight after longhaul flight, sleeping in foreign beds that were always built wrong for my back, being pummelled by jetlag on continents where I didn't know a soul – all those things ramped up my pain. And then to meet the person I'd dreamed could give me my life back and to realise they couldn't was the worst feeling of all. I was Dorothy, risking everything to reach the Emerald City, and pulling back the curtain to find a scared little man instead of an omnipotent wizard. Except, unlike Dorothy, I was alone. And there was nothing waiting back for me in Kansas, either. Each time it happened, the grief hollowed out another part of me, until I was a husk of myself that not even I recognised.

I rarely talked about it. I never told a soul how profoundly every failure affected me. Sometimes I'd joke about it – hahaha guess who flew all the way to China to meet a guy who wouldn't even take her pulse. Sometimes I'd précis what had happened in the baldest of terms, steeling my voice not to crack. Sometimes I'd pretend I wasn't 'ready' to talk about it.

On rare occasions it would explode, like on my 33rd birthday when I'd exiled myself from friends but gone for dinner with my mother at a local restaurant. I'd burst into tears over the main course – 'Where *is* he, how long will this take, how long do I have to keep looking, when am I going to *find* him?' – and it was only when I connected her mortified face to the look of kindness in the waitress' eye (my birthday was the day before Valentine's) that I realised everyone thought I was some kind of poignant *Sex and the City* leftover, and I had just delivered Charlotte's desperate singleton monologue almost word for word.

Later, when I got a lot better and then it started to slip away, I was so out of my mind with grief that I had to call a friend who's also a Samaritan. It wasn't just the disappointment, or the realisation that I was running out of options; it was the blow to my self-esteem. I'd thought I was clever, you see, and a good judge of character – a cut above the people you read about in the paper who sign over their house and life savings to faith healers. But it turned out I was only a step up from the poor sods who believe in true love with a mail-order spouse.

It was such a rollercoaster, this process of hope – I would be fizzing with excitement one day, inconsolable the next – that sometimes I wondered if I was going mad, or if I was undiagnosed bipolar. Again, I kept that quiet – I didn't want to confirm that yes, she is crazy, it's all in her head. Instead, I tried to control it myself. After a Dr Ho or a Ketut Liyer, I would tell myself that there were other people, that this wasn't my fault. I learned to temper my excitement when yet another incontrovertible sign had revealed itself – to remind myself that this might not be it, that the faster something works the more likely it is to be placebo. I tried my best to ride the rollercoaster with context and knowledge, and still I had to grip with all my strength not to fall off.

Now, I wish I'd spoken about it more while it was happening, because I don't think I was the only one who felt this way. Later, in South Africa, I would meet my friend Zee, who told me about his colleague who'd suffered chronic headaches. Like me, Jared had bounced from person to person, doctor to alternative therapist. Like me, the pain had set him on the rollercoaster – the high of excitement when he met someone he thought might have the answer, the slough of despond when he realised they didn't. In fact, it was only when I heard Zee talking about Jared that I realised I wasn't bipolar after all, that the extra weight I'd been carrying for years had never been a part of me. Hearing Jared's story, I realised it was just the pain.

Jared had wanted to get off the rollercoaster, though. He killed himself.

I flew to Italy from China, a work trip after Mr Wong. Grenades were going off inside my arm every time a nerve fired (and nerves fire up to 50 times per second). The pain was so great that I couldn't walk, couldn't hold a fork. When, one night, I started sobbing into a plate of pasta, I was so embarrassed that I told the waiter someone close to me had died. I wasn't strictly lying, either. The moment I'd set eyes on Mr Wong, I had really thought, this is it, here he is, it's been three and a half years but now it's over. I was so sure, that time, that I had dared to tell several people. I'd even put it on Facebook.

Would I rather have left China without meeting him? Would it have been better to take home only the memory of Dr Ho and the man who'd herniated my disc? Possibly. I learned a lot from Mr Wong, and maybe if I'd let him crack my neck or had another session it would have been revelatory. But as it was, the disappointment, once I'd decided without a doubt that he was The One, was almost too much to bear.

There's a fine line to tread between giving someone

unnecessary hope and sucking them dry of it, especially when you don't quite know what's going on, and you don't have a prognosis.

Dr Good handled it beautifully. One day, as we sat in front of another discharge letter from another clinic written by another doctor who didn't think they could treat my pain, I looked at him drily – because I was all cried out that day – and asked, 'How long is this going to take?'

I'll never forget the compassion as he paused. He thought for a second. And then he said, 'I really don't know, Julia. But I'll keep referring you to people who might until we have an answer.'

PRIEZ POUR NOUS

Dim phantoms of an unknown ill
Float through my tired brain
Elizabeth Siddal (1829-1862: chronic illness patient,
painkiller addict, celebrity other half, poet)

Five days after leaving Mr Wong, I was in Rome, wondering whether this time it was time to die. The pain from the acupuncture had redoubled like a tsunami rushing back to shore, and the disappointment had snuffed out my last spark of hope. I had an article to finish, though, and my last piece couldn't be a dud, so I limped out to the Vatican to do the research.

I wasn't looking for divine intervention; I was over religion. For three years now, I'd asked for help from the ether in churches, temples, mosques and synagogues. I'd lit candles, rubbed Buddhas, filled collection boxes; removed my shoes and flipped my stick upside down, handle on the floor, to walk with respect. Over and over again, I'd promised to believe – in whatever, whoever – if I received even the flimsiest of signs. And nothing had changed.

It wasn't just my arm this time. My back pain had returned, that palette knife levering my bones apart. I decided to walk back to my hotel, in case exercise might help, and as I walked, I noticed a handwritten sign: *Reliquie di San Pio di Pietrelcina*.

A modern languages degree and a stint waitressing in the Marche had long instilled in me a yearning to be Italian – in spirit, at least, if not in lumpy Anglo-Saxon body. As a faux Italian, I knew well who San Pio was: Padre Pio, the modern saint famed for his stigmata and magical powers of bilocation. Every Italian loved Padre Pio, his kind face that looked like a nonno; every Italian felt national pride in his status as the best-known stigmatic since St Francis of Assisi. So I had loved him too. When, in 2004, the village where I'd lived had hired a bus to drive to Puglia to see his body, I'd even bought a ticket.

That day in Rome, I followed the sign as much for a Proustian recollection of life before the pain as in hope of a miracle.

It was a typical Catholic church, all glitz and no atmosphere, altars dripping in gold. By the door was a lifesize fibreglass statue of Jesus carrying his cross – looking round, baffled but grateful, at Padre Pio as he selflessly shared the weight from behind.

I sank to my knees in front of a brown glove crusted in blood – Padre Pio had covered his stigmata with fingerless gloves – and for the first time in my life I prayed, really prayed, prayer not as a bargaining tool but as a plea. I don't know what I said and I don't know who I said it to, but I remember the novelty of it and the embarrassment at the tears that, out of nowhere, were suddenly streaming down my cheeks. I left in a hurry.

I had dinner with a seminarian friend that night, and I told him I wanted to die. That the problem wasn't even the pain any more: it was the disappointment, the tiny cuts of defeat and self-recrimination that came with every failure and festered into mortal wounds.

I was exhausted, I told Tommaso, in mind, body and spirit. Chronic pain had rewired parts of my brain I never knew existed: the somatosensory cortex, the glial cells, the amygdala, the prefrontal cortex, the hippocampus, the hypothalamus, the nucleus accumbens, the insular cortex and the anterior cingulate cortex. It had destroyed swathes of grey matter and hijacked the bits that were supposed to control memory, emotion, decision-making, stress management and impulse control. It had given me brain damage and a new personality, aged me a couple of decades and weighed me down by several stone. It was the reason I now ate three cupcakes at a single sitting, wept at anodyne news stories, called my mother the foulest of names when she balked at chauffeuring me around, and passed out after meals. It was why I'd alienated friends and acquaintances, forgetting to reply to emails, turn up to things and blanking all recollection of important life events and babies' names. They call it the 'Pain Brain', this metamorphosis of our body's HQ: a disease in itself. Chronic pain isn't just pain that doesn't stop; it puts your entire body in a chrysalis and morphs you into a monster.

Mr Wong was the tipping point: I was drained, I was angry, I was crushed and in agony. I'd barely slept since I'd seen him because with every tiny movement, even a myoclonic twitch, the pain had stabbed me awake. I had tried. I had tried for three years: I had tried for my mum, for Miffy, for revenge on the doctors, but I couldn't do it any more. I was done.

Like the priest in London who'd offered to send me to Walsingham, Tommaso listened, really listened. He became the second person since that morning in May to hear me, hear what the pain had done to me, to commiserate instead of sitting in awkward silence or paralleling some experience of his own. He didn't even offer to pray for me. He just let me rail.

The next morning, I realised Something Had Happened.

I wasn't completely better, but I was tremendously better. I had slept. I gripped my cutlery at breakfast. The inferno in my arm had cooled to a gentle smoulder. I know my body, I texted Tommaso, and I know its recovery times. This is as if I've hibernated for a fortnight. Is it Padre Pio, or is it Mr Wong? Tommaso refused to commit, but I decided it was probably a miracle.

'Pray to your own god,' Jero Pura had said. 'I don't know your prayer,' Richard Morse or Erzulie Dantour had threatened. I didn't know my prayer either, but I knew I wanted one. Prayer had topped a US survey of chronic pain patients as the most effective painkiller, tied only with prescription drugs.[16] A patient's prognosis is better if they're allowed to share their faith with their doctors – recent research in Jordan showed that incorporating Islam into treatment was central to the recovery of many mental health patients.[17]

A meta-analysis of studies of 32,000 US cancer patients showed that those with a spiritual belief reported better physical health during treatment;[18] religious cancer patients have better coping skills and are less prone to depression and anxiety, according to studies from both Italy[19] and Taiwan.[20] One of my old teachers swore her arthritis was cured by her prayer group. It was the placebo effect, of course, but why were people so dismissive of it when it worked? Herbert Benson, the Harvard cardiologist who popularised mind-body medicine in the west in the 1970s, thinks the placebo effect is a terrible name for what he calls 'remembered wellness'. We all have the ability to improve our health, he writes in *The Mind/Body Effect*. It's just a question of reminding our bodies how things should be.

I applied myself to developing a faith as diligently as I'd applied myself to medical research and weird therapies. I googled the patron saints for my symptoms: Gemma Galgani for back pain, Sts Ubald and Cornelius for misfiring nerves. I made my mother drive me down to a sixth-century well near Penzance that was linked to Madron, the patron saint of pain. On Christmas Day – in Venice for work – I went to mass three times. And then came another miracle. One day, when the palette knife had slipped back into my spine, I'd crept into the nearest church and asked a picture of Padre Pio for help again; the next, my back was better. 'Ti aiuteranno,' said the caretaker monk – a capuchin, like Padre Pio – when I returned for the fourth time in a fortnight, to bid the picture goodbye. He'd asked who I was, this foreigner who kept coming to his church and weeping into his candle wax, and I'd told him everything.

Ti aiuteranno: they will help you, Padre Pio and his fellow saints. But I must trust my doctors too, he warned, because God works through them. I thought of the pastor at the Colorado mega-church who, instead of inviting me to prayer group, had told me to go forth and smoke marijuana. I thought of the priest at Walsingham, right at the start of my journey.

Take your medicine, said my monk; a miracle isn't

necessarily what you think. I didn't dare tell him there was no more medicine and a miracle was all I had left.

On my 35th birthday, I flew to Lourdes on one of those 6am Ryanair flights scheduled to test even the faithful. It's terrible what they do there, said the man pushing my wheelchair at Stansted. I've loaded the cripples on and off for years, and no one's ever come back miracled. They sell the water there, that holy water. It's disgusting.

He was wrong, I soon found out. They don't sell the water there – that would be outrageous. They just sell everything else: the containers for the water, the postage and packing for the water, pictures of the water and the candles that, once you've left, 'prolong your prayer' beside the holy spring.

'Bon anniversaire,' said the owner at the Hotel Adonis, swallowing her confusion at my arrival *toute seule*. She led me to my boudoir, where a crucified Jesus watched over a kingsize bed and Bernadette guarded a bottle of sparkling wine with two plastic cups. Tomorrow was Valentine's Day, and I'd booked the Romance Package because it was cheaper than a single room.

Lourdes was closed for February, apart from La Grotte. The wax museum, the rides, most of the souvenir shops – all fermé. I walked down – all roads lead to the grotto in Lourdes, they even have arrows to it painted on the pavement – past shuttered shops with names like Tourisme et Religion, Palais du Rosaire and (my favourite) Oh Lourdes. It was the lowest of seasons, the sky a grimy grey, pilgrimages suspended till summer, exactly as I wanted it. February was when Bernadette had begun the visions, anyway.

I had lunch at a bistro, a 'pilgrim salad' with a quarter litre of birthday rosé, sitting outside in defiance of the weather. I ate round a pubic hair tucked discreetly under a piece of chicken, and drank the first glass of wine as I looked down the street to the enormous spire in the distance. A coach drove by, and the driver stopped beside me to wave, then mime a blowjob. In the church, people stared at me and my stick – one woman even followed us around. February brought

tourists, not pilgrims, I realised, and I was one of the sights –
'They were all on the look-out for prodigies,' as Zola wrote
in *Lourdes*, his excoriating novel about the grotto. They only
let me off the hook when a man in a wheelchair turned up.

I didn't like Lourdes, I decided. I didn't like the main church
(there were two), its brutal size or gloomy interior. I didn't like
that to reach it you had to climb 60-odd steps or trail up the
equivalent height, a 21st-century Via Crucis for the sick and
weak. I didn't like the vending machines inside the church,
selling medallions stamped with the Pope and Bernadette. I
didn't like the prices: €20 for a mass, €500 for a mega-candle
to be lit beside the grotto. Even the grotto itself left me cold.

There was a queue to walk through it, mainly excited
Italian nonnas rubbing the stone with scarves and photos of
the sick. I stared at the spring – encased in glass, surrounded
by fake flowers – and waited for a solemn young man to
trace his hand up the wet rock so I could copy him. I scraped
the moisture into my palm, licked it, rubbed the rest on my
armpit. I don't believe this, I whispered, but show me I'm
wrong. The rain came in torrents, splashing the thighs of
the faithful who knelt at the grotto. Dinner was chicken and
chips in my room from the supermarché. On Valentine's Day,
I was turfed out of the queue for the piscines, Bernadette's
miraculous baths – too many people, they said, no room
at the inn – and picked up diarrhoea at the only open restaurant in town. Two men on a street corner yelled vaguely
threatening things as I returned to bed and sparkling wine.

Walking back to the piscines the next morning, I was
shaking. I told myself it was anticipation of the cold – they
were tubs chiselled from the ground and filled with spring
water flowing straight from the snow-caked Pyrenees – but I
knew that wasn't true. The problem was that I was unnerved
by my revulsion at one of the holiest places on earth; that I
might be disrespecting Holy Mary Mother Of God if I had
the bath without believing; that if I couldn't find a miracle
at Lourdes, I would never find one anywhere.

At least there was still the placebo effect. In *Lourdes*, Zola acknowledges miraculous recoveries, though he puts them down to mind over matter. Mind over matter was fine by me – in fact it was precisely what I needed. A quick rewiring of my brain to retrain my body was all I sought. *I don't need a real miracle, just a medical one, merci.*

I cursed my inability to surrender as I waited outside, the snow starting to fall. I tried to think of poor Bernadette as we moved inside to the baths, each enclosed by a privacy screen. But she never acknowledged the miracles here, I thought, overhearing prayers and sobs, the odd gasp with a splash as the women went in. When a reporter had asked her about the prodigies supposedly taking place in her grotto, she had known nothing about them.

And Bernadette was chronically ill herself, I remembered, peeling off my clothes behind a screen, a school shower setup with three volunteers and three patients: one undressing, one in the water and one dressing without towelling down because the water is supposed to dry miraculously. She died at 34, after years of pain and illness. She never found a cure.

A volunteer with a weapons-grade bosom and gap-toothed smile came over to fetch me. She'd supposedly been shielding me with a sheet as I undressed, clinical as a doctor in her white overalls, but I could swear I'd caught her taking a peek at my body before she wrapped me in it.

She took the bra that she'd instructed me to hold in my right hand and led me to the bath, stale sweat percolating as she moved. Three steps down, like a full-immersion baptism. I stared at an icon of the Virgin as she told her colleagues to be careful. 'Elle a des problèmes partout,' she said grimly, wringing out a wet sheet – I had warned her not to yank my shoulders – and all three of them, who dealt with women on stretchers, immobile women, women old and young, fat and thin, tall and short, mortally ill and perfectly fine, looked me up and down with terrifying pity.

She gestured at the steps. I crossed myself in florid Italian fashion.

One step. In a split second they wrenched the modesty

sheet from me and slapped the wet one round my torso, ice-cold from the mountain, to prepare me for the ducking.

Two. They were chanting the Lourdes mantra, *Mère de dieu, priez pour nous, Sainte Bernadette, priez pour nous*, and I was meant to join in but I was hyperventilating with the cold and the fear.

Three. They walked me down to the head of the bath, beneath Bernadette, and conferred in French. 'Can you sit down?' Bazookas asked in English, concerned for the cripple. Sure, I said, and angled forward. 'Not on your knees,' she gasped. 'Seet down.'

I hesitated.

'Yes,' she urged. 'Seet down.' And they put their hands on my shoulders, all three of them together, and plunged me into the water that had melted from the Pyrenean ice caps, flowed through the cold rock and emptied into this mighty great bath. I gasped. I was so deep into panic mode that I could see the wet sheet floating open, pudenda emerging to greet the women, and it didn't even occur to me to clamp my legs shut.

I came to as they dug their arms under my shoulders and hoisted me up. 'Non,' I said, breaking free and bending over to scoop up more of the water – because, sitting down, it had only come up to chest level – and slapping it over my neck and my face, head and armpit as the sheet rode up over my bum crack right in their faces. 'Non!' they gasped as one. 'Non!'

'Vous l'avez fait,' said a schoolmarmish one with white hair, dragging me back up. She gave a grim smile. 'Vous l'avez fait.'

Mère de dieu, priez pour nous. Sainte Bernadette, priez pour nous.

She gave me a pitcher to dab on my face, into the few nooks and crannies that hadn't been wetted, and I walked out of the bath towards the youngest of the three, wet white sheet completely transparent. They wrapped me in a blue one, threaded my arms through the straps of my bra – 'Like a baby,' I cried out, and they smiled now and chorused, 'Like a bébé'. As I struggled to peel my jeans over my chapped legs, I realised I was still wet, that I hadn't been granted a miraculous drying. En route to the Adonis, I traced my hand along the stones of the grotto and slicked the rock with my tears.

The odd thing was, though, that on the walk back, I felt a bit better.

After lunch – omelette, chips and red wine, much to the amusement of the OAPs of Lourdes, who were enthralled by the lone foreigner who neither dressed nor behaved like a pilgrim – I asked Dr Alessandro de Franciscis what he thought. How could I capitalise on this slight muting of the pain, turn the spark of hope into a proper fire? I had taken the bath, not believing, and yet I felt better. What had happened?

'I think the baths are the baths,' he sighed, and told me about a man who'd written a book about coming to Lourdes with cancer, right before dying of it. Sandro was head of the Lourdes Medical Bureau, a doctor charged with sorting the wheat of miracle from the chaff of placebo. He suggested I go back and spend some time in the grotto, so after I saw him, I went and sat in the snow. He also mentioned that the only pattern to the miracles was that they tended to be granted to people who'd come to Lourdes to pray for others, so I wrote prayer requests for all the Catholics I could think of and, flying home the next day – studiously avoiding eye contact with a curious family who'd clocked me on the way over – I thought of sick friends and relatives all the way across France. The pain flared back on the coach from Stansted.

Three weeks later, I was in Florence. I'd been sent to Umbria to write about my favourite hotel in the world, Eremito – a modern-day hermitage where guests switch off their phones, eat in silence and sleep in rooms modelled on little monk cells. I had a night in town on the way back, and called in on my friend Pietro.

Pietro was a craftsman, a one-of-a-kind throwback to a golden age. He was a true renaissance man, self-educated and fiercely intelligent. He made exquisite things – earthenware pottery that looked like it was Ming Dynasty. He was a communist, as so many of Italy's intelligentsia are, and an atheist.

I've been to Lourdes, I told him when he asked what I'd been doing. Lourdes, you know, in France. Miracles, freezing baths, the air heavy with misogyny.

Yes, he said, I know Lourdes.

It's mad, I pressed on. Disgusting! Commercialised! You have no idea—

I do, he said. I've been there. He paused.

We took my son.

I knew about Pietro's son. He was profoundly disabled. His wife had cared for him for a quarter of a century. I had always wondered whether he was the reason Pietro spent all his hours in his tiny workshop, labouring over those perfect little pots that he'd work on for days on end and then sell for €30.

When his son was still a child, Pietro said, they had gone to Lourdes, a family holiday that wasn't a holiday. Then he was silent.

'Is your wife religious?'

She had taken their son to countless shrines and priests over the last quarter-century, as any good Catholic would. None of them had made a difference, and the last time they'd gone somewhere, Pietro had almost come to blows with a priest. Because they had been to countless doctors, too, and there was nothing that could be done.

'It's not right,' he said quietly. 'To give people false hope.'

Five minutes earlier, I'd told him of my plan to use the pot I was buying from him as storage for some petals that had fallen from Padre Pio's coffin. (The Pope had summoned his body to Rome, and I had flown over especially and rushed to scoop up the petals, as the women of Florence had done with Savonarola's ashes after he was burned at the stake in 1498.) I had wondered why he hadn't laughed.

Some Russians came into the shop and Pietro slipped on his showman's mask.

'I'm meeting lots of doctors at the moment,' I muttered. 'If I find anything that might be relevant, would you like to know?'

He looked baffled. 'Of course,' he said. 'Of course I'd like to know.'

I took a short cut to the Duomo, down a street that had barely changed since Medici times. It was dark, and the palazzos that looked so grand by day were intimidating at night, their child-sized stones and house-height doors wreathed with spikes. I burned with shame at my flippancy. Guilt that I was chanting half-hearted Hail Marys when others had greater need. Guilt that I'd laughed at something others took so seriously. Guilt that I'd experienced some relief where others hadn't, though they'd deserved it more. Guilt about how I was talking about that relief. Was I giving hope to people who instead needed reality?

When I'd left Eremito five hours earlier, I'd turned on my phone to find a message from Iluh in Bali. We'd been in constant touch since I'd left, but this was different from the photos and emoticons we usually exchanged. Made Reni had cancer, she wrote. The doctors in Denpasar had removed a chunk of her bowel, but there was cancer in her liver, too, and fluid on her lung. Made Reni, who'd been there for me in body and mind when I had started my journey. Made Reni, who'd been so outraged when the bad balian had called me fat. Made Reni, who'd gingerly scraped a coin along my ribcage on the off-chance I had some hot wind that needed to be let out. I wanted to be there for her too.

I wondered if we could get her to Singapore, or if their anthropologist friend in LA could suggest a cutting-edge American treatment. Then I thought, I couldn't pay for any of that, but I could send them enough money to take her to a balian. Should I cover a visit to Jero Pura, I wondered, or Ketut Suwitra, the Munduk man who specialised in internal disorders?

I visualised myself sending the money to Made Reni. Here are 600,000 rupiah, I would say. Buy yourself a top-notch offering with orchids on top and go to Jero Pura on me. Maybe the god will cure your cancer, shrink the secondary tumour in your liver and leach the liquid from your lungs.

Here, have another 600,000 rupiah and go to Munduk as well. Just in case.

I couldn't do that.

I realised that I couldn't act as if I believed a balian could cure cancer, wouldn't minimise her disease by pretending it could be helped by someone flicking holy water on her head. I wanted to support Made Reni but I didn't want to give her undue hope when it was clear there was none. I wanted to support the family, but I didn't want to make them drive her round the island asking for an answer to something that wasn't so much a question as a full stop.

I asked Iluh to send Made Reni my love, told her to contact Mr Robert in America to see what treatment he suggested, and reminded her to take care of herself. I'm here if you need support, I wrote. If you're sad or tired, I'm a WhatsApp message away. Text me any time you need.

I prayed for Made Reni everywhere I went.

Some weeks later, Iluh told me, Made Reni was feeling a little better. They were going to visit some saints, she wrote – not balians, but something different. Her father didn't approve because he didn't believe in that stuff, but they were going anyway.

A week or two after that, Made Reni was better still. They had been to see the saints, Iluh wrote, who'd confirmed her mother had been subjected to black magic. The holy people were helping, though, and her mother had slept through the last two nights. Things were looking up. We sent each other smiley faces and heart emoticons. I told Iluh to take care of herself again, because I wasn't sure I believed in holy people any more. 'We miss you dear Julya,' she wrote. 'Please come to Bali.'

Four days later, I woke up to another message. 'Julya,' it read. 'My mother already dead.'

I was done with saints. I was over religion. I would look for an answer amongst the living again. And this time I would try a woman.

THE LAST ROAD IN SOWETO

But what [the doctor] said to himself was,
'Putting it on, a virtuoso performance,
a daughter of Eve comme il faut.'
Theodor Fontane, *Effi Briest* (1896)

I don't deal with illness, she said. I deal with problems at home, with love, or finances, but not illness. If someone came to me with a broken neck, I swear, I'd send them straight to hospital.

I swallowed. 'But physical problems can be a symptom of spiritual upset, can't they?'

'Usually only when people have a calling.'

This is what happens when you do something on a whim, I told myself, and perhaps it's what happens when you go to a woman. That the men I'd seen had focused on my physical shortcomings was bad enough, but here was a woman thinking I'd flown 6,621 miles for a horoscope reading.

Perhaps it was because I'd been calling the person who would heal me 'my Jesus' or perhaps it was because I'd spent three decades being inculcated by the patriarchy, but throughout my search for a cure, I'd always assumed the person to cure me would be a man. It was an odd belief for a feminist who knew about Yentl Syndrome, and it was odd that the contradiction had never occurred to me, when what the men had said had upset me so much. I'd happily bounced around the world, offering myself to them – *do what you like as long as it helps* – and wondering whether I was making it all up when they said there was nothing wrong with me. I had tried to laugh them off, but I'd internalised their criticism, and although I knew they were ignorant and their diagnoses wrong, on some level their voices had lodged in my brain. Fat. Lazy. Nothing wrong. All in your head. Get a man instead of a cat and all will be fine.

The pain had neutered me when it first arrived – as it does to every woman, as Janet Williams says – and I'd been grateful for the anonymity, the ability to walk down the street without feeling the acrid assessment of my thunder thighs. And although a builder's catcall was the last kind of validation I wanted, the alienation had whittled away at me. But I didn't realise just how much the medical and male gazes had taken from me until I met Thabiso.

That 80 per cent of black South Africans would visit a sangoma, or traditional healer, over a western doctor was my starting point. Then there was Herbert Benson, the Harvard professor, writing in *The Mind/Body Effect* that ngangas – Zimbabwean sangomas – have a better understanding of patient psychology than doctors. After Haiti, I was more convinced than ever that the answer lay in my brain, and I thought maybe a sangoma could reset it better than a COPE psychologist. With minimal googling, I found Thabiso Siswana. She was unlike anyone else I'd seen.

She was 26 years old. She wore makeup, sharp suits and form-fitting dresses instead of flowing robes. She'd done interviews and been on TV. She was of my world, not some esoteric nether region, with a normal job in banking in the Central Business District of Johannesburg. It just so happened that on the weekends she went into a trance, got possessed by her grandfather and healed people.

She was also a she, of course, and after the bad balians, the Dr Hos and the Mr Bloggses, she was a breath of fresh air. When she emailed me back – 'It would be my pleasure to assist' – I felt first-date quivers.

Sangomas are real, said Zee, as we drove through Soweto. Oh, I'm sure, I said vaguely, thinking of Benson, who wrote that western medicine should meet tradition halfway. No,

Julia, he said; they really are real. In touch with another realm.

We'd been introduced by a mutual friend – Zee was a TV producer who moonlighted as a fixer on his days off. Over email he'd seemed competent, and in person he had the kind of gravitational pull that induced intimacy in a matter of minutes, a solemnity and empathy that reminded me of Mr Wong. He'd asked me straight away what I was doing here – why I'd crossed continents to meet a sangoma – and he'd told me about Jared, his friend who'd killed himself because of his chronic headaches. To Zee, I was able to voice things I hadn't dare tell anyone else.

Zee was as cosmopolitan as he was learned – a guy who, at school, had begun his process of studying the major religions in depth before deciding on a belief system. He was a man of technology and yet here he was, believing almost completely in sangomas. He didn't know how they worked, he said; he just knew that they did. He told me stories of friends who'd had callings; of a secret half-brother whose existence was predicted by a sangoma. One day, he thought, science would show how they did it, hooking a Thabiso up to a monitor to show the electricity sizzling between worlds. There was no contradiction for him: science and sangomas could exist alongside each other.

We drove through Soweto as the film guy – a friend of a friend who'd heard about my quest – solemnly zoomed in. We went right to the edge of the township, where the last road in Soweto threaded round open fields, and stopped beside a detached bungalow surrounded by a concrete wall.

She was at the door as we pulled up, the TV blaring from inside. I didn't recognise her at first – this quiet, bespectacled woman who stood five feet to my six and said hello with the air of a grandparent. I'd been expecting someone younger, louder, kookier – a Charmayne or a Dr Ho. Perhaps this was her aunt.

'I'm Thabiso,' she said. 'Come on in.'

She introduced us to her little cousin, Owami, furiously

shy and glued to the TV. I sat on a cream pleather armchair, those first-date butterflies beating feverishly in my stomach. I admired her tattoos, all six of them, and blushed when she approved of my own tiny one. I presented three gifts: a secondhand iPhone, knee brace (she'd had a car accident right before my visit) and bottle of expensive perfume that a client of hers in Yorkshire had asked me to mule. Gold, frankincense, myrrh.

'People come to see me about things that are happening in their life,' she said, explaining what a sangoma does. 'Maybe he's a business person, he's worked so hard, and next thing, things have fallen, you know? Or maybe someone doesn't understand what's happening in their marriage. People having problems conceiving, you know? Things like that.'

'And illness?'

She shrieked with laughter, a joyous, girly laugh. '*Illness?* I'd be, like, are you kidding me?'

My throat tightened.

'It's usually people who want answers to things in their lives,' she said. 'If someone is sick, I'm not going to burn incense; they'd have to see a doctor. Sangomas don't have anything to do with medicine. At the first sight of blood I would faint.'

'But the interviews said that...'

'Yes,' she pronounced it 'yiiz', rolling it out, long but curt, and schoolmarmish – one didn't argue with Thabiso. 'They didn't... that isn't quite right.'

'Oh,' I said, hunching over.

Physical issues were physical issues, she explained – sangomas couldn't treat them. The only exception was if someone had the calling to be a sangoma, and ignored that calling. If that were the case, they would start developing physical symptoms until they accepted their fate – Thabiso, for instance, had suffered migraines before answering her calling. Her aunt's cancer had gone into remission the moment she became a sangoma, and returned years later when she turned to Christianity. The journalists, she was afraid, had oversimplified it.

Owami turned off the TV.

I thought of the money I'd spent to reach her, the three planes I'd sat on to get the cheapest route. The arthritic ache that engulfed my body after every flight did a little flare, as if to say, oh hi there, 6,000 miles and £1,500 and you didn't even bother to check if she could help you. Stupid. Fat. Dumb. Female. Go back to the men.

'Oh,' I said politely. 'How interesting.'

She said that normally before a client came, her ancestors told her what to expect, gave her some kind of clue, but with me she'd had nothing. Normally, their diagnoses were revealed to her in dreams, but since the accident she hadn't dreamed. In fact, since the accident, she'd been angry with her ancestors and had been too upset to communicate with them. She'd gone into her little room that morning to make amends because I was coming and she wanted to help, but they'd stayed mum.

'I've been praying about it actually, because Julia said she has something wrong with her,' she announced, glancing around: Zee, Owami, the film guy, her grandfather watching us from a large frame on the wall. 'And they're not telling me anything.'

Oh come on, I thought, I've crossed continents for this. Can't you at least pretend?

'I feel very heavy, though,' she said. 'I've slept so much today. I just feel tired, like my body is tired. I'm tired. I've got a headache.'

'From thinking about me?' I said. 'I'm sorry.'

'No,' she said. 'I have a headache right now. I'm trying to connect to try to feel what's wrong. Something is wrong.'

'With me?' I said. 'Well I hope you can—'

'Oh,' and she did a little moan. 'I'm feeling a whole overwhelming of emotions. I feel you cry a lot.'

I cry at nothing.

'All the time,' I said.

'You're making me cry because you cry a lot,' she said, tears running down her cheeks.

Hey, not that much, I muttered.

'She was crying in the car,' said Zee, the school sneak.

'No I wasn't,' I said. 'When?'

'You *were*,' said the film guy.

'I cried when you told me about your friend who killed himself,' I snipped. 'And I cried at the elephants yesterday.' Zee had met us at a safari camp near Pretoria where I'd stood nose-to-trunk with a seven-tonne elephant. It had whinnied at the ranger and I'd burst into my usual tears: crying at nothing, crying most of the time. Please, I'd begged the universe – there in the Cradle of Mankind, touching an animal I'd only ever seen on a screen – I've come halfway across the world. Please don't let this be another failure. Please let her be different.

She could not have told why she was crying, wrote Kate Chopin in *The Awakening*, her 1899 novel about a woman's gradual realisation of the cage into which she's been born before she kills herself in despair.

I said to Zee, defensively: 'I don't just cry at sad things, I cry at happy things too.'

'I know,' said Thabiso, sniffing. 'You've got so much sorrow though. That's what I'm feeling from you. So much sorrow. So much pain. That's why I'm feeling so much pain and I'm having a headache. But anyway, I guess we'll talk about it tomorrow.'

'Physical or emotional pain?' I'd deliberately not explained what was wrong with me in our emails because I'd wanted to test her.

'Both,' she groaned. 'Both. It's heavy. I mean, not heavy as in your weight—'

A healer saying I wasn't fat was a miracle in itself.

'But it feels like everything you're going through is heavy,' she sighed. 'It's physical pain, it's emotional pain, it's things that are inside. It's a lot of things that are happening, actually.'

She paused, studied me. 'But let's talk about it tomorrow, because I've got a headache. Your headaches are awful. They hurt.' Headaches are the least of my worries, I wanted to say. What about my arm?

She hauled herself up from her chair, went outside to smoke, and I followed her like a child does its mother. Does your back hurt, she asked, and your legs? Because mine are really hurting.

Probably the car accident, I said.

No, she said, it isn't. Do you have pain there? Because I feel it. I feel terrible.

'Is this how you feel every day?' she said. 'Because I couldn't live like this.'

Not everyone had suffered from Yentl Syndrome or said there was nothing wrong with me. Some of them – Mr Wong, Jero Pura, Jannie the psychologist – had acknowledged my suffering. But feeling it themselves? Nobody had ever said that.

Later, she told me that she knew right away, that first night, the moment she felt my pain.

We stayed until midnight, watching the stars from her patio as she told us of the burden of being a sangoma. She had no time to herself any more. She was tethered to her ancestors. She couldn't travel, didn't have a boyfriend. She hadn't chosen to be a sangoma, but she had to accept her lot.

'Becoming a sangoma means a lot of pain,' she said. 'Sometimes I feel, like, why can't I just be a normal girl?' She sighed, and looked down at the iPhone that hadn't left her grip since I'd handed it over. 'How do I install this Facebook Messenger?' she asked crossly. As we bid her farewell, she was uploading a new profile picture to WhatsApp.

We would go to the river in the morning, Thabiso had declared. We'd arranged to meet first thing, but I awoke to find I'd gone eight rounds with jetlag overnight. The palette knife in my back was plying my torso in two and the autonomic symptoms that came with my Condition – dizziness, feeling faint, shaking – were on red alert. My hands were so weak that the film man had to spread my toast for me; it took three hours to get up and dressed. I hadn't felt this horrific in a couple of years.

Thabiso was looking thunderous when we arrived.

'I'm so sorry—' I started, but she cut me off. She could barely move for the pain – my pain – she said. Her back was breaking, her legs were swollen and her head was pounding. She felt half dead. 'Is this you?' she asked, with an unhinged laugh. 'It's you. What have you done to me?'

I'm sorry, I said again, then Zee piped up that he had a headache, too. It was catching: mass hysteria on a micro level, as virulent as flu, the early miracles of Lourdes or the women dancing the pizzica (or tarantella) in Puglia's Salento peninsula, supposedly whirling out the venom from a tarantula bite but more likely rebelling at their lives, an allergic reaction to the patriarchy.

We went to the river.

The river wasn't exactly a river, more a slim stream running round the outskirts of Soweto, drawing the local faithful. A group of men stared at us – tiny Thabiso in sundress and leopard-print cape, the pallid giant lumbering behind her – as if we'd beamed down from the moon. Two women, sangomas, walked a semi-naked man into the river and poured the contents of a bucket over him: the Baptism in the River, Y-fronts for a loincloth.

'Here,' said Thabiso, crouching on the bank beside them. She lit candles and impepho (an incense-like herb), mixed cornmeal and water into a porridge, laid out Haribo sweets for the spirit guardian of the river. She shuffled close to the water, chanting softly, then started to cry, and then to sob. I thought of Erzulie Dantour, of *The Awakening*'s Edna, the anonymous woman in *The Yellow Wallpaper*. Did Lilith cry, I wondered, or did she only rage?

At lunch, it was my turn to weep.

We were at a Sunday buffet – the South African equivalent of a carvery, only without the Yorkshire puddings. It was in Orlando West, where the eyes of the world had briefly rested during the apartheid struggles – Mandela's old house was here, and 12-year-old Hector Pieterson was killed during the Soweto uprising. Nowadays, this was the touristy part of town, where visitors clustered in white groups chaperoned by single black tour leaders. They photographed the street buskers, then turned away when they asked for tips.

She waited till it was just me and her – Zee and the film guy had gone for a second round at the buffet, and Owami was engrossed in her phone – to ask about my Condition. What did healing mean to me, she asked – to be less restricted by the pain, or to have the whole thing completely gone?

What a question!

'It means someone waving a magic wand and telling me, you're fine,' I said.

'But that's not really practical,' she said. 'At the end of the day, we need to look to reality. We're so busy looking for hope that we don't see things can happen another way. Maybe it didn't work with all those other people' – I had told her about the Charmaynes and Mr Wongs who had gone before her – 'because they were focusing on trying to make this thing go away, instead of trying to figure out why it's happening to you.'

I was lucky to be doing what I was doing, going around the world, meeting people from all walks of life, and she could see that I loved it, she said. Did I want to go back to who Julia was, or did I love who Julia was right now?

Inside me, something drained away. I hadn't had her down as one of the do-you-really-want-to-get-better crowd. 'He alone will die who wishes to die,' wrote psychosomatic medicine pioneer Georg Groddeck in *The Book of the It*, in which all the chapters are dedicated to a female friend, and start with, 'My dear'. *I am a doctor, dear, and I know.*

I don't even know who Julia is right now, I said, but I don't care. I just want to get better.

The reason I ask is that you're always smiling, she said. And I think certain things that happen in our lives are trying to lead us to things that we wouldn't otherwise have done.

The tears dripped into my mashed potato. Owami glanced up from her phone.

'Your condition took you to 20 different people to learn 20 different things,' she ploughed on. 'Do you only care about the pain, or do you want to know the answer to why it's happening to you? Is the answer that you're really seeking where to go from here? Don't focus on a magic wand because I don't have one.'

Owami reached for my hand.

'I can feel what you're feeling,' Thabiso went on, 'and I wouldn't want to feel this every day of my life. It is awful. But I can safely say, I'm not going to take it away, Julia. I want to be the one to give you the answers, to open your eyes and show you there's a reason for you to go through so much.'

He says no one but myself can help me out of it, writes the *Yellow Wallpaper* woman, *that I must use my will and self-control and not let any silly fancies run away with me.*

'At least you can live,' she said. 'At least you can do something that can make you wake up in the morning and get out of bed. You're stronger than what's happening with your life, stronger than what you're feeling, stronger than your pain. You're so optimistic that you're willing to go the extra mile.'

'But what for?' I said, raising my voice. I'd already tried on the brave cripple identity and it hadn't fitted. I didn't care about strength; I was sick of being told everything happens for a reason. Made Reni hadn't died for a reason. Samba El's people hadn't been torn apart by an earthquake for a reason. Mr Bloggs hadn't been a cunt to me for a reason.

'What is it *for*?' I said again. Owami withdrew her hand.

'I don't know,' said Thabiso. And then suddenly she was saying that my grandmother was there, at the buffet with us, urging me to live. All you have to do, Julia, is live, she said. Don't focus on a miracle. Just live, despite the pain.

'It's so sad, Julia,' she said, wiping tears from her eyes, 'because you're hoping for that little magic touch that will take your pain away.'

I wondered whether Zee knew any better sangomas.

'Just because the pain does not go away doesn't mean you failed,' she said, but I knew she was wrong.

She said something under her breath, but the music was loud and there was a margarita swirling in my head.

'Did you say everything is going to be okay?' I said.

She whispered: 'I hope so.' Then she said, 'We'll try, my dear,' and told me about a bar I had to visit before I left Johannesburg.

———

Back at her house, we went straight to the ancestors' room, filled with sacred things by Thabiso, her mother and her sisters, all of them sangomas. Take off your shoes, she said, nobody enters who is not barefoot.

It was the size of a garden shed with a tiny, high-set window. Raised on a concrete platform and taking up about half the room was the sacred space where the ancestors ruled. There was a washing line drawn coyly across it, hung with patterned wraps and goatskins, as if to shield the spirits. There was a photo collage of those same ancestors; candles, matches, little heaps of charred impepho; and shelves and shelves of muti, the magic herbal medicine of the sangoma's toolbox.

I'd been warned about muti. I had read terrible news stories about 'muti killings' of albino children, abducted and dissected for their precious body parts. I'd read that sangomas used parts of endangered animals to concoct their medicines. The previous day – which seemed a lifetime away, now – I'd interviewed a doctor who'd warned me about sangomas: they use black magic, she said, and kill animals to make their potions. We had left her house and made straight for Thabiso, but not before a police car had trailed us through an Afrikaans bastion, watching our car and its odd cargo: black driver, white passenger, Asian with a video camera in the back seat.

There's nothing dangerous here, she said, watching me as I studied her shelves: powders, ground herbs and dried leaves in recycled jam jars. You could eat it all and the worst that would happen would be an upset stomach.

Then she belched.

'Excuse me,' she said. She leaned on the wall, looking pale. She sighed, gulped for breath. She belched again – longer, this time, and more guttural. 'Ooh,' she sighed quietly. 'Excuse me.'

'Do you want to do this?' I asked. 'You look ill.' She smiled weakly, nodded.

'But you look terrible,' I said, leaping up from my chair because even though I felt at a four-year low – POTS raging, joints on fire – she looked worse. She shook her head, looking at me but almost through me, as if the exhaustion had taken her out of my reach.

'I think,' said Zee thoughtfully, 'this is it. She's connecting.'

I stared. She sighed again, a girly, high-pitched sigh. Then from her delicate mouth came the kind of noise a champion speed-eater might make after a hot dog-eating contest. She groaned.

'I'm sorry,' she said, looking embarrassed. 'This is how they come. I'm sorry for the noise.'

We ushered her into the sangoma room and she unrolled two straw mats and dragged a goatskin between her splayed legs. She rolled her head, perkier now that she was in her element. She lit some impepho and I put my offering – 100 rand, or £5 – on the floor, careful not to touch her (she had the same rule as Jero Pura and, when I came to think of it, Charmayne too. Three women, three continents, all in it for the vocation, not the money). She scooped it up and popped it in her 'bag of bones' which was really anything but – a drawstring cloth bag filled with twigs, shells, a few coins and a couple of tiny unidentifiable animal bones that might have come from something the size of a rabbit.

She asked me my parents' names and my mother's maiden name, told me to speak to the ancestors in my head, and blow.

Please, I begged silently, don't let her fob me off. No

more pain-is-here-for-a-reason. Cure it. Please. Heal me. I ran through the names of all the ancestors I could think of – grandparents, great-aunts and whoever had gone before them – then she held her bag of bones towards me and I leaned forward and blew on it, a long, yogic exhale filled with four years of desire.

She slammed it on the ground and started chanting in Zulu, bouncing the bone bag to the rhythm and rotating it slowly 360 degrees. She spilled the contents onto the goat-skin, and rolled her head as she inspected how they'd fallen. She sighed.

'Hmm,' she said quietly. 'Hmmmm.' She drew out another belch.

'They're telling me that what you have is not a burden,' she said. 'They're telling me that what you have' – and she made another swooning noise, straight out of Austen – 'is primarily just an illness right now. What they're telling me is that they're not here to say they can take everything away, what they're telling me is that they can—' she moaned, gasped. 'Ahhh! Really try and find an easier way for you to live the way you are. Ohhh, I'm feeling a sense of—'

She sounded like she was struggling, like the ancestors were using her as the rope in a tug of war. She kept trying to stray off the subject – into finances, love life, career – and each time they would drag her back. 'Ohh,' she kept saying. 'Okay. Oh. Ummm.' She sounded like she was in pain.

'Let's go back to your affected areas,' she said.

She touched the points where she felt my pain. Her knees, her swollen feet, her lower back. My back was heavy, she said, like someone was pounding it. 'Like it's breaking,' she said, smacking her palm on the floor. 'I feel like your back is breaking.'

Yes, I said. That was how I always described it to make people listen.

She went through the pains on my right-hand side: the point where two ribs had been pulled apart by strain-ing muscles, my shoulder, my arm. She talked about the headaches and asked if I had questions – usually, sangomas and their clients work in tandem, guiding each other to what they want to hear – but I refused to make it easier. No, I said, I have no questions.

She said I wouldn't be going through what I was going through if my ancestors didn't think I could take it. Anyone else would have ended their life by now, she said, and in fact, she thought maybe I'd tried to end mine but it hadn't worked out. I've never tried, I wept, I've only ever thought about it.

'They're not allowing you to end your life,' she said. 'That's why it's always going to be a thought.'

I thought back to a grey afternoon before I'd met Kevin. The pain had grown tight as a thicket around me, and I could no longer make out a way ahead. My insurers were ruling me fit to work while I couldn't type or even hold my mobile phone, and I had opened the windows of my child-hood bedroom, climbed over the chest of drawers and sat on the window ledge, debating whether or not to jump. My mum had rushed in and begged me not to, and I had looked at the ground, 15 feet below, at the neighbours' children playing obliviously in their treehouse, and tried to summon up all my courage to do it. I had sat there, hands steadying me on each side of the ledge, the struts from the window levers digging into my fattening thighs, and then she'd changed tack, warned me that I wouldn't die, just disable myself even more, and I had quietly climbed back down and returned to bed.

'You're not going anywhere,' said Thabiso.

I had ancestors here, she said – female ones, strong women who I needed to bring closer to me so they could give me strength (suddenly I remembered Bali, an old woman saying something similar as she spat cold porridge over my arm). 'Let's not say it's part of the healing,' she said, 'but to start the process...' she paused, changed tack. 'They want you to get to a point where you accept that whatever is happening to you is not because you did anything wrong.'

He alone will die who wishes to die. Nobody is ill without

192

wanting to be. Groddeck may have been the first, but he wasn't the last. Kevin had said it. My reiki-giving neighbour had said it. Mr Bloggs had said it. And now I sobbed as she told me I hadn't brought it on myself.

This may not be the answer you're looking for, she said, but think of it as a blessing, not a curse. This is why you're on this earth – to help others.

Why did illness always have to mean something else, I wondered. Why did people with cancer get told it was because they bottled things up, why did people with heart disease have to read that their explosive tempers were to blame? Why was chronic pain in our hysterical female heads? We were already on our crosses – why did they feed us vinegar?

I don't believe in a reason for my pain, I told my ancestors, and I've no interest in helping others, so please just take it away.

'Are you saying I'm not going to get better?' I asked her. And then I added, floundering for something to grab on to: 'Can I get better even if I can't get perfect?' It was the first time I'd imagined a cure might not be a complete one. Congratulations, said the COPE psychologist in my head, you're on the way to acceptance.

'I hope you'll get better,' she said, solemnly. 'But I'm not going to say tomorrow, next month, 2017 or 2018. It's going to take time, it's going to be a process. All I want from you is hope – hope that the little something I can contribute can really help.' And there it was, that infinitesimal spark.

————

I was to return the next day for a cleansing. She paused – was I open to a chicken?

'Yeah,' I said casually. 'What kind of chicken?'

'Not eating it,' she said.

Jesus Christ.

We would slaughter the chicken, she said, not as a sacrifice but as a diagnostic test – with our prayers, it would take on my physicality and, opened up, would show what was wrong with me, an MRI without the mega-magnet. The chicken was white and pure – it would bring light and cleansing, and as it died, it would flap and kick, expelling the bad stuff and hopefully healing me in the process. Afterwards, I'd purge with an emetic, then she'd bathe me in the river and finish with sangoma-style 'injections', cutting me with a razor and rubbing muti into the wounds.

On Tuesday, she said, because today was Sunday, you are going to wake up and get out of bed and be okay.

I chose yellow and white candles to guide me through my process.

She told me I was helping her too, making her do things like go to the river and kill a chicken, things she'd been too scared to do before. She said that my gogo, or grandmother, had sent me to her; that gogo was happy with the process our ancestors had decreed. And we sat there for 20 minutes like old friends, inhaling the impepho as she belched like Linda Blair and showed me how to interpret her bag of bones.

'Can I ask one more question?' I said. Impepho is a mild tranquilliser and I felt two pints down. 'It's something Rakesh said yesterday.'

The previous evening, as we'd been talking, and Thabiso had explained that physical illness was only treatable by sangomas if the sick person was ignoring a sangomic calling themselves, the film man had butted in. Could I have a calling, he had asked, but more importantly, could *he* have a calling? Because he had what the doctors called mental health issues, but he felt it was something else, something more significant.

She'd deflected his question and quickly changed the subject, and I had squirmed at the idea of two poshoes steaming into her front room and claiming they had callings, too. It was cultural appropriation at its finest. And yet ...

Is it definitely not some kind of spiritual thing, I asked – a need to connect with my ancestors or look into traditional English medicine, anything like that? She paused.

'I don't think they would want to do anything to your health,' she said, carefully. 'But your health problem is for a greater purpose.'

My body checked out as Zee drove us home. It had been an overwhelming day: from the difficult start, symptoms on red alert, to the physical exhaustion and mental turmoil that Thabiso had unleashed – that she couldn't cure me, that my grandmother was with me, that the pain was my destiny yet I wasn't allowed to kill myself. On top of that, I would have to kill a chicken in the morning. I had to hold on to the wall as I staggered to bed, and the next day I felt worse than ever.

We left at 7am, just me and Zee. My stick was in the back, in case I needed it, and as we pulled up he told me that if I was black, I'd have integrated it into my look already, snazzing up the leopard print and changing my gait to draw attention to it, making beauty from adversity. We were laughing as we reached the door.

She'd just woken up – her glasses were on, she had no makeup and a little tuft of hair at the front like Little Lord Fauntleroy. She'd thrown a wrap around herself instead of the modern clothes I was used to seeing her in. She looked skittish, with a childlike nervousness about her.

'Oh my god you guys,' she said, jumping back to let us in. 'Here you are.' She paused, looked nervously from Zee to me and back again. 'There's something I have to tell you.'

THEY CAN KILL US

In me was every woman.
George MacDonald, *Lilith* (1895)

'*WHAT?*' I shouted. '*Are you serious?*'

'I am serious,' she said. 'I am dead serious.'

'But you never said that.' I stared at her. 'I was even think-ing about how you hadn't said that this morning.'

'I *know*!' she said. 'It was the first thing – the first thing I thought that night, but I just didn't want to say it.'

'Why?' I shrieked, too loud.

'I just didn't want to put it that way. It sounds absurd.'

'It does sound absurd. It really does.'

My heart had sunk when she'd said she had something to tell us, and potential bombshells had clicked through my head. She'd been lying when she'd said she felt my pain, and couldn't deceive me any more. She hadn't really spoken to my gran or connected with her ancestors. She knew she couldn't help me, and hadn't wanted to disappoint. I would have to kill the chicken myself.

Zee had run to get the camera – he was filming for the other guy that day – and she'd motioned me to sit down, under the watchful eye of her dead grandfather, on the same pleather armchair as that first night.

'You might not want this on film,' she had said, and the bile had started churning in my empty stomach and I'd said it's fine, I don't mind, but all the sounds around me were draining away and I thought I was about to faint.

'Are we still going to do the treatment?' I asked timidly.

'Yes,' she said. 'We still want to do the treatment, but I just wanted to share something with you . . . I got a message from my mum. And what she's saying... basically, it's something that I didn't want to say, so she's like, "I'm going to say it." So I need to play you the voicemail. Because it's completely like...' She squirmed. 'I was just asking her, like... it's impossible, it cannot be.'

Zee had asked me on our grim journey that morning whether I was scared, and I'd said no, more stressed than scared, but now I started to tremble.

'You remember yesterday you asked me a question about whether it's possible for someone who's not of African descent to have a calling,' she said.

'Well, Rakesh said that,' I said hastily.

'Yes he did,' she said. 'But you wondered about it too, because we spoke about it yesterday.'

'Yes,' I blushed.

'So I don't know...' she paused. 'I don't know how I'm going to say this or whatever, but because of your grand-mother's presence, that makes you someone who has a calling. Like I have.'

'*What?*'

'You have an ancestor in you who wants to work and who wants to heal people,' she said.

'*OH MY GOD!*' I screamed.

'So there's something like that,' she went on. 'Because of all your symptoms. When I told her, Mum was like, "Everything that she's going through is pointing to it," and she said that when she communicated with her side, they were saying that they—'

She stopped to look at me, my eyes watering with hope.

'It's not like, here goes the magic wand, vanish,' she said, gently. 'It's just that all those things you were crying about – your aches and everything – those are the things that you could be able to take care of if we were to say... put you through an initiation process kind of thing.'

'Are you serious?' I whimpered.

'I couldn't tell you,' she said. 'It's absurd. Remember when we were talking about how this kind of illness can only happen to African people, or someone who's black. I mean, I couldn't even imagine how it was going to work. But my mum was certain.'

She had cleaved me in two. One side was sounding a fanfare – *this is it! She's going to cure you! You'll never hurt again!* But the other half was ringing the alarm, screaming it's a trap, she wants your money, she wants you to write about her, she wants to be on TV. There was something else, too. I didn't want to be the one who came to sub-Saharan Africa for the first time in her life and promptly declared herself a traditional healer. If I had to come out as a sangoma once I got back home, I might die of culturally appropriated shame.

Her mother was in Swaziland at the moment; they'd been exchanging voicemails on some app that a Luddite like me had never heard of. They'd spoken in Zulu and even now Thabiso was too jumpy to translate herself – she didn't want to say it, she said, couldn't bring herself to give me the news head-on – so we waited for Zee to come back. He looked baffled, creeping in with the camera to find us eyeing each other nervously from either side of the room, as if one of us had just declared an unrequited passion for the other.

'Zee,' she said, brandishing her phone imperiously. 'This is my mother.'

She looked nervous as it played, 30 seconds of a woman speaking Zulu, and I assumed it was because this was a setup, and she felt guilty. Later she would tell me that she couldn't fathom why I was taking it so well, this mighty burden that she'd just wrapped around my shoulders. Didn't you realise I wouldn't care about the burden, I would say. The burden is nothing compared to the pain.

Zee's eyes widened so far that they risked popping out of their sockets. He stared at me, grabbed the phone from Thabiso as if touching it made it more real. 'Wow,' he said. 'Did she just say what I think she said?'

'Yiz,' said Thabiso.

We all stared at each other.

'I couldn't tell her yesterday,' she said. 'And that's what my mum is telling me – you know exactly what this is, and you must tell her – you must tell her, and she will understand.' They turned to me. I was laughing as the tears dripped down my face.

How sublime to be the chosen one, for once, instead of the fat drama queen. How wonderful to have this woman – this woman who had felt my pain and struggled to share her truth with me instead of all the men who'd pocketed my cash and sent me packing.

'It's scary to tell someone they have a calling,' said Zee, looking solemn because he knew what it meant.

'I'm surprised you're taking this so lightly,' said Thabiso. 'In my head, for me it feels … it seemed impossible. Not impossible, but …'

I pulled myself together. 'Yes, it seems impossible, and when Rakesh mentioned it the other day, I cringed,' I said. 'I only came because when I first read about you, it said that you thought physical pain is spiritual pain from the ancestors. I never thought this.'

'Well it is for you,' she said. 'Because you've got elders on you.'

She'd told us the first night that when her gogo came through, her feet swelled up, and when she channelled her uncle, who'd walked with a stick, she started to limp. Come to think of it, she had gone on and on about my swollen feet, and I hadn't taken any notice because flat feet were part of my Condition, and I'd assumed she was just doing a more delicate rendition of the 'you so fat' routine.

'You've got elders on you, so you have elderly people's symptoms,' she said simply. 'When you get swollen feet, that's what old people get. Your back pain – old people have bad backs. You get all these things because you've got elders on you.'

I was comfortable with the idea of ancestors, I said – I had regular one-sided conversations with my grandmother – but I didn't want to be the person who returns from South Africa claiming to be a sangoma.

'Your initiation would just be to heal you, though,' she said. 'You don't have to work as I do. Some people have illnesses they can't explain – headaches, cancers, things like that – they go through initiation and they just get better. They don't have to practise. You just cross the bridge.'

'Crossing the bridge' was the first part of the initiation process – the spiritual side, where you learn to connect with your ancestors, crossing the border into the spiritual realm. That took about a month. To be a full-on sangoma, I'd have to study herbs and traditional medicine for several more months, but that was the part I didn't need.

'It would just be a matter of you crossing over,' she said. 'It would unlock certain things – it would unlock grandma being able to speak through you or work through you.'

We knew which grandma it was, because the previous day at the supermarket I'd had a Proustian moment with a pink-and-white-striped flannel identical to the one my mother's mother used to have. I'd picked it up and, right there in aisle three, I'd smelled her rose glycerine soap and the fog of her warm bathroom. What I hadn't told Thabiso was that my mother's mother had been born in Johannesburg.

So you're saying, I asked, that if I came back for a month – and yesterday at lunch, now I thought about it, she'd suggested I return for a month, had even said I could stay with her – if we did the initiation, my pain would be over?

'Her mum was adamant,' said Zee. 'There was no room for doubt in that message. She said, you *do* have ancestors and that *is* why you have your symptoms and if you *do* do the initiation, you *will* be cured. That was it.'

'We'd heal you as we'd heal an ailment of someone gifted in that sort of way,' said Thabiso. 'It doesn't mean you're going to have to be all obedient – we would take it as a healing process, and help you cross the bridge.'

'Why didn't you say this yesterday?' I asked, because the doubts had struck again.

'Because it sounds absurd,' she said briskly. 'Anyway, I was trying to act normal, but that's the news. Mummy feels we should still do the ceremony today – I was hoping she'd say we could skip the chicken but she said no. Your ancestors chose to bring you here.' In the ceremony room, I stared at the jars filled with old herbs and new meaning. I should feel different, but I didn't. She dressed me in one of her wraps, told me not to focus on being an actual sangoma, but to work out how to translate that into my culture. *Pray to your own god. I don't know your prayer.* 'Worship your own god,' an Igbo ancestor tells a white man in *Things Fall Apart*.[21]

Maybe I would be a psychic, she said, or maybe a healer – I'd have to work it out for myself. But that's what she'd meant the day before when she'd been talking about my being destined to help people, and that was why she'd kept hesitating in the consultation, changing the subject, reluctant to tell me what they were ordering her to say.

———

The chicken was in a crate of chickens by the roadside.

'Choose the one you connect with,' Thabiso was saying, and I looked at the chickens and thought, should I do this to the one I connect with, or should I be sparing it?

'That one,' I said, pointing like a Roman emperor in the Colosseum. I stared at it, and it stared back quietly. It had been standing motionless in the corner as the others clucked and strutted about: me at a wedding, unable to dance.

I'm sorry, I said to the chicken, and it blinked.

It cost 80 rand, or £4.20. It scrabbled to stay in the cage at first, but in Thabiso's grasp it stopped moving and let her dump it in the boot, resigned to its fate. Truly, it was my spirit animal.

I cried all the way to her house. I wept in the ceremony room. I sobbed as it coughed when Thabiso lit the impepho. Suddenly I didn't mind being ill – I could take the pain, if it would save the chicken's life.

The real question, she said, is why you think your life is worth less than that of a chicken.

I laid my hands on my chicken as she untied its feet and settled it in front of the yellow candle. It struggled for a split second, gagged on the smoking impepho, then relaxed as we prayed over it. We asked the ancestors to show what was wrong with me through the chicken, and asked the chicken to take on my ailments. I felt it tremble beneath my hands as it confronted its fate, and I wondered who was more scared: me, the chicken or Thabiso, who said she had a phobia of killing things.

Zee carried it out of the ceremony room to the patio, where Thabiso's brother held a black plastic tub and a machete from the kitchen. I owed it to the chicken to watch my process but I gagged as he brought up the knife so I watched it at one remove, through the reflection of the French windows of her sister's bedroom. There was no sound. I saw Sechaba's arm sawing back and forth and Zee bent over, his back to the reflection. Then there was a flapping noise, the men talking urgently to each other, Thabiso calling an order and I heard the knife clatter to the floor.

I turned around. Gobbets of thick blood were spattered all over the patio and up the wall. They had moved the body round the side of the house in deference to my sensibilities but the head lay on the ground, staring at me, coxcomb flapping accusatorily in the breeze.

Thabiso slapped the corpse on an oven tray. I stared at the severed neck as she set it down on the steps. The wind was picking up and she tucked the edge of her wrap inside itself – she had dressed us both in traditional robes by now – pushed her glasses neatly up the bridge of her nose and picked up the knife. The body was so fresh that it exhaled as she sawed through the ribcage. She peeled it open, delved inside with two-inch nails painted neon pink. She extracted the organs. They gasped, all of them who knew what the insides of a chicken should look like: Thabiso, Zee, Owami, Sechaba.

The liver was three times too big, she said, and the heart was enlarged. Did this mean anything to me?

No, I said. I'd given myself hepatitis at university when

I'd kept drinking through glandular fever, but the liver had regenerated and the hepatitis disappeared. As for my heart, I knew it was healthy because they'd tested it while diagnosing me. My Condition caused my heart to beat irregularly, but there was nothing wrong with the heart per se. Should I get checked out by a doctor, I asked, if the chicken was mirroring my body? She thought carefully and decided no, that though the organs were enlarged, they looked healthy.

That was extraordinary, Zee said. I've killed a lot of chickens but I've never killed one that didn't struggle. Sechaba concurred. It had sat meekly as he'd sliced through its neck, and it was only once he'd hit the spine, right at the back, that it had flapped my pain away. It was as if it had died willingly for me. As if this was meant to be.

She put the organs in the plastic tub, where they'd collected the blood. Owami took the body and dumped it in the kitchen sink. They would have it for dinner.

After that, the purging was easy.

There were about six litres in the bucket – of what, Thabiso didn't know, because she prepared her muti in a trance. I was to drink it all and vomit it back up. She handed me a smaller bowl, for drinking, and a strip of bin bag to stick down the back of my throat. The liquid was dark pink, with undissolved powder coating the bottom, and it was warm.

'Is there blood?' I asked.

'Definitely no blood,' she said. 'Drink it.'

I crossed myself and called on my gogo, stuck the bowl in the pail and took a swig. It was fine, actually – tepid herbal tea with added grit. I downed the bowl and looked at her, triumphant.

'Drink,' she said, proudly. 'Drink drink drink drink drink.' I drank another bowlful. Owami grinned.

'Drink drink drink drink drink,' said Thabiso.

I wanted to make her proud of me after the two days we'd spent together, so I downed another, then another. A huge belch erupted. My ancestors are here, I announced, only partly joking.

'Now make yourself sick,' she said. My phobia of making myself sick was on a par with my allergy to backwash.

I took the strip of bin liner and waggled it daintily in my mouth, gagged, but nothing came up so I drank more and more until it was rolling up my gullet by itself. My eyes watered and my throat hurt, but it didn't cramp – because I was doing it on an empty stomach, Thabiso said, pleasantly surprised that I'd stuck to her rules. A typical medical compliance rate is 50 per cent, meaning half the patients who see any doctor will fail to follow instructions. Chronic pain patients are worse – because nothing works for us, only three in 10 will stick to the rules.

'I fasted too, so we could do this together,' she said, as Owami ruffled my sweaty hair. 'Now hurry up and drink so we can have lunch.' Not only had she believed my pain and felt my pain, but she'd fasted with me. Lots of people I'd seen had said I'm sorry you're ill; others had understood me. But Thabiso was the first to suffer alongside me.

Technically, we should be bathing you in the river, she said, but I don't think you'll be comfortable doing it there, so maybe we should just bathe you symbolically, here on the terrace. I thought of the man from the day before, standing in his pants in the river, and was torn between the biblical image and the mortification I knew I'd feel when everyone stared. The film guy had told me the night before that he and Zee had already discussed my figure and were fascinated to realise that I had an 'African body minus the boobs'. Perhaps, wondered the man who'd spent two days silently inspecting that body through his viewfinder, it explained my calling.

'It's better for you to concentrate on the ritual here than be embarrassed in the river, all naked,' Thabiso was saying.

'Naked?' I squeaked. She looked at me as if I was deficient.

'Yes,' she said, 'Naked. What did you think? The blood has to touch your flesh.'

'What blood?' I trembled.

'The chicken blood,' she said.

'*Chicken blood?*'

'Yes,' she said briskly. 'I'm bathing you in the chicken blood. What did you think I would bathe you in?'

'You didn't know?' asked Zee. 'Oh my god, you didn't know.'

'I thought we were bathing me in the river,' I whimpered.

'You should be in the river, bathing in the blood and the entrails,' said Thabiso. 'Like the man yesterday.' I'd been so busy tactfully averting my eyes that I hadn't seen what they were tipping over him.

I glanced at the guts piled up in the black tub: everything but the major organs floating in the dark blood. Beside it, the chicken head stared at me through eyes still open. I died for you, bitch, it said. Now see this through to the end.

Thabiso picked up the pail of regurgitated muti and poured it in the tub. She stirred it. Bubbles of saliva mixed with clots of blood.

'Come on,' she said, picking up the tub and following the patio round behind the ceremony room. A turquoise towel was pegged to a washing line in front of a concrete wall – she was sure the neighbours couldn't see, but for my privacy, she had put it there anyway. She put the tub on the ground, and the guts slapped against the side like the sea on my Cornish cliffs, suddenly a million miles away.

She disappeared into the ceremony room and re-emerged with a candle and more impepho. She lit both, said a prayer and a pretty chant, and stared up at me. I stood there, mouth jammed open, numb. I couldn't let the chicken die in vain. I couldn't let Thabiso down, either.

'I've done this before,' she said. 'You can do it.'

I undid my wrap.

'Do you have any tips?' I said.

'Yiz,' she said. 'Try not to breathe through your nose.'

She'll think you're fat, I warned myself as I turned my back to her and yanked down my pants. She will see your cellulite and realise why you're in pain. And it hurt me to the quick, the idea that she might change. And then I thought:

no, she won't, because she's not like the others. She believes you.

I stood like a limpet, pressing my nakedness against the turquoise towel.

'Get in the tub,' she barked. It was still warm from the chicken's and my insides, and my feet squelched down on top of body parts. The bottom of the tub was rough with the muti grains and the bits of corn she'd squeezed out of my chicken's oesophagus. I stood there shivering, a rabbit in headlights.

'You must bathe with it,' she said from behind me. 'Bend down and wash your face.' I folded over, arse in her face, and scooped up a handful of gore. Nose and mouth clamped shut, I smeared it over myself. I wondered if she'd let me off if I fainted.

'Now your hair,' she ordered, and I took another handful and ran it through my hair, a shampoo commercial except with chicken blood and vomit instead of a waterfall. I followed her instructions – neck, arms, legs – then stood up as she began to dip a pitcher in the tub and pour it over me, our baptism in the river, her standing on tippytoes, me crumbling in on myself like a foetus.

'Pray,' she said, and I prayed that I would get through this and get better, begged my ancestors and the chicken that had died for me. Then, more urgent, she said, 'Come on Julia, you need to scrub,' and I realised the tiny moans I'd been hearing were coming from my mouth and instead of washing myself I'd been rooted to the spot, gripping the towel.

'Scrub scrub scrub,' she said, and I thought, you've come this far, you're naked in her garden in broad daylight, you're covered in blood and vomit, you may as well do this properly; and I bent over again, giving her an eyeful, and splashed around in the tub, rubbing it into my neck, my armpit, frantically scrubbing the path of the ulnar nerve down my arm until, like the ladies at Lourdes, she said, 'It's okay, you can stop,' and I doused myself one last time for luck and leapt out.

I had to stand in front of the tub and kick till it flipped over, and the gore went everywhere, blood clots the size of tablespoons flying through the air, semi-digested corn stuck to trachea tissue pebbledashing the concrete. I reached for the towel – 'No,' she said, 'the wrap,' so I grabbed the wrap and started to towel myself down and she grabbed me – 'You must air-dry', just like Lourdes – then looked at me maternally. 'Here,' she said, my friend again, instead of my sangoma. 'Let me teach you how to make your boobs look bigger,' and she tied my wrap in a halterneck.

'Will I have to do that again if I do initiation?' I asked. I was sitting on the blood-streaked patio, trying not to lick my dried-out lips as flies buzzed round me; she was coming from the ceremony room with a pack of clean razor blades and a pot of muti.

'Oh, no,' she said, darkly. 'For initiation, it will be a goat.'

I remember Zee playing devil's advocate, asking whether I minded the razors, being cut by a sangoma in the land of HIV – because there were more cases in South Africa than anywhere else in the world. I remember looking at him like he was a simpleton – after I've done *that*, you think I mind *this*? – and telling him the blades were clean. Really, though, that had nothing to do with it – the fact was, I'd have done anything for Thabiso. The past three days – the understanding, the acknowledgement of my pain, the sharing of my suffering, the mothering during the ritual, the fasting solidarity – had bonded me to her. I wanted to go home to process what she'd told me about the calling and the initiation, but whatever I decided – whatever I believed – I knew I would return. I loved her already, just as I had loved Iluh and Made Reni, Lea and Charmayne. The filament of a sisterhood connected us across the continents.

'This is our version of injections,' she said, squatting beside me and pointing to faint scars along her limbs. 'All South Africans have these.' Owami rushed to show me a long, silvery one on her arm. We would be as good as blood sisters.

She cut me down my spine and rubbed in the muti. She

went along my arms and down my legs, making little in-cisions. 'Think of me as a doctor,' she said. 'Tell me where it hurts.' I asked if she could treat my TMJ, and she cut a slice at the back of my jaw, at the exact spot where back home they injected Botox to weaken the clenched muscles.

Zee asked if she knew what chakras were, and when she said no, he pointed to the seven cuts she'd made along my spine, each marking a chakra point. How strange, she said, to share points with the Chinese – or was it the Indians? – but really, it wasn't strange at all. *It's all connected*, whispered Richard Morse in my head – Richard Morse who'd felt wiser than anyone else, Richard Morse who seemed to understand more about the world than I could ever hope to, Richard Morse who may have scared me but had also cared for and about me and given me hope. Then she took me into the ceremony room, prayed with me one more time and picked out some muti: white muti, for a sangoma.

She handed me a sandwich bag of beige powder that smelled of sick. When you have pain, shower with this. Scrub yourself with it as you scrubbed yourself in the tub and try to connect with your ancestors. She handed me two smaller bags – one filled with paler powder, one black. When you feel the pain, she said, put a pinch on each hand, and lick it off. I eked them out over the next few months – the paler one tasted of salt, the black one of charcoal.

That night, I inspected myself in the mirror. Did I look different, I asked my reflection, now that a spiritual truth had supposedly been revealed? I didn't think so, but I took a photo to zoom in on, just in case. Looking at that photo now, I seem more scared than I felt, as if I'm shrinking into myself, away from the blood on my skin, away from the revelation. But I look lighter, too, less haunted and younger – something that had lived in my face before, and had gone into hibernation when the pain had arrived, was back. I'd turned a corner; not necessarily physically – it was still too early to tell – but mentally. Thabiso's acknowledgement of my pain – her vow that she would want to kill herself if she had to live with it – had been more important than I could ever have predicted. Now that someone understood what I was going through, I could mentally move on.

I was tired but hopeful the next morning. I washed my hair four times, the water swirling brown around my feet, but Thabiso still wrinkled her nose when we picked her up: 'I smell chicken,' she frowned.

I was flying home that afternoon and she was supposed to be busy, but I didn't want to leave her and she seemed to feel the same, so we went to Mai Mai, the market for sangomas in downtown Johannesburg, where we bought matching bracelets and wraps. At one shop, a woman asked if I was Thabiso's initiate, and when I looked confused she grinned, pulled out a crumpled photo of a white sangoma in Botswana, and pointed at it, and then at me.

'I'll come back,' I sniffed, hugging her goodbye at Johannesburg airport, her beautiful eyes – for she had eyes like nothing on earth – glistening. As I walked away, watching her watching me, I realised that I meant it. I'd never felt so supported as I had by Thabiso: supported in my health, in my identity, most importantly in my gender. It was pleasant, of course, to think of myself as a chosen one – who didn't like to feel special? – but what had made more of an impact than the revelation about the calling was that Thabiso and her family – Zee, too – were invested in me, genuinely cared about what happened. Thabiso had begged me to give her a chance and trembled as she'd tried to help me. Zee had urged me not to be cynical about my process, not to share it with anyone until I absorbed what had happened.

I thought of Sechaba quietly agreeing to kill my chicken, and reassuring me as he walked past during the vomiting that I was fine, this was normal, that he was going to do it tomorrow because he had a cold on the way and wanted to purge. I thought of Owami, painfully shy to start with ('Hi,' she'd whispered when we'd asked her name), ruffling my sweat-matted hair as I threw up, telling me everything was going to be alright.

Thabiso had offered meaning to my pain, and whatever I would come to think of her explanation – because on one level it made perfect sense, on another it was absurd, and I needed to distance myself from her to work out which side I came down on – the fact that she had done that had helped me. Whatever I made of it, once the rush of holiday romance had subsided, I knew I would never forget my time with her.

I was standing in line to get my passport stamped, studying my razor cuts – raised and angry now as they started to close over – when I realised I was standing.

We'd arrived late, too long shopping, and in my hurry, hurling my bags at the check-in desk minutes before it closed, I'd forgotten to ask for a wheelchair for the first time in several years. I had walked, which wasn't unusual for a good day, but I had also lifted my little case onto the belt to go through security, which I couldn't usually do, and now I was standing in the queue, which should be making my heart beat too fast and risk me fainting. My back was aching slightly, but I was standing tall.

I texted them from my seat, waiting for take-off. I did it, I wrote, I made it to the plane by myself; and the tears dripped onto the screen as I tapped the letters into words, wondering if it was tempting fate – 'tempting God', as Thabiso called it – or whether it was good to think positive. Whether, even, this was the start of something new. But I crushed that thought the second it popped up, because nothing would be worse than being let down by her.

In London, I went straight from the airport to a work meeting, suitcase in hand, and didn't feel dead. I talked about what had happened in Johannesburg but with a carefully chosen cynical tone – enough to show that I wasn't stupid, that I knew it was absurd and that I was laughing too – though whether with or at myself I wasn't yet sure.

When the pain started circling later that week, I leapt in the shower to scrub myself with the muti that smelled of vomit, and prayed to my ancestors as I licked the white and black powders off my hands. I talked to myself out loud, chided Julia for killing a chicken and not taking it seriously, told her that she owed it to the chicken to make sure this worked. I WhatsApped Thabiso saying I was doing okay, because I couldn't bear to tell her I wasn't (it was Charmayne all over again), and I emailed Zee to ask, now that we had 6,000 miles between us, whether he had really believed her or thought she was taking me for a ride.

I believe her 100 per cent, he wrote back. Don't lose faith. Don't tempt God.

I decided I'd return to South Africa once this was all over – for a holiday, to see Zee and to see Thabiso, if not to do the initiation. I realised, as I desperately tried to tread water while sinking back into the slough of despond, that I'd felt better with them than with anyone else since my pain had started – not physically, but mentally, and the hope had been a balm to my body. First I had to go to Brazil – I'd booked it before I'd realised there might be something to Thabiso – and then I had to write the book. But afterwards, if I could afford it, I would try to go back.

Charmayne, Stella, Jero Pura, Thabiso – all had believed in my pain. All were women, yet they were the only women I'd seen. What had I been doing, running to all these men? Why had I assumed they would be the ones to heal me? Why had I believed them over myself?

It wasn't a male versus female thing, of course it wasn't – at least, not intentionally. But the balians would never have told a man to lose weight, Mr Bloggs would never have told a man to stop worrying, my neurologist would never have told a man, it's not the medication, you're just depressed. I'd bet my statutory sick pay that the locum who signed me off that morning in May would have prescribed a man some painkillers with it, that my former GP wouldn't have told a man that debilitating knee pain was part and parcel of turning 30, that my rheumatologist wouldn't have refused a man potentially career-saving physio because he'd already had six sessions on his bum. I wonder whether specialists would have told a male student that his post-viral fatigue was a mental health issue, or that the RSI during his A Levels was stress-based. I don't think they'd have told a 14-year-old boy that his hypermobile circus tricks were nothing to worry about, or that a paediatrician would have told a father that his little boy was squatting on the floor just fine and by the way had he heard of Munchausen's by proxy.

Less likely to get adequate pain medicine. More likely to have our pain dismissed as in our head. More likely to die of coronary heart disease because we don't look like we're suffering. Twelve doctors to spool through before the one who medicates us as they would a man. They can kill us, literally, with their fixed ideas about the female body, yet they say it's all in our heads. *I am a doctor, dear, and I know.*

Thabiso taught me that all those men had been wrong. That I wasn't making a fuss or making it up – that I was in pain, that my pain deserved to be treated, and that I hadn't brought it on myself. It isn't your fault, she had said, and, finally, I believed it wasn't.

Two weeks later, by the time I was going to Brazil, my pain was exactly as it had been before I'd met Thabiso. I would die before I admitted that, either to her or to myself – but as I realised months later, she had done something more important than cure my arm. She had given me back my humanity and my identity.

She had woken me up, made me see that I wasn't a patient, a body part, a statistic, a repeat prescription, an annoyance, a supplicant, a passenger needing assistance or an object of intrigue on the bus. She stripped me of those layers.

She made me remember that I was a person. More importantly, I was a woman.

TEMPLE TO THE SICK

And then the vile, diffuse pain completely flowed out of his head, out of his temples and into her soft hands, and on through them and her body down into the floor, covered with a dusty, fluffy carpet, where the pain totally disappeared.
Mikhail Bulgakov, *The White Guard* (1926)

The reason Herbert Benson thinks a nganga has a better grasp of patient psychology than a western doctor – why he believes western doctors can learn from what he calls 'primitive' medicine – boils down to one basic thing: bedside manner.

We all know it's important – patients like me happily wait ages to see Dr Good because we know the reason he often runs late is because he takes his time with us. When, in 2013, a male doctor diagnosing a patient called Kate Granger with cancer failed to introduce himself, she – also a doctor – launched a campaign to better clinical rapport, called #hellomynameis. Before her death in 2016, she'd won support from 400,000 colleagues and started a nationwide conversation about patient-doctor communications.

But there's more to bedside manner than just good manners. Studies show a good one can help symptoms of chronic illnesses like asthma, osteoarthritis and diabetes – it correlates with better blood pressure, blood sugar, pain levels and weight loss.[22] Multiple studies show that mental illness can be significantly affected by doctor attitude.[23] It can even affect procedure outcome: a recent survey of patients getting lumbar facet joint injections showed that those who chatted to the radiologist had a significant reduction in both pain and recovery time.[24]

When I told Jannie Van Der Merwe, my old pain psychologist, how Thabiso had unleashed something in me – changed me profoundly despite not having cured me – he wasn't surprised.

'If you approach someone with compassion and empathy, that patient will do better,' he said. Thabiso had made it clear, I realised, that not only did she believe me, but also that she cared.

She cared enough to monitor me, both in Soweto and beyond (18 months later, as I write this, we're still in contact). She was professional – she made me complete the ceremony, after all – but she cared enough to hold my hair as I threw up, tell me I was doing great as I stripped naked, and remind me that she, too, had done this as I rubbed chicken entrails into my face. She even cared enough – or so she claimed – to feel my pain.

'That appreciation, that acknowledgement, that validation is crucial,' said Jannie. 'We all have an idea of what our life looks like, and pain stops you in your tracks. It's traumatic. So before you even start to look at treatment, a medical professional needs to express empathy with that, and feel it. They need to do what your sangoma did, and say, "I can feel your pain". More than that, "I'm *prepared* to feel your pain".'

That's behaviour immediately at odds with the modern medical system, of course: the average GP appointment currently lasts eight to 10 minutes.[25] But a shift in attitude doesn't have to take time, and the mounting evidence is clear. Bedside manner goes beyond professional appearance, depth of relationship, simple courtesy or rebalancing the power dynamic in the room, which starts off entirely in the doctor's favour; it means that however knowledgeable you are, however cutting-edge your treatment, if you're not connecting with your patients, you could be doing them physical harm.

Benson reckons doctors could learn 'esteem, affection, sympathy' from ngangas – in fact, in *The Mind/Body Effect* he goes as far as to write that the social positioning of a shaman – the way they interact with their patients – is a 'viable model... for a good modern doctor'. I think of the differences between my doctors and Thabiso: clinical empathy – 'That must be very difficult for you', 'I can imagine you're frustrated', 'Yes, that must be depressing' – versus the rolling up of sleeves, the fasting with the patient and slaughtering a chicken for them. But it doesn't have to be one or the other. There exists a middle line.

———

Francesco Forgione had a bad experience in Naples. Nobody really knows what it was, or exactly what he made of it, but we know that during World War I he spent part of his national service working in a military hospital there, and we know he didn't like it. One person devoted to his legacy told me he didn't like the way the doctors talked to each other instead of to the patients; another said he was horrified by all the admin that detracted from caring for the sick.

What we do have on record is his reaction.

Francesco Forgione never forgot his experience in Naples – nor his experiences as a patient, when, as a sickly youth, he'd been in and out of hospital. So when he became something of a celebrity in Italy, he used his fame to show how he thought it should be done. He decided to open his own hospital: a hospital built by a patient, for patients. People said he was mad – he wanted to build it on a mountainside in one of the most remote, underdeveloped parts of the country, right after World War II when the nation was struggling to eat. He had even less architectural experience than he did medical. And yet he did it. Francesco Forgione's fans sent him money, 400 million lire – enough to build a marble palace on the mountain, a palace so huge, so grand and so defiant that you can see it from the air as you fly into Bari.

It opened in 1956. Sixty years on, Francesco Forgione's mountain hospital in Puglia – still 112 miles from the nearest airport, 25 from the nearest train station – is rated one of the best in Italy, runs on a non-profit basis, and is at the forefront of research into neurodegenerative diseases. 387,000 patients cross its threshold each year; doctors migrate from north to south (which never happens) to work there; patients from all over Italy (and beyond) request to be treated there – and it's feasible, to be treated there when you're not from there, because one of the things Francesco Forgione insisted on was free housing, in real houses, for patients' families.

You eat well at Francesco Forgione's hospital, because all the food apart from pasta, bread and fish – all the meat, the vegetables, the oil, the dairy – comes from two organic farms that well-wishers donated. You feel supported, because although the doctors have many patients to see, there are ancillary staff, there purely to provide pastoral care. And I'll wager that you also feel rather special, more like a guest in a grande dame hotel than a lowly ward patient, because this hospital is unlike anything you've ever seen: salmon pink and white for the exterior, with Corinthian columns and turquoise shutters. Interiors clad entirely in marble and a lobby where emerald columns square off against swarthy black floors and purple walls veined so precisely that each slab looks like a Rothko painting. There's art nouveau-style feathered glass in every stairwell, and views to die for of the pristine Gargano peninsula, the Adriatic Sea and the olive-carpeted plains of Puglia down below. It's more a royal palace than a hospital. And, you know, Francesco Forgione got flayed for that. They said it was unnecessary, unseemly, unedifying opulence for what was only a hospital, what were only patients. But he didn't care – 'I'd have built it in gold if I could,' he said. Because to him, the patient was everything. Not only must the patient be in an environment that makes his soul sing, but the patient must be shown love and compassion, because to Francesco Forgione, the patient was God.

You probably won't have heard of Francesco Forgione, but you'll know his stage name – Padre Pio, Italy's favourite saint. I'd known of Padre Pio for years, but only of his miracles: healing parishioners, predicting the deaths of others, appearing mid-air beside planes during turbulence to guide them safely down to earth. But it was only in 2016, when I'd followed his body to Rome to ask for some magic, that a man watching me watch the relics noted my stick and my tears, my savage glare of hope as I traced my hand over the glass protecting his bloodied robes, and told me about the hospital. Everybody associates Padre Pio with miracles, he told me, but the real miracle is the Casa Sollievo della Sofferenza: the House for the Relief of Suffering, the single work he left the world, a marble wedding cake on top of a mountain, visible from space.

And no matter where you stand on bilocation or stigmata or my back, curiously pain-free after a desperate prayer to a blood-encrusted glove, there's one thing you can't deny. Padre Pio was talking about the patient-doctor relationship and the importance of the hospital environment decades before anyone else.

I wasn't sure what I'd make of it, this temple to the sick ('a temple of prayer and of science', Padre Pio had called it). I worried it would be another Lourdes, fetishising suffering (for Padre Pio believed that the sick are closer to Jesus on the cross than the healthy are). I worried I'd find it as ugly as I do most Italian churches. I worried they'd try to convert me.

But as I walked through the marble corridors, what struck me most was what it lacked. There was no reception desk, no security guards playing spot the abusive patient. It lacked the tang of disinfectant, a smell which provokes a Pavlovian response of fear, in me at least, every time I go through a revolving door – 'It doesn't stink of illness,' as a Vatican official said (because Padre Pio, perhaps fearing another Lourdes, left his hospital to the Vatican). And it lacked a hospital atmosphere – that sizzle of stress, that brooding worry that presses on my shoulders when I normally walk inside one; there was none of the frenetic movement of doctors or patients, hurrying to treat the sick, hurrying to get out.

Calm, it seemed to me. Peaceful and serene. Beautiful, too – everything from the doors to the lift shafts designed to give pleasure. Everything I wouldn't associate with a clinic. I thought of the hospitals I normally go to – that I've been to all over the world, because my Condition has an annoying habit of tripping me up wherever I go. I can think of some I liked – a stylish one in Budapest, a slick one in Singapore, one in London with walls covered in Quentin Blake sketches – but those are all still clearly hospitals. This felt like something entirely different.

You don't have to be Catholic to work at the Casa Sollievo della Sofferenza, but obviously it helps. There are no set prayers or services, but there are two churches where I saw officials in scrubs sitting quietly. You don't discuss religion with your patients, because the nuns do that – they're there purely to chat. What you do have to be is prepared to abide by the founding precepts of the hospital: that you must treat patients with dignity and respect, and deliver love and comfort at the same time as your treatment. Everyone who works at the hospital is given a book to read, some 170 pages, detailing the philosophy of the institution and its founder. You can be the best clinician in the world, at the top of your game, but if you don't communicate effectively with your patients, the Casa Sollievo will sack you.

'The sick aren't just weak physically, but psychologically too,' Domenico Crupi, the director, told me. 'Here, we look after them on every level.' Their 'clima di famiglia', or homely atmosphere, doesn't just make patients feel better, he said; it helps them accept their disease, because acceptance is easier when you're shown love – and for much of modern medicine, acceptance is a cornerstone of treatment. 'I've worked in many hospitals,' he said, 'but I see these things germinate here.' Before I left, he showed me a poster for an upcoming talk on resuscitation, illustrated by a Van Dyck: Cupid rushing to rouse a sleeping Psyche. Did I like it, he asked proudly, and I remembered the NHS poster I'd seen in London the year before – a pair of red stilettos with the caption, 'Yummier Mummy: Breastfeeding mums don't have to spend their money on formula milk' – and said, yes, I love it.

'We have a huge responsibility here,' said the head of the geriatric unit, Antonio Greco, as he introduced me to his newest recruit, Mario: a €4m robot being trained to talk with lonely old people and rehabilitate Alzheimer's patients. Mario was a pan-European artificial intelligence project being trialled in 10 different environments. The Casa Sollievo had been chosen as the sole hospital participant – partly because of their technical skills, he said (psychologist Grazia D'Onofrio, who was firing up Mario, is a world expert in robotics), but also, he suspected, because they had a reputation for care that went beyond the clinical. Dr Greco was from Rome, but had come to Puglia 26 years ago.

'It goes beyond religion here,' he said. 'This dream, this vision – I haven't found it anywhere else. There's a spirit of belonging, and there's a domino effect. People talk to each other.' Later, I would see Dr Greco again, on the main staircase of the hospital, two floors and several corridors away from his department. He'd stopped halfway up to talk to a patient – or maybe, because she was only middle-aged, a patient's daughter – and they were chatting quietly, smiling at each other. It was a sight I never imagined I'd see, a doctor off-duty, talking to a patient like an equal – a person, instead of a body part or the Alzheimer's in room two.

———

Foucault called this separation of body and patient the 'medical gaze'. Remember that psychologist who diagnosed me with crippling social anxiety right before my Haiti trip? Dr Good had referred me because at the time I was struggling. I'd been rattled by Patrick and worried by Colorado, scared that one might have helped me, that the other might not. My pain was through the roof – it was the beginning of the bad back – and he'd said, let's have one more go with CBT for pain. So I'd gone for an assessment, and the psychologist had looked terrified as we'd run through his list and I'd said, sure, I think about killing myself all the time because of the pain, and no, I never go out any more but that's because it hurts too much – can you help with that? And he'd ignored the pain and just seen the anxiety – to him, I wasn't Julia, but Anxiety – because he had tick boxes for anxiety but not for pain. What he hadn't seen, beyond his checklist blinkers, was that Anxiety wasn't a standalone thing, but was made up of Pain and her children: Hopelessness, Despair, Frustration and Banging Head Against Brick Wall.

Modern medicine, according to Foucault in *The Birth of the Clinic*, began with this separation, when the question changed from 'What is the matter with you?' to 'Where does it hurt?' And although modern medicine has bettered the world, of course, this imperceptible change of angle has skewered the part of us that doesn't belong in a box.

'The way modern medicine is billed is undermining doctor-patient relationships,' Herbert Benson told me as we discussed my pain. 'And I think that should be unacceptable, because study after study has shown that a doctor-patient relationship is vital for chronic pain. Doing away with that may be contributing mightily to the excessive use of opioids.' But they don't do away with that, do they? They give us pills and diagnose us with psychiatric problems instead.

For me, the biggest problem with the medical gaze was that I was divided into body parts and dispatched to see a different expert for every one of them. Not only did each expert only care about their expertise – nobody looked at the bigger picture, which is why I was hospitalised with suspected adrenal failure when I'm almost certain it was the medication I was on – but instead of seeing me as a human being whose life had been derailed, to them I was always just a C-list patient. The rheumatologists saw people whose EDS had put them in wheelchairs. The cardiologist saw POTS patients who couldn't stand at all. The gastroenterologist dealt with Crohn's, and the pain people dealt with phantom limbs and the suicide disease. The neurologist – who I'd held out so much hope for, whose rejection brokered my schism with the medical world – spent his days dealing with strokes and seizures. Why would he waste time and sympathy on the weeping woman with the poorly arm?

'Just because you haven't got the worst case scenario doesn't mean you don't have a problem,' Dr Cuong, my acupuncturist who straddles the east-west medical divide, once told me.

The week after I returned from Puglia, I found myself at a work lunch opposite a doctor from a hospital in Ancona. Ooh, I said, flailing for conversation, I was just at the Casa Sollievo della Sofferenza. It's incredible what they're doing there for the patient-doctor relationship.

They're a *Catholic hospital*, she said aggressively – because she was a gynaecologist – and I said yeah, well they wouldn't be my first choice for an abortion, but as a non-Catholic I found the Jesus in the stairwell fairly inoffensive, and as a patient, my god, I've never seen anything like it – how different my life might have turned out had I ever been treated there.

They're a Catholic hospital, she said again, as if the first word cancelled out the second, and as she reached for a slice of bread I caught her shake her head and roll her eyes and give a tiny snort of disgust, *idiot patient*, and I thought, I may not share the same moral code as Padre Pio's lot, but I sure as hell know who I'd want treating me between you and that man on the stairs.

———

People at the Casa Sollievo don't talk about miracles. It may have been founded by a saint, but it's a hospital, after all – a hospital whose founder planned it to be 'capable of fulfilling the boldest clinical needs'. One place where doctors and nurses do happily discuss miracles, however, is Lourdes. Although, even at Lourdes, miracles aren't necessarily what you think.

Four months after my disastrous visit, I returned. I wanted to see Lourdes in pilgrimage season, when groups from all over the world descend on the grotto. Miracle season, too, though by now I was less interested in the idea of miracles and more in the 'Lourdes effect' – the frequent improvement in sick pilgrims' symptoms that stays while they're there but usually disappears once they return home. I'd seen my own Lourdes effect in South Africa, Haiti and Bali. I'd had it emailing Patrick every day for a month; I'd even felt it writing to the strange Tong Ren man in Vegas. It was easy to come by, it seemed, but harder to make it last.

That's not to say the Lourdes effect always wears off. A 1982 study[26] following a group of sick pilgrims showed a significant decrease in anxiety and depression, sustained 10 months after their return home. Huddling from the July Pyrenean rain in the Hotel Solitude (an inappropriate name if ever there was one: the lobby was full, and about 50 wheelchairs were lined up outside the front door), I met Dr Jennifer Klimiuk, Specialist Registrar in Palliative Medicine for North West England. She was a regular at Lourdes, the medical team coordinator for the Salford Diocese, and when we met, she was combing through the findings of a similar study of her own. She wanted to know not only whether quality of life had changed, but also why – was it the holiday, the holiness, or the company? Many of their sick pilgrims – the famous 'malades' of Lourdes – lead lonely lives back home, yet her early findings were that spirituality was a big factor in why they felt their lives had improved.

'I don't think there's anybody who comes to Lourdes on a regular basis who'd deny they see a massive change in people,' she told me. She was talking not about miracles, but emotional shifts – though she said they could be just as profound. She wasn't the only one to say that.

Kerry Jones (as I'll call her) is a nurse at a hospital in the north of England who makes a pilgrimage to Lourdes every summer. We met in a strange way – a preordained way, I would have said at the desperate height of my pain. The day before, five minutes after arriving in Lourdes, I'd walked into a wall, knocked myself out and spent the best part of the night in hospital. The following afternoon, still alarmingly concussed and, thanks to my somatic focus, unable to contemplate anything except my impending death, I'd gone to the drop-in centre at Bernadette's grotto. Kerry was the nurse on duty.

As we'd waited for the doctor, she'd told me that she

regularly witnessed miracles here – small miracles, sometimes physical but more often mental. And when I'd cried as the doctor dispatched me straight back to hospital – because I couldn't stand any more soulless doctors poking me around like the one the night before, and I couldn't spend another night on a trolley in the corridor in a gown that ended halfway down my thighs and didn't close at the back, because I was done with doctors, scarred by doctors and refused to see any more of them in 2016 – Kerry had made me an offer I couldn't refuse. If I went back to the hospital today, she would meet me tomorrow and tell me all about miracles.

'People don't come here for miracles,' she said the next day in the Hotel Solitude. 'They come to get the strength to cope with what's facing them.' Her words spun me back four years – it was exactly what the priest at Walsingham had said when I'd started my search. It hadn't been good enough for me then, but the subsequent years riding the hope-despair rollercoaster had made me wonder whether I shouldn't have capitulated at the start.

'One per cent of their hope might be for a miracle, but 99 per cent is to get the courage to face what's coming in the future months or years,' said Kerry. 'Lots of people come here knowing that they're dying and knowing that they're not, you know...'

She saw things happen all the time, she said, but they might not be what I'd call a miracle. They would be small things, or temporary changes – like the stroke-ridden priest they took from his nursing home, where he lay, mute and paralysed, to Lourdes, where he knelt down and began to pray.

It wasn't a miracle, she said – he'd been capable of moving and speaking for a long time. He'd just chosen not to, until Kerry had bought him robes so he could take part in the pilgrimage as a priest rather than a cripple, and the volunteers had showered him with attention.

'It was the socialisation,' she said. 'Something happened when he got here that changed his whole outlook so he could become the person he was before the stroke to some extent. I think he was stimulated by the fact that people were actually talking *to* him and not *at* him. I think he was stimulated by the fact that he took part in the processions as a priest, not with the sick, so he changed his role. It's not a miracle. It's just that, in the home, he chose not to do it.' As soon as he got back, he reverted to silence.

'It's very easy to be dismissive,' she said of the medical profession. 'Especially if you're in acute medicine. Like your A&E doctor.'

Two nights earlier, the doctor who'd treated my concussion had been a textbook Yentl Syndromer. Initially he'd tried to dismiss my symptoms, saying that my drifting in and out of consciousness was probably tiredness, that the visual disturbance and ringing in my ears were probably normal for me and I should be fine with some ibuprofen. When, filled with the confidence of Thabiso, I'd said no – no, I know my body, I don't have tinnitus, I can usually *see*, and anyway, surely you're not recommending ibuprofen for a head injury, not ibuprofen that'll make my brain more likely to bleed – he'd turned into a terrified little boy, scared of the Lilith in front of him, and commissioned a CT scan. When that came back clear he'd discharged me – except he'd failed to explain that even though I wasn't haemorrhaging, I'd still have symptoms. So the next day, when the black spots were still skating across my eyes and waves of dizziness were still powering over me, I'd assumed I was having a new bleed, gone to the drop-in centre and been whisked straight back to hospital. The new team had taken four hours and splurged on another CT scan before confirming I had post-concussion syndrome: unpleasant, alarming, but ultimately safe.

'That man only saw you as a set of symptoms that needed to be seen, treated and discharged,' said Kerry. 'He didn't see you as a person underneath it all, a person needing reassurance and explanation.'

We were back to the medical gaze.

Later that day I watched the famous procession of the sick: hundreds of people in wheelchairs and little hand-drawn carts being paraded round the grounds of the church before rolling into an underground basilica where they would be blessed. To me, it was fetishising suffering. But then to me, the whole shrine fetishised suffering: backless benches to sit on, a marathon hike to the main church, interminable queues on hard pews for the sacred baths. After four years of pain, I believed in making things as accessible as possible for people. I didn't think pushing them to their physical limits helped spiritual growth.

But what did stand out, watching that procession, was that every sick person was being cared for by a volunteer. Nobody was pushing their own wheelchair; the people in the carts would usually be struggling with a stick. And whatever I thought of them being paraded around (and of course, I was projecting – I'm sure they enjoyed every second), I could see that something special was happening at Lourdes.

These weren't carers being paid minimum wage and no travel time, rushing to get patients dressed and undressed, trying their best but up against the clock. They weren't hospital or nursing home staff, checking on the hour that nobody had died or fallen out of bed. They weren't harried children or spouses, treading water in a bid to keep the household going, or even kind neighbours popping in for a weekly cup of tea. They were people who'd volunteered to push the sick around, talk to them, hang out with them, enable them to do whatever they wanted. No wonder the malades were blossoming.

'This is a place in which there's a very unique relation between caregivers and people who suffer,' Alessandro de Franciscis had told me. 'I think medicine can learn a lot from the relationships: person-to-person relationships, not professional-to-diagnosis relationships. The way you learn here to look in the eyes of a sick person, to call them by name and not by diagnosis or a number – all of this is Lourdes.' I may have objected to the €500 candles and the pressure to do penance by kneeling on the hard ground, but I couldn't deny that in exploding the medical gaze, Lourdes was doing something extraordinary – like the Casa Sollievo della Sofferenza, but for entire communities instead of individual patients.

Miracles aside – and at the time of writing, only 69 have been officially recognised in the shrine's 158-year history – people often get better at Lourdes. Maybe not physically, but mentally: they begin to see their illness in a different light, to accept what seemed unbearable before. 'The pain just disappeared into insignificance,' one patient told researchers, talking about the moment a volunteer held her hand.[27] Just because that can't be measured with a scan or a blood test, doesn't mean it can't be transformative.

I'll never forget that priest in London who asked not how I felt – where the pain was, how long it had been there – but how I was coping. Was I okay financially, he asked within minutes of meeting me. How about emotionally? Did I have support? They were questions that not even my psychologists had asked.

Eight minutes is no time, of course – it's not enough time for a GP to take a history, make a diagnosis, organise referrals and write a prescription, let alone add on pastoral care. But something, somewhere along the line needs to change, because if paying patients more attention can help them clinically, doctors should be doing that. The 'do no harm' ethos isn't confined to medication and surgery. And harm isn't only done with intention. Sometimes, it's done by omission alone.

Because let's face it – the patients spending £5bn per year on alternative therapies are rarely getting cured, but they are, more often than not, feeling better, like the 70 per cent of chronically ill patients who were helped by homeopathy. And until medicine can match that kind of pastoral care – until we ditch the medical gaze and make Padre Pio's patient-doctor relationships an everyday thing – we'll keep going to homeopaths and Tong Ren practitioners and faith healers. If you don't give us what we need, we'll find it elsewhere. Because we know it helps. Even if we know it's probably bullshit.

ACT LIKE YOU BELIEVE

I must heal my Self before I will be well... This
must be done alone and at once... It is at the root of
my not getting better. My mind is not controlled.
Katherine Mansfield (1888-1923: TB patient, writer)

Here's what I thought.

John of God was a fake. I knew he was a fake and for as long as I'd known of him I'd known he was a fake.

At least, that's what I thought. But I still wanted to see him, just in case I was wrong. In undoing my shackles and giving me back my identity, Thabiso had lit a tiny flame of hope.

John of God's name was outrageous and his story was worse. Born João Teixeira de Faria in 1942 in Goias province (now home to the capital, Brasilia, but back then just dusty flyover country), he'd been penniless, an illiterate farmhand, until one day, outside a Spiritist church (a denomination that believes spirits communicate with us from beyond the grave), he'd been possessed by King Solomon and set about healing the congregation. From there, João Teixeira de Faria began to transition into João de Deus, or John of God. At the bidding of his spirit guides, he settled in Abadiania, a tiny village with nothing going for it apart from what the spirits assured him was a vortex of energy, a gossamer divide between his realm and theirs. People started to make pilgrimages. He started to tour abroad. He acquired eight cars. Oprah arrived in 2010.

It had been Kevin who'd first told me about him – Kevin my messiah, whose own life had changed in Abadiania. Kevin's blog – photos of him at John of God's, dressed all in white, smiling beatifically – led me to a Facebook group which discussed João's miracles, offered prayers for the sick, and shared photos of the 'Casa' (John of God's centre was called the Casa de Dom Inacio, named after Ignatius of Loyola, the dead saint who headed up the army of spirit healers). There were photos shot directly into the sun and into streetlights at night to capture camera flare – 'orbs', as the pilgrims called them. The orbs, it was generally accepted, were visual proof of the 'entities' – the thousands of spirits that made up the 'phalanges' (I think they meant phalanxes) of St Ignatius and the other phantom healers of the Casa. When John of God was possessed by a spirit, he was referred to as 'the Entity'. It was a whole new vocabulary.

John of God, his followers said, could cure anything: cancer, HIV, arthritis. He could raise the dead and restore the sight of the blind. From what I understood from the Facebook group and its strange vernacular, this involved prayers, herbs and 'surgeries' where he would scrape the sick's eyeballs with a knife. Sometimes he rammed inches-long clamps up their noses. Both therapies could attain miracles. I wondered if Oprah had braved either.

John of God couldn't be real – if someone this well known really could perform miracles, he'd be feted the world over, not just by the kind of American who thought wearing white (the Abadiania uniform) benefitted chakra flow. But, said a tiny whisper deep inside me, for all these people to believe – John of God's fanbase seemed to be one of repeat pilgrimages, not one-off missions that dwindled into disappointment – isn't it possible for Something to be Happening?

Once he'd taken root in my consciousness, of course, he kept popping up – he'd be mentioned in something I read, someone I met would have gone to him, someone else would have heard of him. Yes, it was confirmation bias, but what if it wasn't? Then, one day, the Facebook group erupted. Medium João, as they called him, had been rushed to hospital for heart surgery. It was soon after Max Beauvoir had died and as I read the news, I knew I had to go. I couldn't not know.

I vowed to leave him as a last resort, because he seemed so outrageously fake that were I to cast aside my last shred of cynicism and leave as ill as I came, I feared it would push me over the edge. So, at some point between Richard Morse and Dr Ho, I set John of God as my deadline, and as each person failed to cure me, I shuddered at the showdown that I knew must come. I was desperately planning other journeys – China, South Africa, Lourdes – when Kevin emailed to say he was returning to Abadiania. Would I like to come?

I wasn't ready, yet in a way I was. By then, it had been 18 months since Kevin had originally sparked my hope. I was in debt, I was exhausted from the travel, I was depressed at the lack of diagnosis and the offensive diagnoses. I longed to call it quits. Doctors and pain specialists would say I was moving towards the crucial 'acceptance' stage of pain management – the moment you stop fighting is the moment you start to bear it, is the perceived wisdom – but they'd be wrong. I was moving towards acceptance that my life was over, because after John of God, there was nowhere else to go. Please don't make me die, I begged the universe. Please let something happen before it's too late.

I was handing my body over to yet another middle-aged man, I realised on the way (Thabiso had thrown off the handcuffs of Yentl Syndrome). I was giving him autonomy I knew he didn't deserve, handing another guy another stick with which to beat me. Worse, I realised that seeing Kevin as fanboy to a fake would probably diminish my faith in the person who'd given me it in the first place. But somehow, I needed the closure I knew that Brazil would give me.

If the journey was anything to go by, though, it would be closure in a bad way.

We were nearly at Abadiania – me, my guru, his taciturn friend Mike – when Kevin asked the taxi to stop. Ninety minutes at breakneck speed along a rollercoaster of a dual carriageway had taken its toll. We were all queasy.

'Sit in the front and focus on the horizon,' I said, my standard response to people made ill by my driving, but

Kevin wasn't car-sick; he was picking up on the entities' energy. 'I felt sick last time, too,' he said, bent double at the side of the road, and as I tussled with the urge to slap him (or possibly me) out of it, I realised it had been a terrible mistake to go together.

It got worse.

'Oh shit,' I said, as we pulled off the main road. 'This looks like it did in my dreams.'

'That's a good sign,' said Kevin proudly. 'It happens a lot. Remember how Mytrae's book talks about the entities sending you messages once you've decided to go?' His friend had written a book about John of God; on Kevin's instructions, I'd bought it, plus several others, too. There were plenty of them on Amazon, and there would be still more greeting me in the Casa bookshop. It seemed writing about John of God was as lucrative a business as guiding miracle-seekers to him (it's free to see John of God, but that doesn't stop guides constructing thousand-dollar itineraries around him).

We drove down the main street past a slew of pousadas, all built in the wake of João de Deus and named after saints and entities. We'd booked the São Raphael, but at check-in they only had single beds, not the double I'd reserved to give my arm stretching space, and I saw my chance to escape Kevin's faith and the end of our friendship. Next door was the Pousada São Francisco, where a woman who spoke no English led me to a concrete block of double-bedded monk cells: slit windows seven feet up, the only view a bathroom the size of a postage stamp.

'It's closer to the Casa, the energy will be stronger here,' I told Kevin priggishly. He beamed at me – Abadiania was his paradise – and I stifled a scream. The Sâo Raphael was full of Americans, whereas there was only one other guest at the São Francisco, I would discover later that evening as we ignored each other over a dinner of boiled potatoes, black beans and indiscernible gristle clinging to chunky bones. Either she didn't speak English or she didn't want to; both were fine by me. I didn't want to talk to anyone.

Abadiania was beautiful – green hills dusted with trees, roads of russet earth weaving amongst them (the town was paved only as far as the Casa). It unnerved me, because it *was* curiously similar to my dreams, but I hadn't told Kevin that my dreams of Abadiania had mainly been nightmares. For my subconscious had predicted what it knew was coming – the breaking of my faith and my body – and had spent the past month throwing up wild dreams in which I died every night.

'There should be an introductory talk at seven,' said Kevin as we swept through metal gates painted cerulean blue. It was humbler than I'd expected: the main hall was concrete-floored and steel-roofed, open to the elements either side with rows of chairs bolted to the floor. Up a slope was the antechamber to the Entity's rooms: more chairs crammed together with walls bisected by paint – white for the top halves, that same sky blue at the bottom. There were pictures all around: Jesus waving from the bank of the River Jordan, Jesus cradling a chubby lamb, Jesus as a Pre-Raphaelite nymph. At the far end, on a low dais, was a wooden triangle about two feet high, its frame stuffed with headshots. This, I knew from the books, was 'the triangle' where pilgrims prayed. People on the Facebook group were always looking for volunteers to put friends and family's photos 'in the triangle'. You wrote their name, date of birth and problem that needed solving on the back of the photo, popped it in the triangle, and the entities would start the healing. Internet cafes in Abadiania would print out photos for 70p a pop.

To the right of the triangle was a portrait of St Ignatius. Above it, next to a picture of Jesus, was a photo of a smiling John of God. To the left, a painting of Jesus hugging John of God. Beyond that, a younger João, slicing open his own stomach during a DIY psychic surgery.

Kevin led me into the reception area where a young woman behind a desk looked up through bored eyes.

'Is the orientation at 7pm?' he said. She waved us away. 'No English.' Suddenly, I missed the zeal of Lourdes.

We went out, past the lanchonete (snack bar) and into the bookshop, which sold crystals, T-shirts, triangles and souvenirs, as well as books in every language on John of God. The woman at the till smiled professionally at us, though Kevin greeted her like an old friend. She told us the introductory talk was at 5pm, and encouraged me to buy a £5 Casa rule book.

We walked through pretty gardens, past a mirador cantilevered over the hillside, to the 'sopa area', where pilgrims were fed free soup, infused with energy by the entities, every day between 11am and 2pm. Roger Federer's doppelganger strode towards us in tight white trousers and a Casa T-shirt, and Kevin looked crushed when he rushed to greet him but Roger seemed less sure. I pretended not to notice, turned my gaze to the kiosk marked AGUA where pilgrims bought their Casa water, blessed by the entities and an integral part of the healing process: 40p for a small bottle, 60p for a large, prices they said in the introductory talk were the same as in the shops, but were actually – because I checked – a nine per cent markup on Abadiania's only supermarket.

'That was John of God's *son*!' said Kevin as Roger strode off. His face was still shining. He was so happy – not just to be back, I realised, but happy to be introducing someone else to the John of God fold. It wasn't the joy of a zealot; it was contentment and love. I realised I must never tell him how I really felt.

I unpacked, changed into defiantly coloured clothes. Although most people dressed in white every day – all the better for reading auras – it was only required on Wednesdays, Thursdays and Fridays, when the Entity was in session, and there was no way I was dressing like a cult member if it wasn't compulsory. It was quarter to five, by now, and two stray pubic hairs on the floor danced to the breeze of a sputtering fan. There was no air conditioning in Abadiania.

There were about 40 initiates waiting for the talk when I arrived at 5pm – chatting and bonding, exactly what I wasn't there for. I slunk to the furthest end of the emptiest table where a ponytailed man sitting alone flashed a shy smile but looked quickly away. I put my head down and started scribbling intently so nobody would try to befriend me.

Fifteen minutes late, there was a rush of energy to the front: one of many foreign volunteers. Even in his white Casa weeds, he was instantly American – closely cropped hair, skin tanned to a crisp, the smile of a televangelist stopping short of wildly staring eyes, a holy Jim Carrey. He made us cram up close, clapping his hands together as if he was herding sheep. He swapped the grin for a look of serious concern and cleared his throat.

'This is sincere business for me,' he said, gravely. 'Because I know that, some of you, your lives are on the line.' Even the birds, which had been singing loudly as we waited for him, fell silent. 'I don't mean, like, you're dying,' he went on. 'Like you're literally, physically going to die—'

Unperceptive, I glowered at him.

'But, like, you're dying spiritually, you're dying mentally,' he said. 'And it's got to stop.'

He stared at us, eyes bulging.

'We're here to make a change, we're here to win, we're here to be successful,' he said. 'And it is my humble hope that if I can say one thing, the smallest thing, the biggest thing, anything – any joke, any story – anything that can help you … please, God' – and he raised his eyes heavenward – 'Let me say that thing.'

As he talked for 90 minutes like a third-rate motivational speaker, I formulated my plan. Instead of the week I had booked with Kevin, I would stay two, hanging on to look pious when he and Mike left. I would save money (the alternative was a week in Rio), reassure myself that this was all bullshit and assuage any anger that might come from Kevin when, inevitably, I let slip my real feelings. He could be irritated if I didn't believe, but he couldn't be hurt if I'd tried.

I saw them that night when I wandered up the street to Frutti's, juice bar and nightlife hub of 'Aba', as the John of Godders called Abadiania. I stood in the darkness, watching white-clad freaks – because what else could they be? – bond merrily without the aid of alcohol. (There were no bars in Aba, because bars were places where negative spirit attachments could hop on us.)

They were emerging from John of God's crystal shop, each brandishing two big bottles. Kevin waved. 'It's the blessed water,' he said. 'You should get some.'

'I'm exhausted,' I said, desperate to avoid a chat, desperate not to disappoint him.

'Yeah, the energy here is overwhelming,' he said. 'Everyone is always tired the first day.'

'Well I've been up since 4am and my body's still on UK time—' I started, but even in the dark I could see the disenchantment in his eyes.

'It's the energy,' he said pointedly. 'You should sleep. Be in the first-time line before 7am.' He turned to Mike. 'We should be there by six.'

Back in my cell, I had a cold shower – it would be day 12 when I worked out how to turn the hot water on – and rummaged for my pyjamas under my new white wardrobe. I closed the tiny windows, shutting out miscreants, mosquitos and entities, and put in earplugs to blot out the John of Godders filing past my room to hunt for orbs around the Casa gates. Before I nodded off, I had a perfunctory cry. I could feel the bruise of despair inside, and it was spreading.

———

I awoke to the sound of a hushed march: dozens of white-clad John of Godders drifting quietly past my window. None of them talked, most smiled into thin air, and some carried parasols – the mark of the spiritual intervention, because for eight days after you'd been operated on, you weren't allowed in the sun. It wasn't yet 6am.

I watched them through the bars of the window over breakfast, the flow swelling now – hundreds of them shuffling to the Casa in their identical clothes and silence, the start of a horror film. What if this is a cult, I asked myself, stomach churning. I was so desperate for a cure that I didn't trust myself not to get sucked in. *Get the fuck out of there*, my new spirit guide Richard Morse whispered in his soft drawl.

Back in my room, I changed into my white uniform – I'd worn a coloured dress to breakfast because I was determined to be rebellious to the last. It was 7.45 – Kevin had said to get there before 7, but I knew that not only did the lines open at 8am, but there were four lines to get through, and the Entity called them in no particular order. There was no need to make the ghosts complacent.

At 7.55 I walked to the Casa in my new clothes: white linen trousers, white vest, super-sized white T-shirt chosen because it skimmed my thighs and covered my new M&S granny knickers (since white was transparent and my sickly fat body was an international disgrace, I'd gone for coverage over style). The clothes were all at least two sizes too big, and utterly shapeless. I was 14 again.

The hall was packed with what must have been at least a thousand people. Every seat was filled and a crush of pilgrims hovered in the aisles, bottlenecking at the front as they gunned to be first in line. Every now and then, a volunteer would climb onto the dais and talk to us – in Portuguese, French, German or English – leading the Lord's Prayer or the Rosary, explaining the procedures or gently shushing the remarkably quiet crowd. When they prayed, everyone held hands.

In the corner by the main reception stood the translators who wrote your requests in Portuguese on little slips of paper that you then took to the Entity. You could make up to three requests. I remembered the list I'd drawn up for Dr Ho, the laundry list of symptoms Thabiso had picked up on, and started to panic. How to edit it down?

I thought about what was preventing me from living life to the full right now. It was my arm, primarily – it stopped me working, lifting, carrying, travelling, using public transport, wearing certain clothes – but that stemmed from my neck. Then there was my lower back pain, which stopped me from standing and made me constantly shift my weight from foot to foot as if I had a recalcitrant bladder.

There was the POTS (or POTS-like symptoms, depending whether or not you believed the diagnosis), which ensured that even if my back pain cleared up, I wouldn't be able to stand for more than a couple of minutes at a time. POTS meant that I couldn't do anything that involved queuing, couldn't go to a gallery or museum, or stand at a bar. It crippled my social life, but it didn't affect my work so much, and getting my life back started with getting back to work. Maybe I should leave it out, I thought. But then I remembered that POTS was also responsible for the permanent exhaustion that crushed me, the thick clouds of fog that wrapped round my brain and joints and never burned off. POTS did affect my work, and it needed to stay. Then something else popped into my head, probably because of the white clothes: the weird, messy, mortifying periods Mr Wong had picked up on, the menorrhagia that had arrived out of nowhere a year into my pain, and kept me indoors for two days a month. Maybe it was stress, maybe – as a friend had helpfully suggested – I was perimenopausal, my life over before it had really begun. Whatever it was, it bothered me, this being controlled by my womb.

The list of things that needed to be addressed came to seven, but I found a way to whittle it down without losing any of them. I wrote:

1: Right arm, neck and spine (pain in arm and shoulder comes from neck)
2: Postural Orthostatic Tachycardia Syndrome: fainting, dizziness, fatigue (parasympathetic nervous system)
3: Period problems

I reassured myself that if John of God was for real, the entities would already know what needed healing. One of the people on the dais – half American, half Brazilian, she'd made herself a comfortable life guiding people in Abadiania

– had already warned us to be quiet because the entities were around us, listening to our every word, reading our every thought and working on whatever process needed to be started.

An American woman stood in front of me: young, blonde, pretty, healthy-looking. Her hair was braided into culturally oblivious cornrows, her smug smile one of someone who has their chakras firmly in order. 'I just want, like, clarity,' she told the translator. He wrote something down, and pointed at her list again. 'Oh!' she laughed. 'Basically, I sprained my ankle, like, a couple of years ago, and sometimes if I'm, like, running or something, I get a twinge.' I walked away, boiling with rage. When I returned, the translator was finishing up with a middle-aged lady who looked pleasingly distressed.

I handed him my piece of paper and explained what was wrong. 'I don't know if I asked for too many things,' I said anxiously. 'If I did, let's stick to the three in the top one – right arm, neck and shoulder. They are the most important. The others can wait.'

'It's fine,' he said without a smile, and started writing. He hunched over, so I couldn't see what he'd written until he handed it back and turned immediately to the person behind me.

In capital letters, like a placard at a Hyde Park rally, it read:

PESCOÇO & COLUMA
&
FADIGA CRONICA!
MENSTRUAÇÃO!

He looked surprised to turn from the next person to find me standing there, rictus grin on my face. I didn't speak Portuguese, but I didn't need Portuguese to understand what he'd written, and Thabiso had polished my inner steel.

'I don't want to be rude,' I said to his glare. 'But I think what you wrote is not correct. The reason I'm here is the

237

pain in my arm. I think it comes from my neck but I'm not sure. I don't want the entities to only work on my neck if the problem is my arm.'

'It doesn't matter,' he grunted. 'The entities already know.'

'Yes but I would feel more reassured if you included my arm,' I said firmly.

He ground the pen into another slip of yellow paper.

'Also,' I ventured. 'You've written chronic fatigue, but my condition stems from my heart and nervous system. It's more than being tired.'

He shook his head, repeated that the entities knew what to do, this was just part of the process.

'I know,' I said. 'But for my process, this must be correct.' I smiled winningly. The John of Godders liked rules.

We had a tug of war over his original list – him eager to throw it away, me desperate to keep it. I won. I folded it carefully and put it in my bag. I would carry it around with me for the rest of time, I'd already resolved. Every time I doubted myself, every time I thought a man was dismissing me because I deserved to be dismissed, I would pull it out and look at it – *chronic fatigue! Menstruation! Hysteria!* – and remember I was valid, my pain was real, and I had a right to seek help for it. If Thabiso hadn't cured my pain, she had cured my self-hatred. She taught me that anyone would struggle with my burden, and that I deserved a cure. That if men hadn't been part of the problem, they certainly hadn't been the solution. She was, as Kate Chopin would have put it, my Awakening – unlocking my cage while, unlike poor Edna, I still had time to escape.

Back in the hall, every seat was taken. Normally, I'd have brandished my stick – *I am not lazy or mad, I'm legitimately ill* – but I'd left it at the pousada that morning because John of God had a habit of commanding people to step out of their wheelchairs or throw away their sticks, adding them to the pile in the display case off the main hall, even if afterwards they had to buy a new one. In the taxi Kevin had said to me, 'If he takes your cane and throws it away, let him,' and I had said, 'The thing is…' and he had cut me off and said, '*LET HIM*.'

I squatted on the floor. In front of me stood six Americans, all in a line, holding hands. The translator led a Lord's Prayer, *Pai Nosso, que estas nos ceus*, and one of the women – fifties, blonde, white clothes that looked demure yet carefully flattered her figure – started to convulse.

They called the intervention line first, and I wandered over to the bookshop to buy a crystal bed session – an elective part of the Casa programme, where you lay on a bed and had crystals lined up over your chakra points, recharging them with rainbow light at £12 an hour. There were 13 rooms, but I'd heard Kevin say the energy was best in Two.

'If you like it, you can buy one,' said the man in charge of the beds, conspiratorially. 'Only 11,000 reis.' My own crystal bed, just £2,500.

'If you pay in cash, that is,' he said. 'With credit card, it's 12,000. My boss, he is the son of John of God.' He gestured at Roger Federer. 'He can ask his father.'

'I'll think about it,' I said. 'I'm not buying a crystal bed until I know it works.'

'He can ask the permission anyway,' he urged – he was French with a Clouseau accent. 'You do not 'ave to buy it. But it's good to know you can.' I stalked back to the hall, gravitated to a Brazilian man in jeans and a striped shirt. Where the foreigners had rolled out their Mykonos linens, the locals wore whatever they had: bedazzled cream tops, beige trousers, once-white Havaianas. Perhaps he hadn't known, perhaps he couldn't afford new clothes, but this man looked mortified, eyes fixed on the ground, and I wanted to hug him, to tell him he was every bit as worthy and as curable as those of us who'd capitulated. Wearing white was, the booklet explained, a sign of respect towards the entities, but already I was shrivelling at the apartheid it seemed to breed.

They were calling the revision line.

I paced around, checked my email (the Casa had wifi,

239

a 21st-century apple of Eden) and tried to meditate, but I couldn't. I walked past the crystal bed rooms that urged silence via a huge smiley face with a finger to its lips, down to the sopa area, where, 14 hours before, Jim Carrey had lit a loathing in me towards John of God and all his followers. I went to the toilet – huge, industrial bathrooms to cope with all the pilgrims, the same mass of cubicles as I'd seen at the Vatican, Lourdes, and a Tuscan spa whose health-giving waters doubled as extra-strength laxatives. I closed my eyes in the cubicle and tried to connect with the entities. I hated everyone, I explained to them, but that didn't mean I didn't want it to work. When they called the first-time line, my stomach dropped out beyond my root chakra. It was show-time and there was no escape.

I hung back till the end, then started to panic. What if the last in line had spiritual significance? What if he spent more time with me? What if we had a Moment with a thousand people looking on? Jim had said that most people are waved past the Entity, some got to speak or receive a pearl of wisdom, and a lucky few got to touch him (we were only to touch him if he initiated it, just like the Queen). When people had quizzed him – just how much can we speak? Can we hold both his hands? – Jim had laughed and told us not to get excited, we would probably just be in and out. In and out. That was all I wanted. Give him a split second but don't get too close. Don't surrender too much hope.

As we walked at a snail's pace through the hall – the speed dictated by the rate at which people were passing in front of the Entity – I had the distinct feeling that I was en route to the scaffold.

St Ignatius guarded the sky-blue door to the Current Room, or Entities' Room, or Entity's Room, depending on what you wanted to call it. I begged him for a sign but nothing came.

Another woman sidled up behind me so at least I wasn't last. We handed over our first-time tokens as we entered. There was no turning back now.

We stood in what I would come to know as the Mediums' Room, a chapel-like space lined with benches. John of Godders on them, eyes closed, meditating. Some looked blissful, others in pain – they'd been there nearly three hours by now. Holy muzak piped through the air and a woman in white stood at the front, urging them on. The first-time line is nearly through, she was saying, keep the current strong, your brothers and sisters need you. I wondered what would happen if I threw up, or made a break for freedom.

There was Kevin: in the front row, his body shifting in discomfort but his face radiating bliss. This is why you're here, I told myself, because Kevin loves John of God and you worship Kevin. Kevin gave you your life back, you'd be dead if it wasn't for Kevin, stop thinking you're better than him and give his guru a chance. His eyes were closed, but I knew he felt me. As I came towards him, his grin broadened and he stretched his palms towards me, directing something that he could feel but which I couldn't believe in.

The second room was larger – the Entity's room, where only the more experienced pilgrims could sit. Beyond the pews were two lines of thrones – comfy chairs with backs and cushions, where the top mediums, the 'brothers and sisters of the Casa', sat. One woman had rolled back her head, eyes half open, in what looked like rigor mortis.

The line was moving slower – or was time slowing down? – and the panic was expanding inside my chest. Beyond the mediums were man-sized crystals. At the end of the room, in an armchair, sat João Teixeira de Faria and whichever entity was currently in possession of his body.

My breath quickened. Richard Morse was screaming now, *get the fuck out of there, get out get out get out*. I bent round the woman in front of me to try and study him, calculate the threat, and suddenly he twisted round in his chair and locked eyes with me.

I didn't care about the pain any more; I wanted out, to be at home with my mum and my Miffy. I could feel the woman behind me shifting from foot to foot with anticipation. Have my place, I wanted to scream. Take it and let me go.

The man two people ahead of me reached the Entity. The Entity glanced at me again as he knelt before him.

The woman in front of me flung herself at the Entity's feet and took his left hand in both of hers. She spoke to him with her head down, and he seemed to talk back.

She exited stage left, weeping, and I stood for a split second, as he stared at me and I stared back at him, and then something kicked in and I walked up, and as I was stepping towards him he was already writing a prescription – with a pencil, on a scrap of white paper, in a language that wasn't human. I stood there and looked down at him, and he looked up at me – I remember his eyes being huge, but I don't remember their colour, because his eye colour changed depending on which spirit was inside him – and I handed him my yellow piece of paper: *Pescoço & columa! Fadiga cronica! Mestruação!*

He glanced at it, placed it delicately in a basket of yellow slips at his side, and turned back to me, holding out his left hand. I took it and we stared at each other for what felt like minutes but was probably less than a second, fingers entwined like Dante's Paolo and Francesca, locked together in the second circle of hell. He looked gravely at me, not welcoming but not unfriendly either, it was almost sad, and as he opened his mouth I realised that I too was going to get the special treatment that Jim had told us not to hold out for, and he held me in a vice of eye contact and spoke to me, just a sentence, in a low, quiet, matter-of-fact voice, the calm voice of a doctor, and I stood there, mouth agape, rooted in horror, until one of the ushers beckoned me away and then took a step towards me to manhandle me off because I was still frozen, and John of God was peering round me to the next person, and I tiptoed over to the usher, and he whispered sharply, 'Corrente?' and I said, 'What?' and he said, 'Corrente? Current? Intervention?' and I said again,

'What?' and he hissed, 'What did he recommend for you, what did he say?'

And I started to cry and I whimpered to him, 'I don't know, I don't know what to do,' and I wasn't having a spiritual crisis, I really meant it, because I had spent four years leading up to this moment, flown 6,326 miles to Abadiania and put my life on the line and he had spoken to me – John of God, the world's most famous healer, had pronounced something that from the tone alone was pregnant with meaning and guidance and a possible cure, and from his face and his voice I knew it meant either the beginning or the end of something, and yet I had no idea what he'd said because I didn't speak Portuguese.

———

'What do you mean you don't know?' hissed the usher.

'He talked to me in Portuguese,' I wailed, if you can wail in a whisper. 'I don't speak Portuguese.' And then I said, wildly, 'I assumed he'd speak English.'

'Why didn't you ask for a translator?' he said, and I took a breath to explain that the idiot Jim hadn't told us, that I'd had no idea the translators were inside as well as out, that I'd come all this way, spent all this money and energy and emotion to find that the John of Godders had ruined it, ruined my entire life for me – but he must have seen the tremors and known the eruption that was coming because before I could say it he put his hand on my arm and said, 'It doesn't matter.'

He glanced at the Entity, as if he was wondering whether he could take me back, but we both knew that was impossible.

'I think you should sit in the Current,' he said.

'What if he prescribed an intervention?'

'He wouldn't have given you the herbs,' he said, ushering me to the door. As I walked, I thought, I'm sure he didn't prescribe me Current, this is all wrong, he told me something that would slot everything into place and cure me in an instant and I have lost it. I sat in a pew alongside everyone else, everyone who'd had their problems solved and answers translated, and began a new mantra – *You fucking idiot, you fucked up John of God, you'll never get better now, you fucking idiot* – when they said, 'Abram os olhos, open your eyes,' and cast us out into the sun.

'What did the Entity say?' Jesus was asking. I was on a bench beside another triangle and a childlike pencil drawing of a face: King Solomon. Under it sat a woman – ironed blonde hair cascading down her back, Kate Middleton's wedge heels under a pretty white dress, English rose through a self-possessed Swedish filter. There was a nervous-looking middle-aged couple, muttering to each other in French. Then there was Jesus.

'So,' he said. 'What did the Entity say?'

Chestnut waves down to his shoulders, tidy facial hair, Jesus sandals.

'I have no idea.' I felt heretical.

'Did you have someone translate for you?'

'Nope,' I snapped.

'No problem,' he said. 'That happens regularly. Not to worry.'

Not to worry? They regularly dashed pilgrims' hopes when they'd spent hundreds of pounds and thousands of prayers to get there? I was speechless with fury: Lilith, Medea and Erzulie Dantour combined.

'Whatever you're feeling,' said Jesus. 'Maybe it's disappointment, maybe you're sad, maybe' – he squinted – 'you're *angry*, that's our work. The Entity will do half, and we need to do our half.' Jim had said the same last night: this isn't a holiday or a magic wand, you have to prove you want it too. 'So maybe feel sad, disappointed, *angry*. Those emotions are telling us more about ourselves, so invite it in.'

I wanted to crucify him.

'I'm not sad,' I spat. 'I'm just worried I haven't done the right thing.'

'Okay, so observe that. Observe the worry. That's what

we want to see. Everything is fine, everything is perfect. This happens all the time. Did they give you herbs?'

I waved my prescription drearily and he told me how to take them: cash in the alien prescription at the Casa pharmacy, take one capsule three times a day before food, excise all spicy food, fertilised eggs and alcohol until they were done. They were passiflora, he said. Medically ineffective but spiritually infused and calibrated precisely for me.

'What this means is that this afternoon he wants you to sit in meditation, in the Current.'

How dare he, I thought, how dare Jesus try to tell me what to do? The Entity's tone hadn't sounded like an instruction; it had been a reflection or an observation. It had been spoken by him but had come straight from a spirit – and not just any spirit, for John of God channelled everyone from King Solomon to St Ignatius of Loyola, Francis Xavier and a soul which wished to remain nameless but was clearly – at least, everyone here hinted – the actual Jesus. You didn't go to the Delphic Oracle, not hear what she said and go, eh, never mind, that's probably what she meant.

He gave me instructions for the Current room: get in line at 1pm, close my eyes at 2, meditate until it was over. If I needed a toilet break, I should raise my hand and Kate Middleton would arrange my escape. I should sit in Current that afternoon and twice the next day – it would help me connect to myself. Then I should return to the Entity on Friday for my intervention.

'I don't want an intervention,' I snapped. Kevin had told me in the taxi that my fear of having my eyeball scraped was a sign that I *really* needed to have my eyeball scraped. I'd said, carefully, that it was more likely to be a fear of being blinded, and he'd said, *exactly*, love, you have so much fear in your life, you just need to surrender.

But there were two types of intervention, said Jesus: spiritual and physical. Most people opted for spiritual; the physical surgeries – eye-scraping, nose-ramming, real incisions – had started because some people refused to believe they'd been healed unless they saw blood. Just like Dr Ho's patients, who felt better if they paid for their tea.

'I just want to be sure I'm not doing it wrong,' I whimpered.

'There's never a wrong thing, you know,' said Jesus.

'No, I know that,' I began wearily, because I had read the books and knew that in Abadiania whatever happened was meant to happen. But what wasn't meant to happen had already happened.

'It's all a process—'

Kate Middleton saw the rage crackling through my aura.

'Even if we do the so-called "wrong thing", the Entity will correct it later.'

'Really?' Two syllables that oozed desperation.

'Yes,' she giggled. 'Don't worry about it.' She seemed nice. I reckoned she would let me skive the Current.

Current sessions could run for hours, I'd read – they started before the lines went in and wrapped up when the last person had gone through. You sat there, eyes shut (aiding concentration and protecting you from evil spirits), arms and legs uncrossed (crossing them broke the energy flow), meditating hard enough to buoy John of God and his septuagenarian body with energy.

Quite apart from the fact that I hadn't ever made it past a 15-minute meditation on my mindfulness app, my sitting tolerance was currently at around 20 minutes. Three, four, seven-hour sessions might well cripple me. I was terrified of the Current.

I don't want to disturb the other pilgrims, I said, gunning for a sicknote, but I have *various medical problems* – I kept them hazy and threatening – and can only sit for about 20 minutes at a time. Oh!, she said, no worries, just sit on the aisle and raise your hand every time you need to leave. Then come back when you're ready.

But I don't want to *disturb* the others, I pressed. Right, she said, so sit on an aisle.

'Ask the entities to help you sit,' she said. 'You know, there are amazing things they can do, and you might be surprised. Things happen here all the time to improve people—'

There would be no sicknote.

'So don't go in thinking, "I can only do 20 minutes"; see how you go. Also, in the first discomfort, maybe don't just run out, because it might be discomfort from them working on you. You might be sad, or worried, or *angry*, or have physical pains that you're already experiencing from your medical situation, but try to sit with it a little and do your best.'

'The idea is that you don't leave at the first sign of resistance,' Jesus interrupted. 'The idea is to sit with that discomfort and see what's going on, because the pain is trying to tell you something about yourself. Pain is a message saying, "Hellooo! Can you spend a little bit of time here?"' He waved at me. 'Be there with it.'

'Yes, but—'

'You don't want to go and run off right away.'

'Yes, but—'

'I realise it may not be comfortable and it may be painful, but that's what we do here.'

'Yes, but I have *medical issues*.' He looked at me, as nonplussed as a balian, a Dr Ho, or a Mr Bloggs.

'All I'm saying is, staying with it is part of the process. The idea is to face the pain.'

I fantasised about the pain I'd like to inflict on him. Punch him. Kick him. Give him misfiring nerves that wouldn't switch off. That'd wipe the pious grin off his face. Part of the process? Try staying with that, you fucking *man*.

'It may not be comfortable, but that's what we're learning here, to see what it's trying to tell us about ourselves.'

'Yup,' I said politely, seething inside. I went for post-Entity soup: thin strands of spaghetti swimming in water the colour of vomit. Whatever energy the entities were sprinkling on it, they'd left out the seasoning.

Current began at two but the John of Godders lined up at one like Ryanair eager beavers. I stood there with them

– inability to stand without fainting was part of my Condition, but from the moment I'd set foot inside the Current room that morning, my dizziness had faded to a shadow of what it usually was. Obviously it was the adrenaline – I'd been in full fight-or-flight response mode – but I must have been more worked up than I realised for it still to be pumping now. I'd been standing for 40 minutes, instead of my usual four, when they opened the doors. Kate Middleton was already waiting for me.

She led me to the back of the room, where, in the gloaming, a pew was jammed against the wall. The legroom was endless and I could lean my head back – a boon because everyone else was arriving with pillows and cushions to bear what was coming, and I, the neophyte for whom a 10-minute bus journey felt like a car crash, had arrived with nothing. It occurred to me that Kate Middleton wasn't just the first person to be thoughtful to me in Abadiania; she was one of the few in the past four years who hadn't dismissed my pain.

Fecham os olhos, close your eyes. Uncross your arms and legs. Stay upright – hunching over breaks the chain ('corrente' in Portuguese). You're here not just for John of God and the people in the lines, but also for yourselves. The entities are healing you as you hold the Current. *Pai Nosso, que estas nos ceus*. She turned on the music, and it began.

I'd show willing, I decided, and wait a bit before leaving. For her sake, I'd try what she'd suggested. It wouldn't make a difference, because I'd already tried meditation for pain – where you're supposed to dive into it, follow and observe it, and watch as it gradually unravels – and every time the pain had remained coiled tightly round my nerves. But I would try.

I remembered my mindfulness app for the first few minutes: focus on the breath, expand the belly not the chest, observe thoughts as they come in and let them go. Acknowledge that hatred of your heavy-breathing neighbour, and let it burn off. Recognise the heat from his thighs on yours and let it go. Feel the guy in front shifting around – the keffiyeh-wearing, ponytail-sporting, privilege-oozing gap yah kid in front – and—

I couldn't meditate. Instead, I thought.

I thought dark thoughts about my neighbours. I thought about how I could stop the rupture with Kevin that I knew was steamrollering towards us. I thought for a bit about why I was so allergic to the John of Godders – I'd deliberately turned away from the medical profession in the hope that an alternative person could help me, and yet I despised all alternative people. I wanted so desperately to believe – I wanted nothing more than for John of God to pat me on the head and declare me cured, exactly the same as I had wanted from Thabiso, from Mr Wong, from Patrick, from Charmayne, from the Walsingham priest, from every doctor and specialist and physiotherapist I had seen from the start. So why was I resisting? Why was I refusing to surrender, as Kevin had urged me to do? Why couldn't I trust them, even for a minute?

I told myself it was because before I believed, I needed a reason to believe. I looked down on the John of Godders because they saw orbs where there were camera flares, miracles where there were none. Jim had said he was at death's door when he'd come to Abadiania, that John of God had *literally saved his life*, but he'd also said that in America he'd been purposeless, miserably single; a heavy stoner who felt electrical charges in his brain and foamed at the mouth. He'd stopped eating and drinking, yet within a day of reaching Abadiania he was eating and drinking three full meals a day. *It was a miracle*, he said, but that wasn't a miracle. It was offensive to God and John of God to call that a miracle. It was offensive to Made Reni and Pietro. And it was offensive to me.

How I hated everyone who believed Jim and believed in John of God. The people who came for spiritual growth, happy and healthy in the white clothes they could afford to buy. The couples sitting thigh-to-thigh at the mirador, seeking permission from the Entity to copulate (sex was banned for 40 days after your first intervention) and naming the resultant child after the spirits. The attention seekers who stuck their heads in the triangle in front of us all, praying for an audience instead of an audience of one. The truly sick who'd come with terrifying faith: scarves wrapped around bald heads, spines propped up in wheelchairs. Their hope was like a mirror, and I hated them for it.

I put my hand up when the pain meant I could concentrate on nothing else. Kate Middleton ushered me out; the Entity observed my limp of shame. Outside, I lay on a bench, stretching my spine into the unyielding wood, groaning quietly as the muscles began to relax. After a while, I checked my phone. I'd been in there an hour and a quarter.

I'd told Kate Middleton I'd have a quick stretch and come back, but a voice in my head (definitely mine) said, pace yourself, else you won't manage 10 minutes tomorrow. That wasn't just an excuse – if your body feels pain at, say, a mile's run, the next time you go for a run it'll sound the alarm at three-quarters of a mile, before you might conceivably damage yourself. It does a fine line in self-preservation.

That night, after snoring my way through a crystal bed session, I bumped into Kevin.

'You didn't have a translator?' he said, appalled.

'I didn't know,' I said uselessly.

'But what did you think would happen?'

'I don't know,' I said. 'I guess I thought a man who's been dealing with English-speaking people for 40 years might speak English, or that a ghost who was Spanish or Italian might speak Spanish or Italian.' I had a point – why would all these foreign ghosts only speak Portuguese? Why wouldn't an omnipotent Entity be able to communicate in every language?

'But it was in Mytrae's book.'

I thought, I can't tell you I was too busy plotting my escape and wondering if your guru was Satan to remember what the book had said, so I said, 'You know my Condition has given me brain damage.' And then I added, viciously,

'Jim never told us anyway.' You hurt Kevin, I told myself as I stormed home, but a temporary drawing apart was better than a rupture.

I had never felt so full of bile as I did now, lying in my stifling room on the lumpy kingsize mattress, weighting the sheet with my tears. I despised them all, I even despised Kevin, but most of all I despised myself.

'Don't focus on having a magic wand,' Thabiso had said. I hated myself for the hope that had brought me here.

Kevin told me things get worse before they get better.

It was Friday, the morning before my intervention. Two days in Abadiania had transformed me, but not in the right way: my back felt like I'd gone under a horse, my thoughts swam through treacle and my arm was flaming steadily.

I'd planned to go to Current, I really had, but I'd been too ill to queue up, and by the time the queue had filed in, the room was full. So I'd walked to the bookshop to reserve a crystal bed and there they were.

'Did you read up on angel numbers yet?'

On Thursday, he'd asked me the time and I'd pulled out my phone. It was 11.11am, and he'd gasped: 'I just got chills.' 1111 is the most powerful of angel numbers, he'd said – it means seismic change is coming. Look it up.

'I've just been so tired.'

Mike slunk off.

I hadn't planned to say anything but he asked how I was doing and I told him the truth, right there in the bookshop, in front of the woman manning the till who smiled nicely every time I bought something but suggested I buy the Casa guide every time I asked a question.

'You get worse before you get better,' he said. 'You have to surrender.'

'I *have* surrendered,' I said, and then I corrected myself: 'I've tried to surrender. But it's hard when I'm in so much pain.'

'But, but, but,' he mimicked. 'You have to stop saying but.'

'Yes but I'm in pain,' I said, trying to stay calm. He led me out into the sun and the POTS – which, come to think of it, had improved since Wednesday – rolled over me. He told me that only those who want to be ill are ill. He'd said it before, and I'd always tried to shove it to one side like a maiden aunt's casual racism, not letting his unpalatable views mar my love for him.

'I need to sit.' I sank down under a statue of some Croatian Virgin.

'You need to surrender,' he said.

'I'm trying!' I said. 'I'm staying on an extra week, aren't I? I'm trying to take it seriously. But—'

'Stop fucking saying but!!!' he yelled. 'JULIA. FUCKING LISTEN TO ME.'

'Oh god,' I whimpered. 'I made you say fuck.'

'It's my *fucking* decision to say fuck, okay?' he shouted. I studied the ground as horrified pilgrims hurried by.

The sun was pounding on my head and I was close to passing out – from the dizziness, from the pain ravaging my back, from the guilt of making Kevin swear in his holy place, from the dehydration as the tears sluiced down my cheeks.

'I'm trying,' I sobbed. 'I'm trying so hard.'

'Julia,' he shouted. '*Listen to me.*'

He told me nobody was ill who didn't want to be ill. Pain, cancer, arthritis – all diseases we brought on ourselves. He told me that things get worse before they get better; that my symptoms weren't signs that something was wrong, but signals to look inside, to see what they were trying to say. That I didn't have to take past patterns into my future (when I'd said, at the São Raphael, that I'd injure my arm in a single bed, he'd looked meaningfully at me and said, 'Not necessarily'). That the pain would go away if only I wanted it to.

I yearned to roll back two years to when he had saved my life, when he had shown so much compassion.

Your pain is getting worse because you want it to, he said,

my every sob stoking his fury. It will stop the moment you let it go.

Certainly, my pain was multi-layered. There was the generic pain of my Condition: permanently sore muscles like I'd run a marathon, minor stabs as the joints clicked in and out of place with every step. There was the dull pain of fatigue that sometimes made washing my face or cleaning my teeth feel as insurmountable as Everest, the numbness that struck my hands, feet and gums every so often and no doctor could pinpoint the cause – I'd have to pump my feet up and down and make fists over and over, stretch my mouth into the Joker's grin before the sensation would tingle back.

There was the vice-like pressure around my jaw that locked my mouth shut daily, ground my teeth together at night and, on bad days, felt like hornets under my ears. There was the low-level headache that never strayed far but sometimes came closer, lancing a temple or lassoing a retina. There was the pain that felt bony – arthritic in my second toes, icy on the backs of my knees if I'd been standing too long, or hyperextended my knee joints (which I did naturally – to stand without knee pain was a conscious decision).

They were the daily pains, the low-level ones that I'd survived for decades. I could cope with those.

Then there were the acute pains from the injuries that my Condition made me prone to and my Pain Brain ramped up to exaggerated levels: tearing a rotator cuff as I vacuumed, scoring a knee tendon when I fell over because my everyday proprioception was that of a drunk, the alarm-level swelling if I walked into a bed, headbutted a door or slipped down the stairs as often happened. What would cause someone else to yelp, rub and move on would torture me for weeks, as my poisoned pain circuits would send my nociceptors into overdrive. The summer Miffy died, in America, I'd tripped over my feet and checked into the ER three days later because I could no longer manage stairs. I could get head, neck and arm pain from a train journey; braking for a traffic light or stop sign could feel like a knife attack.

And I could even cope with the acute pains, disorientating as they were.

But then there were the pains that had come more recently and would be the death of me: the sack of bricks on my lower back, the palette knife easing my vertebrae apart. The saw inside my neck. The fire crackling under my right shoulder blade and electric circuit in my arm.

Those were the pains I was here to cure. But it didn't mean I wanted to make the others worse in the process.

'Medically, I can't be sitting that long, that still, in the Current,' I said, using the line that had silenced Jesus and stirred Kate Middleton's empathy. 'My doctors say you have to build things up gradually, otherwise you go backwards.'

'Oh yeah?' he said. 'Your doctors say that? And how's that working out for you? *How much better have your doctors made you feel?*'

I put my hands to my head and sobbed like a toddler, but he had a point.

'Fuck the doctors,' he shouted. 'Fuck the doctors! What the fuck do they know?'

Well, I began silently in my head, because I still respected doctors, for all they had failed me.

'How long have they been treating you?'

'Nearly four years,' I whispered.

'And are you better?'

'No,' I howled.

'So don't you think it's time to try something else?'

His anger hurt him too, I could see, and he did have a point. The only thing the medical profession had managed in nearly four years was to tell me I would never find a cure, feed me drugs that made me suicidal and shit myself, and decimate my self-esteem. At least Kevin had returned me to work and life part-time. And if he'd done that through angels or entities, it was time to give them a chance.

The tension between us was that he needed me not to hope but to believe, and I needed proof to believe. You couldn't really believe in a four-leaf clover until you found one for

yourself, after all. You couldn't know for certain that antibiotics were going to cure your pneumonia until your snot
turned clear. You couldn't be sure a plaster cast had really
knitted your broken limb back together until it was sawn off.
I wouldn't be sure my grandmother was talking to me until,
under the guidance of Thabiso, I slaughtered a goat and was
able to talk back.

I didn't say any of this.

'You're right,' I said. 'You're right. I'll surrender.'

He hugged me good luck for the intervention. Pray for
me, I said, and he said: I have been. They say, 'Tell her to
surrender.' Surrender, I told myself, as I waited for my guide.
I disapproved of guides, of course, peddling the myth that
John of God could heal us in return for our money, but
desperate times called for desperate measures. I couldn't
afford to go wrong again.

Plus on Thursday afternoon, I had dragged myself to Abadiania's only supermarket and mistakenly pushed in front of
a young, mop-topped man at the till.

'I'm so sorry!' I'd gasped.

'That's okay!' he'd said in an American accent. 'I'm in no
hurry.' I'd flushed scarlet as the communal gaze fell on my
purchases: crisps for my fat belly, mega sanitary towels for
my troublesome mestruaçao, food for the stray cat which
had attached itself to me upon my arrival. He had offered
me his card.

'Matt Hills, life coach', it said. On the back, it read: *Expect
a miracle today!*

He would take me to the sacred waterfall, life-coach me,
and guide me through the intervention line for just £35.

There were three bridges, he explained at the waterfall, in
a whisper because talking was banned. One represented the
past, one the present and one the future. You crossed them,
letting go of your past, your present, then embracing your
future before cleansing yourself in the flow.

I followed two women – the sexes had to go separately
– down a path cut into the hillside. The waterfall was in a

wooded gully, chipping through the same ruddy earth that you could see from the mirador. It dropped from a flat ridge, pelting down in a perfect curve and eddying delicately across rocks before sweeping under the bridge of the future. It was, I had to admit, beautiful.

'Blessings,' smiled one of the women as she left the water-fall, and instead of smacking her in the face I smiled back and begged the entities for change. Forgive me, I whispered, I surrender. I looked at the rainbow shimmering in the foam, held on to the railing and stepped in. I cleansed three times: past, present, future. I stuck my arm in till the water wrapped itself around it, and then pushed my head through so it pounded on my back. I felt calm, maybe a little differ-ent. I was still terrified of the intervention, though.

'You'll be receiving a surgery,' said Matt, calmly. 'It's just that you're not in the hospital getting operated on by a doctor with physical tools. Many people have reported having cuts afterwards, having scars afterwards – it all depends on what you're asking for, and what they feel is the best way to treat it.' My throat closed in on itself. I hadn't realised that even with an invisible surgery – where you just sat in a room and meditated – the entities could slice and dice you inside.

Matt had originally been like me, he said – appalled by the idea of physical surgery – but the longer he'd stayed in Abadiania, the more his faith had grown. The interventions were miracles, every one of them, because nobody suffered long-term damage. Sure, some people talked of week-long nosebleeds, and Jim had cried blood for days after his eyeball was scraped – but that was nothing. The nose job should be fatal – the forceps were long enough to penetrate the brain – but the fact that it had yet to kill anyone was proof of what was going on.

'The general belief,' he said, 'is that the clamp morphs into divine energy once it hits your nasal cavity.'

'I believe the spiritual surgery demonstrates more faith,' I said piously. 'I'll stick with that.'

So I would go into the small Current room and meditate.

If I was here for a physical issue – *yes*, I squeaked – I would lay my right hand on the place that was the problem. If I was here for multiple issues, I could just put my right hand on my heart. The entities could heal nine problems at once. Make a list, he said, and keep thinking of it once you're in there.

The intervention could take anything from two minutes to 45, or longer. I might feel waves of bliss, hands on me, scalpels operating inside me, or pain. Then I'd return to the pousada and rest for 24 hours. That would be easy, I told myself, for someone who mostly lived, worked and travelled alone.

I looked at my hands, and they were trembling. Perhaps that was a good thing – Matt said people who doubted were often granted some kind of sign. He himself had been sceptical until a group of entities had shown him their faces as he lay on a crystal bed.

'If you have doubts, they will show you something that will make you believe,' he had said.

Surrender surrender surrender.

My knees buckled as they called us. 'See you in 45 minutes,' he chirped.

I had a panic attack in the intervention room – without Kate Middleton looking out for me, I was ordered into a middle seat. Other people were filing into the room and I remember the tears streaming down my cheeks as the panic built, the battle inside over whether to jump up and leave, come back another day or never come back, catch the next flight back to Rio, because there was always Thabiso, there was still that month with Thabiso. I remember glancing through semi-closed eyes at the people around me, seeing the white-clothed ushers shuffling round the pews, hissing at us to *fecham os olhos*, close our eyes, and Richard Morse or my instinct screaming to me to *get the fuck out of there* – I hadn't felt terror like this since that night in Port-au-Prince. I remember my arm burning as I brought it to my heart, wondering whether I would do irreparable damage holding it up like this, a pose which never failed to bring flare-ups.

I remember sitting still, trying to meditate as the Current music piped through the room. I remember going through the steps of my mindfulness app: feel your bodyweight on the pew and your feet on the ground, feel the heat of your hand on your chest, hear the music and your neighbours' breathing, focus on your breath, in and out, in and out. I remember feeling calmer once escape was no longer an option. I remember sitting there, waiting for the hands and the blades inside me, slicing my nerves, rewiring my brain, possibly rejigging my spine and neck vertebrae.

I remember a male voice – deep, sonorous, kind – saying a prayer in Portuguese. I remember the disorientation when they told us it was over, to get up and file outside, the realisation – my god – that Something Must Have Happened, because I only remembered about a minute of meditation. I remember the flash of delight that I was one of the sceptics who'd been shown proof, whisked up to nirvana while my earthly body was operated on down below, and blinking in the sunlight as I came out to find Matt standing next to Jesus. And I remember the plummet back to earth as he grinned, 'That was quick!' and I checked the time. The intervention had lasted less than three minutes.

Jesus went through our post-intervention instructions: bed, no activity, stay with it whatever happened. No waterfall trips for three days, no exercise or direct sunlight for eight. No sex, healing or energy work for 40 days. We must get a taxi back to our pousadas, unless we were in the one next to the Casa.

'What if we're in the one next to the one next to the Casa?' I asked. I wanted so desperately to follow the rules.

'Hmm,' said Jesus. 'How do you feel?'

'I feel fine,' I said. 'Normal. Maybe a tiny bit tired.'

'I *think* you would be okay to walk.' He looked me up and down. 'Having said that, you have physical issues, right? Could they have worked on anything that could affect your walking?'

I bloody well hope so, I wanted to say.

'Yes,' I said.

'It's up to you,' he said. 'I *think* you'd be fine but only you know what you asked for so if you don't want to risk undoing anything, get a taxi.'

I didn't know what I'd asked for either, I realised. I'd been so tight with panic that I'd forgotten my list. The only thing I remembered asking was to stay alive.

In the taxi – £2 to drive 10 metres – I thought about one of the last things Jesus had said to me. He must have seen me looking dazed – *nothing*, I'd snapped, when he'd asked if I'd felt anything – and after he'd given our little group instructions, he'd turned to me, the first moment of empathy between us.

'Really no writing?' I'd said. 'Not just a little email as I lie in bed?'

'No.'

'Not even reading a book if it's about John of God?'

'No.'

'Oh.' The reality was sinking in – living alone was not usually living with your thoughts.

He'd looked concerned. 'If you don't know whether to believe, act as if you do,' he'd said, solemnly. I'd let that sink in, pondered it a little. It seemed reasonable.

Act like you believe, I told myself as I threw myself on the bed. Surrender surrender surrender, I believe I believe I believe. I lay there for a few minutes in the baking room, and picked up my phone. Surely one email wouldn't hurt?

Act like you believe.

I put the phone down and stared at the ceiling. The adrenaline was ebbing away and I was suddenly very tired. When I woke up, three hours had passed.

SURRENDER

With the hook of life still in us still we must wriggle.
Virginia Woolf (1882-1941: mental health patient, writer)

You're jealous of them, I told myself. *You resent their unwavering belief, their trust, their faith, because you envy it. You're jealous because you're scared to surrender.*

Maybe on one level, I thought back – in that 24-hour silence, my head had never been noisier – but on a more important one, I'm not. My scepticism is very precious to me.

And how's that scepticism working out for you? How many years is it that you've been a cripple? Four, right?

Three, not four. Three years and 11 months.

Three years and 11 months on the sidelines as my colleagues had moved up the ranks, my friends had bought houses. Countless promotions, several marriages and a few babies for them; two and a half stone, 10,000 grey hairs and a creping neck for me. Three years and 11 months of plans squashed and friendships lost, work undone and parties unattended. Three years and 11 months of debt, squeezing ever closer like a car compactor. Three years and 11 months of identity obliteration.

Surrender surrender surrender.

Act as if you believe, Jesus had said, so after that first nap, I'd picked up my phone and switched it off.

I'd lain there quietly, listening to pilgrims tramping past my windows, and counted everything that could be a sign – scrappy little twigs individually but which, if you rubbed them together, might produce a spark.

I'd been lying on my favourite crystal bed that morning when I'd felt a pressure on my forehead. I'd swiped at it but there'd been nothing there. We were given eye masks on the crystal beds, so it was probably referred pressure from that. But maybe it wasn't.

That particular bed, I'd noticed that morning, had a portrait of Dr Augusto de Almeida on the door. He was one of the main entities here, and as soon as I'd read about him I'd felt drawn to his name and his face – a bearded young man with a hint of Edward Norton. I'd instantly decided he was my favourite, and soon afterwards I'd read that because of his previous life – he'd been a surgeon in a time before anaesthesia – at the Casa, he often treated pain.

On the Thursday night, after most of the John of Godders had left, I'd walked into the main hall, crept up to the dais and put each hand on the bottom corners of the wooden triangle. Please, I'd whispered, give me a sign, and I'd shoved my head through the triangle onto the grease-stained wall, and for a second it had felt like gravity was pulling me in, trapping me in an eddy. It was all in my head, of course, but maybe it wasn't.

I had sat for over an hour in the Current, and although it had left me feeling shit, I could have felt a lot worse.

I'd felt peaceful at the waterfall, and maybe it was just because it was quiet and green, but maybe it had been the special energy.

Kevin would have labelled all this evidence. 'I'm getting chills,' he'd have said, running a hand up his biceps to feel the goosebumps. But however hard I tried, it wasn't enough.

Surrender surrender surrender.

I'd broken off for dinner, and when I'd returned to bed I had asked myself why I loathed everyone here so much, because it was unusual for me to be so full of hate.

You're jealous of them.

Hate was the word of a four year old. I didn't hate them; I just despised them.

'But you don't despise everyone,' I said.

Correct. I despaired of Kevin's credulity, but I still loved him. I didn't despise the man with the ponytail who had smiled at me during Jim's talk. He'd introduced himself at the end – Mike from Minnesota, here for spiritual growth. He wasn't smug like the others and he wore hospital scrubs, not holiday clothes, because they were the cheapest white things he'd found on Amazon. I didn't despise the woman at my pousada, either: the smiley Brazilian with a gammy leg who came here regularly for spiritual sustenance, not physical change, like the sick who returned to Lourdes year after year. These were the people whose faith I coveted – the ones who looked no different to you or me, yet gleaned something more important than physical transformation from their pilgrimage. The people who still believed when their god let them down again and again.

Surrender surrender surrender.

I tried to tell myself that I'd felt something in the intervention – a heat, a tingling, a spectral hand deep inside me, moving joints and rearranging nerves. But I knew I hadn't.

'Nobody is ill without wanting to be ill on some level.'

'It's okay to be depressed.'

'I'm afraid you're better served by another doctor.'

I thought about my pain and my relationship to it. I went over that May morning in 2012, combed through it to find some evidence of intention in the reach for the tepid coffee – an embrace, on whatever karmic level, of the fire – but there was nothing. Yes, I'd hated that job and myself for doing it – and as a Harvard psychologist would later tell me, job dissatisfaction is one of the main predictors of whether an injury will turn into chronic pain. But I'd loved my career and had wept for it daily. Being stripped of my identity had made me want to die. And the constant assumption that there was some psychosomatic process going on – that I secretly enjoyed moving back in with my mother, that I somehow preferred £344 a month statutory sick pay to a £40k salary – had, in a way, been more upsetting than the pain.

'Do you want to get better? Really, really better?' they had asked, and I'd wanted to throttle them, every single one – of course I wanted to get better, of course I wanted my life and my independence back, of course I didn't want to be in pain all day every day, the multiple levels of pain – chronic, acute, misfiring nerves – all interlacing to create a mid-level circle of hell.

Yet at the same time, there *were* benefits to the pain. Being given a seat on the bus, albeit often reluctantly. Boarding trains and planes early with staff to handle my luggage. A wheelchair at airports to whisk me through interminable security and immigration lines. Those were all side effects of the pain that I liked. But then again, if I wasn't in pain, I wouldn't be affected by their lack.

There's something else.

No there isn't.

Yes there is.

It was the thing I'd been trying not to say for nearly four years, and because I'd said everything else by now, I made myself say it.

It made me feel special, the pain. I hated it, of course I did, but I also clung to it.

In journalism we're taught to have a niche, and in a grotesque way, the pain gave me a niche in life. In a way, it made me a victim, assuaging my guilt for being white and middle class: I may have gone to Oxford and fannied around in Italy as part of my degree, but I, too, was a minority. I had a burden. I was disabled.

On a literal level, of course, I *was* disabled. And sometimes that label was necessary – being stamped as disabled by the rehab woman in order to qualify for insurance payments was obviously a good thing. If I got another office job, I'd happily alert HR to the need for them to make reasonable adjustments. Legally, all 'disabled' means is having a physical or mental impairment that has a substantial and long-term negative effect on one's ability to do everyday activities. If you look beyond the visible, there are many more disabled people than you realise.

But when I was describing myself as disabled, it was rarely

to an apparatchik who might buy me a special keyboard or a laptop stand. I was cladding myself in another identity.

'Because I'm disabled,' I liked spitting at people asking why I was asking for a seat when there were no seats, to skip the queue where there was a long line. I liked shaming those who thought there nothing wrong with me. I hurled my diagnoses at them – chronic pain, heart condition, malfunctioning nervous system, brain damage – and luxuriated in their embarrassment when they realised they'd made a faux pas, possibly breached the Equality Act 2010, made someone cry. Why did I cling to the thing that had ruined my life? Maybe it was some kind of primal female guilt, I thought. Maybe we grab at all these labels because we're excusing ourselves for not being the have-it-all women our generation had expected to be.

As I sobbed into the thin sheet, John of Godders chatting happily outside now their spiritual duties were concluded for the week, I thought back to something Kate Middleton had said during the Current. Every so often, when the 'energy level was dropping' (more like when people were nodding off), she would speak some kind of exhortation or encouragement – *the last line is coming through now, you're doing great, keep this wonderful energy going*. She'd follow it with a line she'd adapted from Rumi, the 13th-century Persian scholar. '*KEEP GOING*,' she would call out. 'The wound is where the light comes in.'

Keep going, I told myself in the Abadiania heat as the fan coughed air at me. The wound is where the light comes in.

I realised that every time someone accepted my self-definition as disabled, every time I wrung an apology from a company or a human being for assuming I was able-bodied where I was not, I felt the validation that the doctors and those closest to me had failed to give. I *was* ill, I *was* suffering. I stuck knives into strangers and corporations because I couldn't stick knives into the people who didn't give me the validation I needed, the doctors who told me I was depressed, the friends and family who acted as if my life wasn't over, as if I didn't want to die, as if we all have pain and I was making a big deal about mine. The friend who, when I cancelled drinks because my pain levels were too high, said 'I know how you feel, I'm really tired today.' The cousin who, at a family gathering, practically short-circuited at the idea that I could permanently be in pain – 'But not right now you're not, you can't be, you're talking to me' – before slinking off to take out his confusion on a sausage roll.

Keep going. The wound is where the light comes in.

I hated the pain, but in a way, it was an outlet for everything I hated about myself. I could blame my character flaws – explosive temper, terrible memory, selfishness, laziness – on the pain, and although it was true that the pain had exaggerated them all, they'd still been there in the first place. It excused my shortcomings: I wasn't editing a magazine because of the pain, not because I wasn't capable. I was single because I was in too much pain, not because I was too fat and mad for anyone to go out with. I'd lost friends because of the Pain Brain, not because I had pushed them away. As long as I was ill, I'd be unhappy and defeated, but I wouldn't have failed. You can't explain away failure.

Looking back on it now, I know I didn't want to be ill. I didn't enjoy it, ever – I was just appreciating the thinnest of silver linings in the tonne-weight storm cloud. I know now that I wasn't inventing the pain, subconsciously wishing it on myself or revelling in the misfiring circuits that made me wish I was dead. That evening, though, after the intervention, I was so desperate for relief – so desperate to see whether the Kevins and the doctors had a point – that I played along with it.

Okay, I said, I surrender – I admit it. I want to be ill, just like Kevin said. You win, now please make me better. It was a little after 8pm and for the fourth night running I cried myself to sleep.

––––––

I woke at 6am, as groggy and disorientated as if I'd crossed 12 time zones. Had that really happened?

Before sleeping, I'd asked Dr Augusto and his crew: heal

me, please, but please don't scare me. Others had talked of entities visiting in the night, of orbs hovering over the bed and heavenly faces at the window; of hands working on them and the healing happening in real time. I don't want any of that, thanks, I told the entities. I prefer my healing invisible and intangible.

And then I'd surfaced in the darkness with a sound on the headboard: three slow knocks, the Black Rod of Abadiania demanding my attention, before I'd drifted back down. Of course, it was probably a dream.

Then, as dawn was breaking, I'd been jolted awake by an almighty kick to my lower back. I'd lain there in the aftermath, on my side in the foetal position – the perfect pose for an entity to have delivered a blow. Was it restless back syndrome, a magnesium deficiency twitch or a myoclonic jerk? Had I dreamed it all? As I lay there wondering, I'd gone under again.

Did that really happen, I asked at 6am. I didn't know. But I felt a tiny flare of hope, like the wet match that flickers if you strike it enough times, until eventually it bursts into flame.

Then I realised there were nine more hours to go.

Keep going. The wound is where the light comes in.

I'd gone as deep as I could into the pain, I reckoned, so I decided to churn through the rest of my life, looking for clues. Sitting in the Current doesn't help only you, Kate Middleton had told us repeatedly; it helps two generations back and two generations forward. So I examined my relationships – family, friends, colleagues, exes and obsessions. I thought of the dead. I went through the people who'd supported me through the pain and those who'd abandoned me. I thought of childhood bullies and work enemies and John of Godders. I thought of the doctors who'd condemned me to a living death and the healers who'd stripped me of my self-worth, all those men who'd chipped away at my identity. I tried to forgive, to send love to them all, and then I tried to send it to myself. And that was the hardest part. Because beyond the hatred of the faithful and the anger at my caretakers, I'd saved the real poison for myself.

It's so obvious now, looking back. Reading the notes I incessantly made in Abadiania to make sure no one dared speak to me, I see it in every stroke of the pen, as clear as Jack Nicholson's typewritten pages in *The Shining*. Underneath the antipathy towards one person, the contempt for another, lay an unremitting self-loathing instilled by three decades of gaslighting.

No, the doctor had said in one of my earliest memories, as I squatted on the floor, legs bunched up like a crab: there's nothing wrong.

No, they'd said at the musicians' clinic, bending my teenage thumb to forearm and folding my hands in prayer between my shoulder blades: there's nothing wrong.

No, the GP had said, inspecting the knees that were giving out after 10 minutes on my feet: there's nothing wrong.

No, the neurologist, the rheumatologist, the anaesthetist had said: there's nothing really wrong.

Try to get on with it. Try some antidepressants. For your glandular fever, for your ME, for your RSI, for your misfiring nervous system, for your chronic pain. It's okay to be depressed. There's no stigma. Try these.

Hysterical yet depressed, overweight yet endangered by exercise, feeling pain that wasn't there yet crippled by a genetic condition for which there was no cure. Do pilates but not yoga, walk on the beach but not in the street, take these pills to cure the symptoms even if they provoke entirely new symptoms. Ignore your pain or zero in on it, build up your typing or stop typing lest you hurt yourself, don't work but try a little bit of work, you're not fit to work but we're stopping your sick pay. You have POTS but now you don't, you've got EDS but you're not hypermobile, your arm is just nerves misfiring but also you've a trapped nerve and two ribs spliced apart by muscle tension, here's a thyroid tumour but your thyroid's fine, you're passing out after meals so go on a diet. Why are you so anxious when we've been recalling you for tests for 18 months? Just stop worrying, you're absolutely fine.

Was it any wonder that I hated the Julia they'd created?

I lay there, going through it all, for nine more hours, then extricated myself from sheets stiff with dried sweat and tears at half past three. I felt alright as I showered – better, but not transformed, as good as I'd expect to feel after a 24-hour rest and a cathartic weep. My arm still burned but I thought of Black Rod and the foot in my back, and cupped my hands over the glowing ember.

I ventured back to the Casa that evening, and the next day. I did crystal beds and sat by the mirador. I scrawled in my notebook with less violence. I sat and stared at the triangles in the main hall and the King Solomon area. I meditated. I stuck my head inside them and prayed. I printed out photos of family and friends and put them in too. I still refused to talk to any of the other pilgrims, but I didn't actively dislike them. I got annoyed when a woman followed me into the main hall one evening, just as I was trying to talk to the entities, but I didn't leave.

Beaten was the word: I hadn't converted, but I was no longer capitulating to things against my will. I wasn't sure what I believed any more, thanks to the events of those 24 discombobulating hours. My pain was still blaring away and my POTS symptoms – which had dissipated in that first encounter with John of God – had resurfaced after the intervention. Physically, I felt a little iller than I had on Friday morning when I'd gone to the waterfall.

But I had finally surrendered. I was neutral: show me what you can do, I said now, rather than prove you can do it. The words were similar but the intent was different. When I felt the pressure on my forehead again on the crystal bed, I still put my hand to my face to check nothing had fallen on me, but I did so minus the assumption that it had.

I was glad Kevin had gone; without him, I no longer felt the pressure to do well for him. I could make up my own mind which crystal bed I preferred, which triangle I found more powerful. Instead of telling myself I had to like the woman in the shop for Kevin's sake, I told myself that she might be a cow but she wasn't an entity. I spent £7 on one of the silly blue cushions that everyone bought to make sitting in the Current slightly more tolerable, because I was determined, in week two, to sit through an entire session. I was still panicking about everything that had gone wrong, but now it was a constructive panic, not an aimless, angry floundering.

On the Tuesday night, I returned to the introductory talk. The man with the ponytail was there again and nodded at me. Jim had been replaced by a man called Diego. And despite myself, I liked Diego.

He talked us through Spiritism and channelling, told us that it was important, if we were attempting communication with the dead, to do so in a place like this, a spiritual hospital, where the clothing was white, the intentions pure, and the abilities of John of God were off the scale.

He told us that going in front of the Entity was a moment with a spirit that could transform our lives. He said that if we didn't hear what the Entity said, we must not leave but must ask him to repeat it (this is where I groaned). He told us not to ask what the cause of our illness was, but ask, rather, for it to be taken away. There was no talk of blame, karma or secretly wanting to be ill. I hung back at the end to ask his advice.

I had blown my meeting with the Entity and had a run-in with Jesus, I told Diego. My pain had stopped me from attending a full Current session, and after the intervention, during my 24-hour rest, I'd secretly sent one email and read three paragraphs of a book. Now everything hurt and I had cocked up the entire trip. What should I do, I asked, voice wavering.

He told me to go back to the Current.

'And if you're sitting there and things start to hurt, ask for help,' he said. 'If it doesn't help, leave. But don't do that until you've asked for help at least once and then let it go.'

Nobody had said let it go before. They'd said focus on it, observe it, stay with it till it goes. After all that, I could just let it go?

'If you keep holding on to it, they won't be able to work on you,' he said. 'Literally, when you say let it go, just give it to them. If you do that and just hang for a minute or two, it should... something should... happen.'

'But when will it happen?' I said, voice breaking.

It was the same question I'd asked myself with each healer on every continent I'd visited. Whose faith could withstand the *it* not happening instantly? Who would keep praying, meditating, connecting with the ancestors or buying things for the loa, keep rubbing bile-perfumed muti over themselves and getting their meridians skewered till they screamed in pain? It was easy to start, it always was, but how did one know when to stop?

'Sometimes it happens in a moment and sometimes it doesn't,' said Diego.

You're impatient and selfish, a John of Godder had told me, sternly, over the weekend, when she'd collared me outside the lanchonete and I'd confessed my doubts in a tight whisper. Matt had promised me that people who don't believe are shown a sign, I'd said. *How fucking long do I have to wait for my sign?*

She had looked at me in horror and asked how I dared challenge God, what made me think I deserved a cure before everyone else. And I had said: I don't. I think, if there's a god and the entities really are omnipotent, we all deserve cures. She had said that was proof I wasn't ready, that my faith wasn't strong enough, that I wouldn't be healed until I believed, I had to wait until I was worthy, and I had said to her in a strangled cry, but I've been all over the world looking for a cure, *how am I supposed to know who to trust?*

My life was finite, as were my funds. If I gave everyone and everything the time they thought they deserved, I'd be 50, suicidal and still adrift in the aspic of pain. If any healer or therapist or doctor or physio could show results in a week or two, I would happily devote the rest of my life to them. But they had to be quick.

It only takes an instant, said Diego, but it happens when it's time for it to happen. If he'd said that a week earlier, I'd have jumped on the next plane home, but it was post-intervention and I had surrendered.

'But what if I lose faith in between?' I asked. And he told me to be kind to myself, to forget what had already happened, and to start again.

'Just keep putting one foot in front of the other,' he said, and I thought, fine, I'll do that till Friday, but then I'm done.

'Do what you need to do to take care of yourself, and everything else will take care of itself,' he said. 'That voice inside you that tells you what to do is the one driving the whole process. What I said before' – he had urged us to spend time alone instead of socialising – 'I meant it. Cultivate yourself – listen, sit, find out who you are inside and what that "you" wants you to do. Because you know what? It knows. See, God is in you too. And God shows up as you.'

And I wasn't sure about the god part but I did, by now, realise that, deep down, I was more in touch with my pain than any doctor or healer or John of Godder. I realised that every fobbing off had chipped away a part of my identity and muffled that voice inside me, the one that told me something was wrong but I ignored because I knew I was just fat and lazy. 'Trust the body of yourself,' Mr Wong had said and, there with Diego, I realised I still hadn't done that. I wondered whether that meant the only person to have a fighting chance at dispatching the pain was me. Because if it was going to be me, we were going to need a bigger boat.

I had four days left in Abadiania. I'd felt a little better and then a lot worse, but something had changed in me. I was less angry, more desperate; and I still felt despair, but it didn't feel like the despair would kill me any more, it was no longer the final showdown. See what happens here, I thought, but there's always Thabiso, that month with Thabiso. And there was always, I thought in a flash, acceptance, but I smothered that down the second it appeared.

I took it seriously that second week: up at 5am, on the crystal beds just after 7, mornings in silence on the Casa grounds. In the afternoons I went to Current. I drank the blessed water and didn't rail about the price. Taking my herbs before every meal became as routine as washing my hands; life without booze in the land of caipirinhas seemed natural. I tried to pray a little, but mostly I talked: to the entities, to God, to myself and my ancestors – because I believed Richard Morse, now, that it could all be connected. I thought about the pain and how I could separate myself from it. I was still holding out for John of God to whip out a wand and magic me better, but I also accepted that maybe I would have to play my part, too. The entities only do half of the work, they said. The rest is up to you.

I hoped.

On the Thursday afternoon, I made it through the whole Current, only going out once. At dinner, swallowing ibuprofen along with my herbs, I stared at another guest, a fortysomething blind man. I'd noticed his pristine white clothes at the Casa: smart, short-sleeved shirt, slacks carefully ironed and probably new. He towered over his white-haired father who led him everywhere by the hand.

I'd noticed him because he hadn't stopped smiling.

He'd smiled in the queue for the queues for the Entity. He'd smiled as he waited in the interminable first-time line. He'd smiled in the afternoon, waiting for the Current to open. Afterwards, he'd sat outside the São Francisco's entrance on a little fold-up beach chair, dressed in a basketball vest and shorts, still smiling. At dinner, he'd seemed the life and soul of his table.

The following morning he was back at the Casa, in white again. He'd smiled as his father manoeuvred him into place, his stick catching on a stranger's foot.

I stared at him now, chatting to the others in his group. Part of me wanted to go over and scream at him – this is your only chance! Go listen to yourself and meditate! If you've had an intervention, lie down!

But I was enthralled by the lightness with which he was treating Abadiania. I was acting as if this was a life-or-death situation, I, who'd flown halfway across the world to get here, I who could see, I who could pass as normal, I who was working part-time. Here I was, acting like I was going to have to kill myself if John of God didn't do a Jesus on me, and yet here he was – a man whose father had to lead him to the bathroom, a man with presumably no job, no wife, no 'independence' as society would term it – and yet he seemed as if he would be happy whether or not he left Abadiania with his eyesight restored.

I want what he's having, I said to the entities, staring at him across the dismal buffet. And then I said: forget me. I mean, I'd like you to heal me, but I want you to help him first. I mean, if you're omnipotent, of course, you should be able to handle us both but... it's okay.

I'll be okay, I found myself saying. Help him first. If you do that, I will believe.

There were others I had seen: a French man in a wheelchair being pushed to Frutti's every night by his aged parents, a blind little girl in a pretty white dress, sitting by the mirador on her mother's lap. I'd made similar entreaties to the entities to help them too. But this was the first time I'd said, I don't matter, heal that other person. At least, it was the first time since I'd begged Patrick to save Miffy.

The only pattern for those who receive miracles is that they were all people who came here to pray for others, Alessandro de Franciscis had told me at Lourdes. But that wasn't why I said it.

On the Friday morning, I collared Diego. A woman who'd aggressively befriended me over the weekend – she who'd diagnosed me as selfish – had said that John of God was absolutely for real. He's the greatest healer the world has ever known, she'd said, and he could cure you at the drop of a hat. He just doesn't want to, because then you'd go home and forget all about him. This way, with your fate in your hands, you're obliged to keep the faith, keep refining yourself spiritually.

But I need something now, I had groaned. Something to give me faith in the first place.

So tell him you're a journalist, she'd said, simply. Because although he channels God, he is but a man, and he's concerned about his reputation. Tell him you're a journalist, and he will heal you – she clicked her fingers – *just like that*.

It wasn't cheating, I told myself, because I was writing this book. In a way, it was ethically imperative.

You need his permission to write about him, Diego said, and I thought, excellent, this is how I bribe him.

The unhelpful translator wrote me a note asking permission from the Entity to write about my experiences at the Casa. As I stood in the revision line, shuffling slowly through the Current, I started to have doubts. You should be focusing on your healing, I told myself – this is your first chance to speak to him since the cock-up, your chance to put things straight, sod the writing, you can always email for permission afterwards. But we were already in the main room – his throne was in sight – and there was no time to get another piece of paper.

I raised my hand when I was 10 pilgrims away from the Entity and the translator sauntered up – the process seemed so simple now it wasn't life-threatening. I hissed that I wanted to know the next steps for my health, too, but he ignored me. We reached the Entity, and the Entity held his hand out to me again as the translator crouched down and murmured in his ear, but I held back because I was scared he would shout at me or curse me or call security to escort the interloper out.

I couldn't hear the translator, but I could hear John of God, and I could understand enough Portuguese by now to know what he said.

'But what kind of book?' he asked, looking as irritated as he looked bored, his hand dangling in the air as I refused to take it. And as the translator murmured something, presumably along the lines of, I don't have a clue, João, I've exchanged as few words with her as is humanly possible, he pulled back his hand and looked at me listlessly.

'If it's the truth,' I made out, and the translator got back up and ushered me away.

'He says you can write what you like as long as it's the truth,' he said. I'd thought he might sense another Oprah moment, might point at me there in the Current room, unleashing all the energies of heaven. But he hadn't. I had gambled, and I had lost.

He'd stuck out his hand and was about to tell you the thing that would have changed your life, I told myself at lunch. And you rejected his hand and asked if you could write about him instead. You silly little girl. You stupid bitch.

I was still tearing myself apart as I went into my final Current session.

You are going to sit through this, I told myself, adjusting my buttocks on the thin blue cushion, taking off my shoes so my feet could feel the cross-tiled floor (rumour had it that the Casa was built over a bed of energy-giving crystals). You will sit through all of it. You will not leave this place without seeing at least one thing through to the end, without not cocking up just one afternoon.

Mike from Minnesota sat down in the pew in front of me. That is a sign, I said to myself, a sign that you will sit with Mike until the end of the Current. Fuck your pain and fuck you for capitulating to it. Now sit the fuck down.

Kate Middleton was nowhere to be seen – a Brazilian woman was leading the session. Keep going, I told myself. The wound is where the light comes in.

Fecham os olhos, close your eyes. *Pai Nosso, que estas nos ceus, santificado seja o Vosso nome*. The muzak started. After maybe 15 minutes, maybe more – eyes closed, it's hard to tell – the pain arrived.

Please, entities, I said silently, could you take it away? I'm letting it go.

I'd practised Diego's trick in the last two Currents and both times I'd been amazed to find that it actually seemed to work. For a while, at least; then it would return, about 10 minutes later. But I'd have another wheedle, and it would disappear again – until the next time. Appear, entreat, disappear, appear, entreat, disappear. It was as predictable as a child in a car saying are-we-there-yet every other mile.

Please, could you take it away? I'm letting it go right now.

It went. It came back.

Please, take it away, I'm letting it go.

It went.

We were on a seesaw, me and the pain, throughout the final Current, and I was determined that when the session finished we would land on my side. I shifted my weight about, moved the cushion from my back to my bum to my neck to under my feet. I sat on my hands to stretch my spine, folded over a few times, even though leaning over would break the current. When I got claustrophobic I slit open my eyes to count the white legs filing past (*close your eyes*, one of the monitors shrieked, when I dared to open them a bit more obviously). I felt a stab of loathing for the voluntary interventions – the people asking to have their eyes scraped, nasal cavities penetrated, flesh cut – how selfish they were, making us all wait for them as we sat in distress and they took centre stage in the narrative they would soon be telling at home. I worked through my hatred until the pain popped up again and I swallowed it down like a Hungry Hippo.

The pain was coming back every couple of minutes now – I was letting it go and it was circling straight back, faster and stronger, like the rhythms of labour – but I reckoned we were on the last line by now and I refused to leave. It wasn't the last line, of course, but then finally it was, there were no more white feet shuffling past and we were being told that this was our time, when the Current and the entities were working only for us. It meant 10 more minutes of silence, then communal prayers, a stretch and a stand, a calculation of how much damage I'd done to myself, and a hobble towards the mouthful of blessed water that was doled out to all pilgrims who made it through to the end.

Come on, I told myself, keep going, the wound is where the light comes in.

I was in agony.

Take it away, I'm letting go, thank you, please please help me.

The wound is where the light comes in, take it away, please, give me something, just one sign before I leave.

Footsteps came towards me and I jumped as a hand patted my arm, and opened my eyes. One of the volunteers, as easy on the eye as Dr Augusto himself, was thrusting a pot of white chrysanthemums into my lap.

'For you,' he whispered.

I looked around at my neighbours, locked in prayer.

'What?' I hissed.

'For you. From the entities,' he said, and turned to go.

'WHAT?' I wheezed.

He smiled. 'The Entity tell me for you,' he whispered. 'Close your eyes.' As he walked off, I started to tremble.

The tears were streaming down my burning cheeks as the Pai Nosso sounded. What does it mean? Is it a sign? Was the woman right? Has he done it? I opened one eye to find another monitor tossing a single flower at everyone in my quadrant. Shit – and I blushed even deeper – I was supposed to hand them out, not claw them to my breast like a harpy knocking over everyone else to grab the bridal bouquet.

'Abram os olhos,' came the command. 'Open your eyes.'

I hissed to Mike from Minnesota: 'A man gave me these. I don't know what I'm supposed to do with them.' But Mike was so blissful he hadn't even noticed his own buttonhole.

We stood up and stretched. 'I don't know,' I said, to no one in particular.

'Your colleague gave me these flowers,' I said awkwardly to the woman doling out the blessed water. 'Am I supposed to hand them out to the others?'

'What did he tell you?' she asked, and I was too embarrassed to say he told me they were from the Entity – I couldn't bear the hubris if she said, 'Yes, from the Entity to give to the others, you stupid smug bitch.'

Two other pilgrims eyed my flowerpot as they sipped their blessed water.

'There he is!' I said. Mike followed me over.

'What are these?' I demanded from the Dr Augusto lookalike. 'What do I do with them?'

He looked confused. 'For you.'

'But for me to keep?' He winced with embarrassment. 'Or for me to give to other people here?'

'Sorry,' he said. 'My English very bad.' He turned away.

'No!' I grabbed his arm. It didn't end like this. '*What do I do?* Porque flores? Para mi?'

'Sorry,' he began. And then a monitor who'd annoyed me from day one because she was ravishingly beautiful – slim, jet black hair to her bum, eyes you could catch fish in, a voice that made Portuguese sound like a song – walked by. I knew she spoke English because, going into my first Current, she'd made me remove the sunglasses that were sitting on my head because they were blocking my crown chakra.

'The entities want you to have the flowers,' she translated. 'They told him to give them to you.' The man beamed.

'The entities or the Entity?' I asked, but either their English or their willingness didn't extend to semantics.

'He say, "Congratulations",' said the man suddenly in English, and I felt the blood pounding in my ears.

'Why congratulations?' I said.

'I don't know,' he said. 'He just say, congratulations.'

'What am I supposed to do with the flowers?' I said, grasping for signs.

'If you don't want,' he laughed, moving to take them.

'I want! I want!' I shrieked.

'Congratulations,' said the siren woman. 'Now we are closing the room.'

We stopped outside in the main hall for me to get my stuff together: bag, blessed water, cushion, flowerpot.

'I don't get it,' I said to Mike, waiting for him to say, 'You're the chosen one, Julia, your miracle will be along soon.'

'Do you think he did this because he knows I'm a journalist?' I said, screaming inside, *no, he did it because THIS IS IT and he's going to fucking cure you.*

'I don't know,' said Mike. He was a serious John of Godder and was still in a post-Current reverie, blankly beatific.

We stood there for a bit, looking at the triangle, and it hit me.

'Oh my god,' I said, to the portrait of St Ignatius. 'Oh fuck. Fuck me. *Fuck*.'

Mike pretended not to hear.

'I'm standing,' I murmured, mainly to myself. 'I'm standing here. I walked out.'

I checked my watch. We'd spent over five hours in the Current, a mammoth session by normal Casa standards, and I'd sat there for all of it, me with my 20-minute sitting tolerance and chronic pain they'd said would never get better, and I had got up at the end of it and walked out. Not stretched for a couple of minutes, then hauled myself up by the pew arm and dragged myself out, all my weight on my stick, barely able to carry my cushion as I'd done yesterday; *I had walked out*.

I didn't feel dizzy, either. And my stick was hooked onto my bag, dangling in the air, as I carried it on a good day when I didn't need it right now but was taking it out just in case I needed it later.

'Oh my god,' I said. 'Oh shit.'

Then I said: 'Maybe it's the adrenaline.'

Mike was one of those people who'd rather let you talk it out than talk it through.

'What does this *mean*?' I groaned, looking up at the painting of Jesus embracing John of God. Mike shrugged. I saw another little gaggle of pilgrims staring at my flowers, trying to contort their envy into happiness for a worthy recipient when we all knew I was the least worthy recipient in Goias province.

We drifted across the courtyard and into the bookshop, where all the staff looked up as I walked in and their gaze followed my flowers as I scoured the shelves for answers. The woman who always tried to sell me the £5 rule book looked like her eyes were about to pop out of her head.

'Where did you get those?' snapped the French man who'd tried to sell me a crystal bed on my first day, and again at the weekend, when he'd taken me into the back room to give me the hard sell, told me he had an in with John of God's son and if I wanted the bed, all I had to do was say the word and Roger Federer would get permission from his father. I'd told him I'd think about it, and as I'd walked over to the bookshelf I'd heard him telling Roger in Portuguese, *I think she's interested.*

'Did He give them to you?' he asked.

'Yes,' I said. 'At the end of the Current. He gave me the message: Congratulations.'

He looked at me like I was Oprah.

'What do you think it means?' I said, triumphantly, and he said he didn't know, but this time he didn't try to sell me a crystal bed.

Back at the pousada, I called my mother. It was past midnight back home, and her voice was thick with sleep and worry as she answered the phone.

'You're not going to believe what just happened,' I said, and I heaved as I spoke, three years and 11 months' worth of memories barrelling into me in slow-mo as the rollercoaster slowed down. It hit me as I told her: the hope, the despair, the showdown, the evaporated career, the disappeared friends, the life I'd nearly thrown away too many times to count. Had it all ended so suddenly, so easily, with some meditation and a pot of chrysanthemums? Was this it? Could it really be over?

'What will you do with the flowers?' asked my mum.

The coach was by the pousada, engine running, the last stragglers climbing on. Where is he, I called out. *Donde esta el señor?*

He looked bemused for a second, tracing his fingers over the petals, and then he unfurled his beautiful smile, his father grinning beside him.

'Obrigado,' he said.

Tell him they're from John of God, I told the woman from the hotel in mangled Spanish. Tell him I have kept half and given him half so we can share my luck. Tell him I hope they can help him as they have helped me. He shook my hand and wished me a safe journey back to England, and I said to the woman: tell him I prayed.

Later that night, when I was the only guest again, she told me that she'd lived in Abadiania 30 years and had seen many strange things, unexplained things, miracles if you will. So you think he's for real, I asked, and she looked at me as if I was a dunce and said, 'Claro'.

Before I went to sleep, I looked at the picture of Dr Augusto that I had bought for 50p in the shop from the woman with the bulging eyes, and I told him: I believe.

FORTY DAYS IN THE DESERT

Pain that comes back is like a viper.
It turns round to bite me even deeper.
Gabriele d'Annunzio (1863-1938: chronic pain patient, writer)

Two days after devoting my life to the entities, I received a life lesson: that the only thing worse than praying for a miracle and not getting it is praying for a miracle, getting it, and having it taken away again.

I'd spent the Saturday parading around Abadiania like the Queen of Sheba, buying all the souvenirs I'd sworn I wouldn't buy, back when I was a non-believer: chakra-tuning crystals, a silver triangle pendant, facewash which promised to realign you with your higher self. It was £10 a bottle, but was made by the woman who'd been monitoring the Current in which I had received my miracle.

I'd told her what had happened, and she had looked at me solemnly and told me I'd been granted a rare and wonderful thing, and now it was my responsibility to work out why: why I had been given my life back and what I was supposed to do with it.

I'd collared Diego and he had smiled a Mona Lisa smile and warned me not to question it. I'd bid farewell to the bookshop people with genuine tenderness. I'd seen Matt in the street, and told him I'd been healed – 'Whoah,' he'd said. I was like the miracled women who strut about, proclaiming their fortune in Zola's *Lourdes*: 'Completely cured as if by medicine,' they say, reclaiming their identities. Like the 'tarantate' – the Salento women who finish their frenetic pizzica dance whole and cured, and walk quietly home.

Don't tempt God, Thabiso would have said. And then it happened.

Three continents, five stages of grief.

Denial at Brasilia airport as I declined the prebooked wheelchair, jogged a mile to the gate and felt a spurt of familiar electricity – barely perceptible but perceptible nonetheless – shoot through my arm as I put my case into the overhead locker for the first time in four years.

Bargaining as I awoke at Iguaçu Falls with my arm burning – a fraction of its normal levels, but burning nevertheless. Bargaining as I practised my COPE course's distraction techniques by standing on a platform cantilevered over the water, Jack and Rose on the prow of the Titanic, 450,000 cubic feet steaming past my feet every second. Bargaining as I slept between Dr Augusto's portrait and a chunk of Abadiania crystal. Please take it away. I'm letting it go. I promise I believe.

Depression in Rio as I realised that although I was a lot better – 'transformed', as a friend there announced – a miracle meant not an improvement but a cure. Depression as I realised that if it wasn't a real miracle, I must have done a Zola and the miracle must have been in my head. Depression in London as I came through Arrivals with the carving knife hovering around my armpit – not *in* it, but testing its point against it, which meant the same thing: failure. Depression as I quietly packed away the crystal and the portrait and vowed not to speak about Abadiania again.

Anger in Los Angeles where I flew to house-sit, planned before Brazil as a space to recalibrate after the disappointment I would surely face – a return to the city of angels and hope where Kevin had saved me two years earlier. Anger at fate-the-universe-coincidence when it paraded my former muses, Banquo-like, in front of me during my 40-day healing ban: breakfast with Kevin on day 32, Patrick San Francesco popping up on Venice Beach on day 36, an acupuncturist who'd obliterated a friend's arthritis on day 27. Anger at myself for having believed it, believed anyone could help me when the doctors had promised me nobody could – anger so corrosive that I called a Samaritan friend to talk it through. Anger at myself for not having enjoyed it when on day 34 I had a rush of POTS dizziness and it occurred to me that I'd been 90 per cent symptom-free for a month, but I'd been so fixated on the elusive total cure that I hadn't appreciated that for the first time ever, I'd experienced life as others do, and now it was gone.

Acceptance in Joshua Tree – at least that was the plan. Acceptance that it was over, acceptance of the pain. Acceptance that the COPE people and the Walsingham priest had known better than me. Acceptance, the one thing I couldn't handle. Acceptance, that made me want to die. I rented a cabin in the middle of the desert, landlords within screaming distance, my only real neighbours a family of wild hares, jackrabbits and a cream-and-pink-coloured snake. Forty days in the desert, minus the miracles.

I'd been back to Joshua Tree several times since that first visit, and I had grown to love it like nowhere on earth. I loved the heat unravelling my joints; I loved the residents, people who'd upped sticks and come here because the land spoke to them. I loved the quiet dirt tracks, the thin desert air and the lucid blue skies. I loved the ladies at yoga, sighing happily as they stretched into their poses as if nothing on earth could bring them more pleasure. I loved Charmayne. I had seen her again in the intervening years, and although she hadn't helped the pain, each time she had delivered some insightful messages from the celestial beings. Some hope.

More than anything, I loved the desert itself: boulders created millions of years ago, rocky hills formed by the rub of tectonic plates, centuries-old Joshua trees, a landscape so still and barren, but teeming with life if you only shut up and watched. The cabin had glass walls and I sat at the kitchen table, trying and failing to write – because the book was due and everyone knows books have happy endings, but every sentence reminded me that mine hadn't come and I wished I was dead. I felt overwhelmed with emotion every time a desert rat would scale a cactus, balance on the spikes and tug at a flower until it detached, and it would put it in its mouth and run home for dinner.

On my third day at the cabin, I'd been up for a couple of hours, aware of a thought that was tickling the back of my mind, yet just out of reach – had I missed an appointment, forgotten an email? – when it struck me.

I was healed.

I had bounced out of bed instead of hauling myself up, brewed the normal eight-cup pot of coffee but only drunk half. I'd whipped through my emails with astonishing speed, combed through the sidebar of shame on a trashy gossip website, and set my alarm for work: 20 minutes, because sometimes I could do more, sometimes less, but 20 minutes would usually at least not damage me.

After four years it was routine: alarm sounds, get up, stretch, make tea, apply pain-relieving lotion, procrastinate, swallow ibuprofen, reset for 20 minutes' time.

I was on my third break when I realised I was stopping out of habit, that sitting and typing was provoking absolutely no pain. That, actually, there was no pain, no fire kindling, anywhere in my arm. That – wait – there was no pain in my back, neck, head, anywhere. I stood up, and I wasn't dizzy. I scanned my body, somatic focus honed after four years of constant monitoring: there was absolutely no pain, no discomfort, anywhere.

Holy shit.

I inspected myself in the mirror but it appeared I was still Julia, just Julia from another dimension.

It happens when it's supposed to happen, Diego had said. It only takes an instant.

The hope sprung up in my throat like a jack-in-the-box and I slammed it back down. Not again, I told myself. Not until you're certain.

By the evening, the only pain was in my fingers, exhausted after their first workout in four years.

That night, I spoke to Dr Augusto again.

Five days later, I opened the jack-in-the-box and allowed the hope out. I emailed Mike from Minnesota – he'd been routinely checking in on me, assuring me that I was healed, that my relapse was merely my 'false core' at work. He'd asked me to flag him once my 40 days were up so that he could send me some healing, and I hadn't replied because I was heartbroken and done with all that.

I should reply, I thought, and I should let Mike in on my new secret: *I don't need healing because I appear to be healed, though I won't say no if you want to send some more.* If healing was allowed by now, that was – I should check. I pulled up the calendar on my laptop, counted the days. Forty-five days since my intervention: Mike was therefore allowed to help.

I went cold, counted again.

My pain had vanished 1,464 days since that morning with the tepid cappuccino, and exactly 40 days after my intervention in Abadiania.

NO SUCH THING AS CURE

I wonder if I've been changed during the night? Let me
think: was I the same when I got up this morning?
Lewis Carroll, *Alice in Wonderland* (1865)

'You're definitely better,' said Dr Cuong. He had taken my
pulse for the first time in two years and as he unwrapped the
needles he was about to stick in me, I was telling him what
had happened.

'Your body's not struggling,' he said. I froze with excitement. This was it.

He told me that in the past – both during my pain and
before my pain – he had struggled to find my pulse (the
pressure pulse he took before acupuncture rather than the
normal pulse he took in his GP surgery). But this time, it
was pretty good.

I had always pretended that I'd avoided Dr Cuong –
even though his treatment made me feel better – because I
couldn't afford him, but it wasn't just that. I'd been ashamed
to see him because of something he'd said to me a couple of
months before the coffee incident, something I had ignored
at the time but been haunted by ever since I reached for that
cold cappuccino.

'Julia,' he'd said solemnly one day, feeling for my pulse.
'You're killing yourself.' Something had to give, he'd said
– I must stop working so much, rest more, eat better, calm
down, stop burning the candle at both ends and from the
middle – because he could feel my energy flagging every time
I came to him. I could feel it too – my normal pain levels
were through the roof in the months leading up to the coffee

incident, and I was fluey with exhaustion – but I had done my best to ignore it.

Shit, I'd thought, that's scary. I'll have to start meditation or something, next month. I'll start cooking instead of living off sandwiches next week. I'll stop working 16-hour days tomorrow. Every day, I'd vowed to change the following day. And then I'd reached for that cup of coffee, and there had been no more tomorrows.

'Yes, I remember,' he said now. 'I saw you as a person who was being pushed towards the cliff edge. I was telling you that all along, that you were pushing yourself to the edge and one day you were going to fall over.'

Why didn't you listen to him you stupid twat? It was the question that had haunted me for four years, along with 'Why did you reach for that coffee when it was cold?' and 'Why did you keep working when you were signed off work?' and 'Why are you such a useless lazy bitch?'

He talked about the difference between western and eastern medicine as he saw it, straddling the two. Western medicine works from the outside in, and eastern from the inside out, he said. He likened my body to a house: if the foundation is strong, the house stands; if it's weak, cracks appear. Western medicine reacts by filling in the cracks, treating the disease, attending to the symptoms; eastern medicine stabilises the foundation. My DNA was the same, he reckoned; John of God hadn't changed my dodgy collagen. But my foundation had stabilised, so I could cope with my genetics.

'Health is mind, body and spirit,' said Dr Cuong. 'The mind has to be right, the body's got to be strong. And the spiritual side is not just about your religion; it's all about your conscience, your internal belief, yeah? We all have our own belief.'

Four years earlier, I would have spat at anyone telling me that my health depended on my mind and spirit, but now I thought perhaps he had a point.

It was in Joshua Tree that I realised that although I was myself again, I was also slightly different. It wasn't an entirely new personality, like the one the pain had foisted on me; it was me, but angled a couple of degrees to the side. I was still neurotic, anxious, uptight and judgemental, but I had changed. You think I should try a soundbath for this sore back? Fabulous idea! You cured your endometriosis by loving your womb? Fascinating. Maybe you're right and those ley lines in the desert really *do* attract aliens. The new Julia was softer – not credulous, but open. I took massages from a woman called Kate, and when her cat leapt onto my shoulder and started kneading right where the fire had always kindled and she said it was because he could feel the energy, I said: yeah, could be. When Kate suggested I might tackle my bizarrely tabled periods by writing in my menstrual blood to embrace my femininity, I thought, what's the harm in giving that a go? (I didn't need to, as it happened; at some point that summer, they followed the pain away.)

If I'd spent the past four years slowly dying of Yentl Syndrome, with man after man telling me to stop worrying, there was nothing wrong, nothing I could do although I could definitely do with losing weight, here in Joshua Tree I began to recalibrate my self-worth in a community of extraordinary women. There was Kate, who dispensed such wisdom that her massages were therapy as well as bodywork. There was Ray Jayne, who led the yoga classes where I went into a semi-trance state as the others sighed with delight.

There was Jenny from the Grateful Desert, the herbalist whose essential oil-filled shower gel had first led me to Charmayne. There was the woman in the petrol station whose name I never got to know, always feisty and cheery, even when it was 46 degrees outside. There was Wanita, a redoubtable 88-year-old hypnotherapist who vanquished my writer's block and helped me trust the body of myself, as Mr Wong had urged me to, in a single session (she was in LA but I spoke to her from Joshua Tree, so she counted).

And, of course, there was Charmayne.

I had gone to Joshua Tree to make a hermitage out of the cabin I was staying in, to try and figure out who I was, what had happened, what I believed. I'd seen her sticker-sheathed car a couple of times while I was buying food in town, but hadn't stopped to say hello. She'd played such a pivotal role in what had gone on that I didn't want to see her until I'd worked out exactly what had happened and what part she had taken. On my last day – 10 weeks in, having extended my rental twice – I came down from the desert, ready at last.

You're better, she said. You don't need the celestial beings to say it, but they're saying it anyway.

She laid a hunk of labradorite on my belly, pressing down into my guts to extract bad energy as she made her noises. She wore a stomach brace, these days – 'I got a hernia from sounding,' she said – and when I asked whether she should still be doing this, she said, simply, 'Gots to do it.'

As the noises came forth – the grunts, the snarls, the screams and the barks (Rolly no longer lived with her, but she finished each sounding with a neat yelp) – I felt my face, all hot and soaked with tears. Tears of anger for everything that had happened – we should really clear that anger, Charmayne said, and I thought of dear Mr Wong, who had noticed it too – but also tears of relief that it was over, tears of joy and gratitude for having found my way back and for who I had become. I lay there, keening, until she asked if there was anything else I wanted to work on and I said no. We had closed the circle.

In the bad old days when I would beat myself up as magnificently as an Opus Dei initiate, demanding over and over whether I liked my pain, whether secretly I wanted it or cradled it – because that's what I took from every man I saw – I would ask myself, would you miss it? If it disappeared tomorrow, would you grieve for it? Would you pine for your victimhood? And I was so full of doubt that I didn't know the answer.

But now I knew: of course I didn't miss it. There was no sense of loss – there couldn't be, because it had never been part of me. It was a cancer that had been cut out of me, weights lifted off my shoulders and peeled from my ankles. It had always been an intruder, and now it had been expelled. Its lack had made me whole again, now that I was cured.

But was I cured? Or was I, rather, healed? Had I been miracled or was I just better? Recovered, over the worst, or regressed to the mean? Semantics I'd never considered suddenly became all-consuming. John of God had done nothing for my OCD.

'You got your miracle!' Kevin had written when I'd told him what had happened, and I had felt a rush of nausea. Having obsessed over it for four years – craved it, begged for it, prayed for it, hoped for it – I immediately excised the word from my vocabulary. It wasn't a miracle because it couldn't be a miracle. Miracles were the stuff of god-squadders and hippies. Miracles happened to the pious, not to me. I had gone out looking for a miracle, and something had happened, something that could easily be described as a miracle, but I couldn't call it that.

Isn't it funny, a friend once said, paraphrasing a Tim Minchin song, that miracles only happen to white first-worlders? I didn't agree – if I'd learned anything on my search, it was that inexplicable recoveries happen in every country, every environment, to people of every culture, colour and every religion. Patrick, Jero Pura, Richard Morse, Mr Wong, Thabiso, Padre Pio, the waters of Lourdes – I believe they've all cured a lucky few. But miracles don't happen to everyone. And that was what I couldn't handle.

Dr Cuong counselled against my using 'cured'. He hauled me up mid-sentence when I slipped it in.

'Let me correct you,' he said sternly. 'There's no such thing as cure.'

'Don't,' I said, crossing myself mentally. 'Don't say that.'

'"Cure" makes people think that whatever they're doing to themselves is acceptable because that thing won't come back any more,' he said.

It's not true, I told my brain. *Ignore him. It will never come back.*

'I look at it like you're strong enough to keep your body

at bay because the body's designed to heal itself and you're strong enough to start healing yourself.'

He's lying, I said. *It's gone forever. It's dead.*

'You've found your balance,' he said. 'Now it's up to you to maintain it. But there's no such thing as cure.'

I tussled with the words: in California, in London, in Lourdes, in Cornwall. Cure, heal, restore. Cure, heal, regression to the mean. Cure. Heal. Miracle.

I thought: I still have EDS. My joints still sag backwards. My back still has a tendency to soreness. I'm a thousand times better than I was, and my body is unrecognisable but I'd still rather sit down than hover at the bar, I still wouldn't volunteer to carry someone's suitcase up the steps of the Tube, just in case. The pain they'd said would never go away had gone away, and the symptoms of my incurable genetic condition had flatlined. But I had the same DNA. And I still had occasional reminders of what had happened – when I knocked myself out in Lourdes and plunged six feet onto the floor, my back ached and a phantom knife tingled in my armpit for about a week afterwards. So could I really qualify as cured? If my nerve pathways had been turfed over rather than obliterated, could I really claim I was better?

But then I thought of something else Dr Cuong had said, something that Mr Wong had said, and Jenny Klimiuk and Jannie, as well as Charmayne and Kate and the wonderful women of Joshua Tree.

Only you know how your body feels. Only you can hear what it's saying.

And it was saying – insisting, even – that it *was* cured. Or, rather, that my pain was. That 'heal' and 'cure' is different – one implies comfort and improvement, the other is definitive. It was saying that yes, okay, my body and mind may only have been healed, my DNA was still the same, but the pain was something else. It had gone, and it wouldn't be back. It was cured.

The only question was who or what had done it.

AN UNSTOPPABLE PROCESS

Sometimes I think illness sits inside every woman,
waiting for the right moment to bloom.
Gillian Flynn, *Sharp Objects* (2009)

Three weeks after my pain had vanished, I was on a plane
to Boston to meet some of the world's top pain specialists.

The irony wasn't lost on me, especially because, even when
I'd been bouncing from healer to healer, I'd long suspected
that the real miracle would be found in a research lab. I
could wait decades for cutting-edge research to filter down,
I thought, or I could collar the experts direct.

So the minute I signed the contract to write a book
about pain, I wrote to them: doctors, scientists, consultants,
psychologists, pain specialists, placebo experts. I even tried
Derren Brown and Penn from Penn and Teller in case cold
reading could help me psych myself out of my pain.

They said no, all of them, sometimes with emails patronising enough to make me blush. Whether it was my lack of
scientific background, my openness to anything outlandish,
or – as I came to wonder as the rejections rolled in alongside pats on the head about 'worthy projects' – my gender,
nobody wanted to talk.

And then suddenly I remembered I had a personal connection at Harvard Medical School, and, just like that, I was
in. (That's not to say the people I met would have rejected
me had I approached them blind, of course – I hadn't asked
them because after the laundry list of rejections, I'd given
up in despair.)

I was in Brazil – that first, angry week in Abadiania –
when they agreed to let me sit in on a conference for pain

specialists, and I imagined that our interviews would be consultations by the back door, appointments in which the puzzle was finally pieced together and I'd find my cure. By the time I met them, it was no longer a life-or-death situation but a mesmerising glimpse across enemy lines. Because they thought it was a battlefield, too – I could tell from lecture titles like 'Disabled or Deceiving: Disability Evaluation', 'Getting High or Getting Better: The Dope on Medical Marijuana' and 'An Addict or a Patient in Pain?' – and yet there were also lectures on the mind-body connection and complementary approaches to pain management. Eight weeks on from my stints in the Current, I found myself sitting with these doctors, serenely meditating – the only difference was they called it 'attaining the relaxation response', and talked about the health benefits (lower blood pressure, decreased oxygen consumption, genetic changes in the production of insulin and telomeres, altering the body's inflammatory response) in concrete terms. Harvard was, after all, where meditation had entered the mainstream – Herbert Benson, the mind-body pioneer, had researched it here in the 1960s.

I looked around as Professor Benson told other eminent doctors that the relaxation response could benefit sufferers of infertility and cardiac arrhythmia, that it could ease the side effects of cancer treatment and AIDS therapy. I thought of everything I'd tried and the doctors who'd scoffed and rolled their eyes if ever I'd dared tell them, and I thought: the tide is turning. Maybe my journey hadn't been so ridiculous after all. Perhaps I was just ahead of the curve.

The talk I'd flown in for was about the future of pain medicine, given by Dan Carr, one of the most eminent pain specialists on the planet. Surely he would have my explanation.

Dan Carr told us that chronic pain was an adaptive, advantageous process gone awry, a disease in itself, but also a social process. Evolution was governed by the need for pleasure, and for millennia there had been a link between pain, stigma and marginalisation. Pain activates the same part in the brain as rejection by a friend or lover. Pain patients were outsiders, and society devalued their experiences. Treating them as they were treated at the moment was 'not wrong, but incomplete'.

My god, I thought. Where have you been these past four years?

He talked about why chronic pain could develop: prior sensitisation (if you've had one injury, a follow-up – however mild – can send your pain networks into overdrive), and abnormal sodium channels, a genetic cause that could predict a patient's susceptibility to chronic pain by about 50 per cent. I started to connect the dots.

If there was a genetic tendency towards pain, I hardly needed a test to confirm it. Not with rheumatoid arthritis running rampant through the generations, my mother with RSI in her arm and nerves crackling down her legs, my grandmother with POTS symptoms and a great-grandmother who'd been exiled to the Hospital for Incurables (now the Royal Hospital for Neuro-disability) when she'd woken up one day mysteriously paralysed. As for prior sensitisation, my arm had packed up for my A Levels, then my dissertation, then my finals, and stayed problematic throughout my career, well before that morning in May. I'd always wondered why writing about wine cruises had tipped the balance. Suddenly a hippy in Joshua Tree who'd told me that my arm hurt now because the tissue remembered all the times it had hurt before didn't sound so crazy after all.

Dan Carr ran through new treatments and forthcoming treatments, things that would replace the narcotics, anticonvulsants and COPE courses of the future. He talked of ion channels and epoxide inhibitors: kinase, NGF and CGRP. He talked of stem cells, of Botox and cannabinoids; of angiotensin-2 receptor antagonists. I had heard of some of them – my forward-looking jaw consultant in Cornwall was giving me Botox for my TMJ – but not of most of them. It didn't matter, though – the science was irrelevant. All I needed to know was that they were finding ways to tackle the pain without wiping the brain alongside it.

It was unfathomable. Here was a doctor saying stuff that no doctor had said to me before. That chronic pain can be genetic, predictable, even nipped in the bud before it kicks in, using a *Minority Report*-style SWAT team for nociceptors. That the current drugs on the market don't do an adequate job. That pain is stigmatising and demoralising and that doctors don't do enough about its psychological effects. That it hadn't been in my head. That I hadn't been hysterical. That I wasn't lazy, or a benefits scrounger, or a fantasist. That it hadn't been my sub-optimal personality type. That it hadn't been my fault.

I listened, choking back four years of tears, telling myself: it wasn't your fault. It was never your fault.

Four years of self-recrimination – 30, if you counted the failure of anyone to diagnose my EDS. 'There's nothing wrong with how she sits,' at four years old, the GP to my mother; 'You're making it up,' at 16, when I'd gone to the dentist, jaw locked shut from the TMJ; 'If you'd only stop worrying, you'd be absolutely fine,' from the endocrinologist at 35. Three and a half decades of gaslighting.

I felt the anger blistering in every cell, metastasising through my body, shutting down my system with boiling rage. And I told myself: let it go. Let it go and listen to what Dan Carr is saying.

He was saying that it wouldn't always be like this; that I had suffered, but my daughter, if I had one, might not. That they would check her genes if she had an accident and medicate her accordingly; that they would prep her for operations differently if she had a genetic propensity to pain than if she didn't. That if she had pain that wouldn't go away, instead of telling her she was getting older or depressed or batting her away with Nurofen, they would precision-target her pain, work out where it came from, twiddle her sodium channels or inhibit her epoxides. And they would also monitor her psychologically – not because they thought her a hysterical woman, but because they knew that feeling marginalised would be her normal, human reaction.

Perhaps my generation was where it ended. Perhaps, in 100 years, people would look back at our stories with the same horror with which we read Fanny Burney's account of her anaesthetic-less mastectomy. There was hope – but only as long as we held on. If I'd jumped out of the window that day when my mum had begged me not to – when my pain had peaked and my doctors were saying I'd never recover and my rehabilitation consultant was suggesting I change professions, *think of something that doesn't involve your hands* – I'd never have heard this.

I thought of my doctors. Why didn't you tell me? Why didn't you throw me a bone of hope? If you didn't know, why didn't you make it your business to know?

And I thought, you didn't make it your business to know, because unlike your brain tumours and your heart arrhythmias and your Addison's diseases, you thought I wasn't dying, and I wasn't your priority. I was an annoyance: one of Janet Williams' chronic pain personalities, one of the 'unhappy people' neurosurgeon Henry Marsh describes in *Do No Harm*, the patients who 'limp dramatically' and speak 'angrily', whose tears 'stream down' their faces. The patients about whom he writes, 'All I can do is to sit quietly, trying to stop my eyes drifting away out of the window, over the car park ... as [they] pour out their misery to me, and wait for them to finish.'

I knew that look: the quiet indifference, the polite impatience. I had seen it on so many faces – of the anaesthetists and rheumatologists and GPs and physiotherapists and counsellors and psychologists and nurses and orthopaedic surgeons. On the neurologist's, most of all. He was the one who'd promised not to let me down, right before letting me down.

I pictured him now with his fair hair and glasses and pleasant bedside manner: friendly but brisk, reassuringly distant, then awkward the last time we met, trying to look sympathetic as he suggested in public schoolboy vowels that I was depressed, and avoiding eye contact as he discharged me.

I know I wasn't a brain tumour, I thought. I know I wasn't your priority, I know you thought I wasn't dying. But if you'd swapped your medical gaze for a human one, looked at me for a second as a person rather than a symptom – not another chronic pain or an EDS, but Julia – you'd have realised that, actually, I was.

I hadn't died, and I had no intention of dying now, but if I had, it would have been on their watch.

———

Ronald Kulich is a professor of psychology at Massachusetts General Hospital who advises the US government on public policy about pain and opioid risk. Most of his work revolves around predicting who might become an addict, and whose pain will turn acute to chronic. But he can also predict who might get better.

'There's a difference between being cured of chronic pain versus managing it,' he said. We were sitting in his office at the Craniofacial Pain Center at Tufts School of Dental Medicine, a modern tower block looming over the low-rise buildings of Boston's Chinatown. Newly pain-free, I'd brightly asked how to predict which of his patients would end up 'cured', and he'd batted me straight back to reality.

'But those who have successful management – which is a different phenomenon from cure – tend to be more resilient, and they tend to be able to develop the opposite of all the risk factors,' he said.

At the start of our chat he'd been very clear that, despite what his colleague Dr Williams had said, there was no such thing as a pain-prone personality. There were, however, risk factors. The risk factors depended on the pain disorder, he said, but were largely trauma, substance abuse history, job dissatisfaction and family factors. Certain personality disorders could be problematic, as well as patients who become 'overly somatically focused': in other words, obsessed with their symptoms.

The people who win back supremacy over their pain, in his experience, are those who turn those tables. They process their trauma: art therapy, of all things, can be better for this than verbal therapy.[28] It's what the UK and US armed forces offer soldiers with PTSD.

They change jobs or deal with employment issues – 'work itself is considered a treatment,' said Kulich. Once a person has been off work for two years, it's statistically unlikely that they will ever return,[29] but return they do. They learn to disassociate their pain from other people's interpretations of it – to trust the body of themselves, as Mr Wong would say – and try to detach themselves from their every twinge.

There are two other hallmarks of a successful recovery from pain. One is switching your locus of control – your belief in what's controlling events which affect you – from an external one to one that's internal. Lying back and expecting someone else to cure you – whether that's your surgeon, John of God or your god – doesn't work. Taking charge of your process, on the other hand, does.

The other crucial component to recovery, he said, is my bête noire: acceptance.

Nearly four years earlier, I had slunk out of the church in Walsingham, frightened by the priest's suggestion that a miracle was the bestowing of acceptance, rather than a lightning-bolt cure. Acceptance had always felt like a snow-drift beckoning me in to sleep – acceptance meant meek assent, acquiescing to my butchered existence, making a life from the scraps the pain had left me with. Acceptance also required a strength I didn't have. Why take up your cross when you can tantrum like a four year old?

Accept your pain because it's trying to tell you something, Thabiso had said – you can't move on until you listen to it. And although I hadn't wanted to accept it – because it still felt like accepting defeat – I could see that I was ravaged by the fight. Resisting was exhausting.

I knew more about Lourdes, by then, where pilgrims came to the grotto for comfort, trusting not that they would get better, but that their faith would get them through what was to come. And it seemed to be the same in Brazil. All the sick in Abadiania were hoping to be cured, of course – that's why they were taking their passiflora caplets, eschewing pepper and booze, and waking at dawn to meditate – but most of them, at least outwardly, seemed more mellow about it than me. They seemed to trust that what should happen would happen – 'for the higher good of all', was their motto. One of the Casa pilgrims I'd found most unfathomable was a young man from Russia who'd come to Abadiania with an inoperable brain tumour and smiled all the time. 'That's faith,' I'd said to Matt when he'd told me about him, but what I'd meant was, 'That's stupidity.' He died shortly after I left, seizing at the airport as he tried to get home – and it was only when he died that it occurred to me that maybe he'd never believed he was improving physically; maybe he'd been looking for something else. Maybe his calm smile hadn't been one of hope, but of acceptance.

Psychologists don't see acceptance as surrender as I did. Studies show that a greater acceptance of pain correlates with lower pain intensity and less of the 'pain plus' symptoms, as Jannie Van Der Merwe calls the weights that attach themselves to the pain and drag you into their mire: *pain plus* depression, *pain plus* anxiety, *pain plus* disability, *pain plus* avoidance behaviour.

'When patients find their pain unacceptable, they are likely to attempt to avoid it at all costs and seek readily available interventions to reduce or eliminate it,' wrote Lance McCracken in a landmark study on acceptance in 1998.[30] 'These efforts may not be in their best interest if the consequences include no reductions in pain and many missed opportunities for more satisfying and productive functioning.' In recent years, acceptance and commitment therapy and acceptance-based behavioural therapy have been gaining popularity on pain management courses. I tried to get referred onto one myself when CBT failed, but of course because I'd already done the CBT, the computer said no.

'I think recovery from chronic pain is a combination of resiliency, teaming up with doctors who don't make you worse, fewer risk factors, and addressing the risk factors that you do have,' said Ronald Kulich. 'Are we ever going to take away all chronic pain? I'm not convinced. But there is science that suggests that certain interventions have *some* effect.'

Not that intervention has always been a good thing. 'Some things we've done over the last 10 years have had a negative effect,' he said. 'Some things in the last 20 years, too. It used to be in the 1980s that everybody with a protruding disc would get a laminectomy, and it turns out that doesn't work – surgery has the biggest placebo effect. By the time the 1990s rolled around, it used to be that everybody in pain would get a big bag full of opiates. Turns out that doesn't work either. I think people acknowledge that psychological treatments have significant limitations as well, if you actually look at the data. It's not a whole lot better than the medications.'

I asked him what he would do if he got chronic pain.

'I hope I would do at least three things,' he said. 'Maintain my activities, use medications rationally, use surgery rationally' – because he had treated, he said, one patient with 47 surgeries under their belt, one on 37 medications and another on an opioid dose equivalent to 700 5mg Percocet pills per day. Sometimes the wealthiest patients are the worst off, he said, because no doctor dares tell them no.

'I would try to consolidate my medical care so I don't have nine people telling me nine different things,' he said. 'Utilise my social supports. Keep working. Those are all the resiliency things you should do. The biggest problem is when people stop doing things.'

So by doing those things if you had an injury, I said, presumably you wouldn't even have the acute pain turn chronic in the first place.

'Or I would manage it better,' he said. 'At least, that's

statistically ... I believe I would manage it better by doing this.'

He paused for a fraction of a breath.

'Whether I could do those things or not is a different story.'

———

That I found my Jesus after I'd received my cure was perhaps ironic, but that I found him back where I'd started, in California – after Kevin, after Charmayne, after my Joshua Tree rebirth – was at least fitting.

He didn't heal me, of course – I didn't need healing by that point. But he did tell me how he cures pain that others call incurable. Not manages it, not teaches people how to accept it, but *cures* it. (He doesn't say 'cure'; he insists on saying 'help'. But cure is what he does.)

He was unlike any of the healers I'd met, because he was a doctor; but he was unlike any of the doctors I'd seen, because he treated people with a method that hasn't – yet – cleared the hurdle of evidence-based medicine. He didn't believe in entities, but he did think there was something to John of God; didn't believe in the healing power of crystals but thought that touching a crystal could heal you. He was as tall as Richard Morse and dressed in Patrick's studied casualwear; he had the empathy of Dr Good and Thabiso's joie de vivre. Yes, I thought, this is it, here is a man for whom I could put down my nets and follow. His name was Michael Moskowitz, and he was a psychiatrist from San Francisco. He was an atheist, too, and his cure – the cure that had eluded me for four interminable years – was neuroplasticity.

Neuroplasticity is what makes us, after all. It's the process in our pliable brains that forms new connections and circuits in order for us to learn new things: riding a bike, speaking a foreign language. But it also breaks us – neuroplasticity is what turns acute pain to chronic, grassing over those neural motorways of chapter one and carving out new B roads that never end. And neuroplasticity works fast. Of the 1,000 trillion synapses in our brains – microscopic gaps between nerve endings which pass messages up the chain, facilitating the rewiring – we change 7.5 trillion per week. I had learned about the carnage that my synapses had wrought early on in my pain. My doctors considered neuroplasticity an unstoppable process.

Perhaps it was because he, too, had been a pain patient – he'd shattered his femur and struggled psychologically with the return to work, and the minute he'd got that under control, his brain had resurrected pain from a dormant neck injury six years earlier – but Michael Moskowitz, pain psychiatrist, didn't share the narrative that people with chronic pain are lazy, work-shy or hysterical. He was aware of the irony of preaching pain management while his own pain stalked his body like Hamlet's dad on the ramparts of Elsinore. He was an expert in neuroscience – in how chronic pain hijacks the brain – but, like every other doctor, it didn't occur to him that neuroscience might be the key as well the padlock, so he continued to talk of coping strategies. And then one day in 2007, a mouthy patient for whom nothing worked – not meditation, not CBT, not even morphine – said to him, 'Why don't you quit writing about what goes wrong and figure out how to make it go away?' Right there, on the spot, he improvised a visualisation technique, describing exactly what happens on a molecular level when pain gets bad and when it gets better. Neurons firing messages up the chain. Synapses awash in neurotransmitters. A needle suddenly lodged in the groove – synapses stuck in the 'on' position, an endless loop. New circuits laid down and worn into the brain. And then, the opposite – how, in an ideal world, those circuits would be broken again.

His patient got nothing out of it at all. But when he finished the exercise, Michael Moskowitz's own neck had stopped hurting. In technical terms, he had switched off his misfiring synapses, turned his long-term potentiation into short.

Neuroplasticity was not, he realised that day, an unstoppable force. It was more of a wild mustang: seemingly out of control but ultimately tameable. He could lasso it, force it to retreat the way it came, and set it back on those original pathways, and he could do that in exactly the same way as it had first arrived. It was obvious, really, and it worked – not on that first patient, maybe, but on 90 per cent of the others, to varying degrees. Half his patients have decreased their medication; a fifth have come off them entirely. That doesn't sound groundbreaking, but out in the big bad world beyond the offices of the Bay Area Pain Medical Associates, the average pain management programme only reduces the average patient's pain by 20 per cent.[31] 'Before I did this, everyone I treated still had pain all the time,' he told me. 'I really didn't have anyone whose pain I got down to nothing. But I see that a lot now.'

Statistics say that the longer you've been in pain, the less likely you are to get out of it. Once you've been off work for two years, we know it's unlikely you'll ever go back; my resurrection, after four years, is disconcertingly rare. But not for Michael Moskowitz. He reckons anyone can get out of chronic pain. And he thinks the current model – the insistence of management over cure, of telling patients that their pain is unerasable and inevitable – is the reason great swathes of us aren't recovering.

If you're wondering why no one else is doing this, why my COPE instructors were caught in the management loop, it's down to the cornerstone of modern medicine: clinical evidence.

'I base my treatment on the best I can come up with, looking at the science and interpreting it past the current limits,' he said, thrusting a bottle of peppermint oil under my nose (we'll get to that later). 'I can sit here and look at the science that leads to the conclusions that I've come to, and I can come up with all these cool things: sounds and vibrations and creams and sprays and peppermint and all that. I can give you good reasons why these should work, and I've seen them work in a lot of my patients, but someone could come by and say, "Well, that wasn't a controlled trial." And I can't say that they're wrong. But I can say, that's fine, but you're wearing the emperor's new clothes because you think that the randomised, double-blind, placebo-controlled trial is the highest level of evidence and, actually, it's the lowest.'

This is why you won't find Michael Moskowitz on a COPE course.

Modern medicine – evidence-based medicine – is about cast-iron proof. A treatment doesn't work until it passes a randomised, double-blind, placebo-controlled trial. For more accurate data, you take a meta-analysis to average out the results from different randomised control trials. Systematic reviews – essentially meta-analyses of meta-analyses – are the gold standard. And of course that's important. Evidence-based medicine is why catastrophes like thalidomide are few and far between these days, why you know that whatever your GP prescribes will most likely work, why we don't use leeches any more. But according to Michael Moskowitz – and to Dr Cuong, who'd used a similar line about acupuncture – the RCT is so controlled that it has little connection to real life.

'It takes one circumstance and tests that in a very controlled way with as many variables removed as possible,' he said. 'That level of control has very little to do with the people who walk into our offices. That has to do with a very rare group of people that you select very carefully to have as uncomplicated a picture as possible, and then you test a hypothesis based upon that very uncomplicated picture. But you're a complicated person. You've got a lot of things going on. You're not the same as the people coming into this study and getting a pill. Test them for six weeks or test them for 12 weeks – what does that tell you about a chronic condition? Nothing!'

It reminded me of a blog I'd once read by a doctor talking about Cochrane reviews, the top rung of systematic reviews. It started from the basis that 'in my experience' is the most lethal line in medicine, because it means what you're saying isn't evidence-based – it makes assumptions, it extrapolates, it leads from the heart not the head – and I remember thinking, maybe that's true, but that's also a great way to shut patients up, to shut out what they're telling you, because the only thing your patients will ever be able to talk about is their experience. You're a complicated person. And your experience counts.

'So no,' said Michael Moskowitz. 'It's not great science, it's actually lousy science, and it's taken over medicine.'

In 1983, a report in the *Journal of Pediatrics*[32] looked at 86 studies published in obstetrics and gynaecology journals. In 90 per cent of cases, the data in the report didn't back up the conclusions of the report.

In 2001, the *BMJ*[33] looked at 53 Cochrane reviews and found that in 17 per cent of cases, the data didn't support the conclusions drawn.

Evidence-based medicine works best for testing drugs, says Moskowitz. It has spawned what he calls 'insurance company medicine'.

'You've created a situation where doctors don't make any choices outside of the ones that are laid out in front of them – they basically become drug mules and procedure hawks, doing things based on these studies. And then the study changes – and then it changes again. I've watched spine surgeries change dramatically over the last 20 years. People say, "We know better now." Yes we do. But look at the crazy shit you did to all those people before!'

In time, his neuroplastic methods will be proven, he says. But he's not going to wait until then. He's going to carry on making his patients feel better. As he says: 'Whether or not we're right about what it does, who gives a shit?'

Would I have given a shit if, in between the CBT and the drug lectures and the exhortations to stretch and the lessons in how to talk to doctors, the COPE people had given us a talk on neuroplasticity and said, the science is sound and the results are great, but we must warn you this hasn't been proven with an RCT? That's a rhetorical question but the answer is no.

But back to that peppermint oil.

The Gospel of Moskowitz rests on simple precepts. What's fired is wired. Use it or lose it. Every new connection is made by breaking an old one. Persistent pain is not a symptom but a disease in itself. And the way to reverse it is through counterstimulation.

You must counterstimulate the pain every time it rears its head. Every twinge, every crunch, every neural flare: react. Tell your brain it isn't needed, that it's overreacting. Distract it by firing up your pleasure pathways – just do *something*. If you can keep that up, constantly shouting the pain down, neuroplasticity dictates it will start to retreat. It must – that's how your brain works.

Visualisation is the bread and butter of neuroplastic pain reduction – whether that's imagining your synapses switching off, turning off the Christmas tree lights of your misfiring circuits, or simply telling it, as I do now when I injure myself, 'you're okay, shut up'.[34] But there are other ways to lasso your mustang, and they're even more unorthodox:

Aromatherapy, because peppermint essential oil blocks a major pain neurotransmitter, Substance-P, and sparks up pleasure circuits – which in turn block pain circuits and soothe the monkey brain.

Tibetan singing bowls (or Moskowitz's pain-tailored recordings of them), because playing them at certain frequencies – frequencies which mimic nerve cell rhythms – slow down, and then switch off, overactive synapses, powering down the alarm system.

Touch, because a gentle massage or vibration can start to unravel the chronic pain takeover process (allodynia – the reason I couldn't bear any scratchy clothes on my arm – happens when nerve endings on the skin which used to report touch or pressure are pressganged into becoming pain receptors). Touch, because even stroking a cool piece of crystal, like the one I brought back from Abadiania, can distract and soothe the brain.

And taste – specifically, raw cacao nibs, three times a day, because they contain anandamide, a 'bliss'-generating neurotransmitter that reduces inflammation in the body and sparks up the brain's cannabinoid receptors, just like smoking weed.

It sounds too easy – so easy that, as a friend whose EDS is far more severe than mine said churlishly, it can't possibly work. It seems crazy. It blasts acceptance theory out of the water and hones your somatic focus, but you might be surprised. It takes effort, the constant counterstimulation – it was six weeks before Moskowitz noticed a clear reduction in his pain levels, though he says a colleague smashed his entirely in four – but even if it does nothing, the worst that will happen is that the cacao might give you wind. Compared to ibuprofen, with its increased risk of stroke, heart attack and kidney disease, isn't it worth a go? Compared to the chronic problems sparked by other treatments – the spine surgery that leads to another, the gateway pill that turns into an addiction – shouldn't you give it a try? Even if it's a placebo, who, in Michael Moskowitz's words, gives a shit?

I was better by the time we met, of course, during my summer of Joshua Tree, but although my pain had gone, its pathways were still there – grassing over, but still navigable. When I did something I'd never have dared do before – swing my heavy case into the overhead locker, drive for more than an hour, a downward dog – I would feel a twinge, the thud of the mustang's hooves seeking out its old routes. But every time I tried Moskowitz's techniques – slathering peppermint oil on my philtrum, telling my brain to calm down, having an aromatherapy bath if all else failed – it would back off.

I still had EDS (or whatever my underlying condition was) – the entities may have reset my brain but they hadn't changed my collagen – so I would still be more injury-prone than most. I suspected my sodium channels made me more susceptible to pain and unless, for his next trick, Dr Augusto could change my DNA, they weren't going anywhere. But the pain had gone, and now I knew what to do if it ever came back, I wasn't scared any more. The first time we met, Michael Moskowitz told me I'd eventually reach a point where I was excited by flare-ups – I could play with the pain, try out new techniques – and I'd felt the cramp of panic and thought, no way, I'll die if it comes back. Today, now that the intractable pain is firmly locked in the past, just a memory (an emotional one, not even a perceptual one any more), I know what he meant. It fascinates me, when I put my neck out cleaning the shower or hear a clunk in my arm scrubbing the bog, to tell my brain to shut up and feel it respond.

Michael Moskowitz believes that experience is important as well as science, and that it's not just the professionals bringing knowledge to the table. 'We doctors are highly trained in a lot of information that's partially correct, and then the real experience of working with people should train us the rest of the way,' he says. 'But a lot of doctors aren't open to that experience – they're only open to what the book says, or what the image says, or what this says or that says. And when they say something like, "That's not possible," they're idiots. Because it's the making what-they-don't-understand "impossible" that screws people over.'

Being told that our pain has shacked up with us and shackled us for life screws us over. Being told to accept this new sliver of a life screws us over. Being treated as if we're making a fuss over nothing, as if we're at fault, screws us over.

Researching this book, I came across a brochure for the oldest pain management programme in the UK, run at the Walton Centre in Liverpool since 1983. It was full of testimonials from patients, with phrases like 'What matters now is adjusting to life with the condition I've got', and 'People with chronic pain can enjoy a good quality of life despite their condition', written in gargantuan letters as pull-out quotes, supposed to be encouraging.

Reading it, I felt a familiar bubble of panic swelling in my chest, the old flap of butterfly wings on my stomach walls, saliva pooling in my mouth. Suddenly I was crying and then I was sobbing, partly as the Pavlovian response to a reminder of my four lost years, partly out of relief that it was over, partly out of anger that they were still saying these things – still stripping the hope from sick people, snuffing out their belief that it could end – partly because the defeat lacing the brochure read like cyanide. 'Despite', 'manage', 'acceptance', 'adjustment'. I was safe, I felt well, I wasn't in pain, I was happy. I was at a stage where not a day went by without feeling a hot burst of gratitude for the life that had returned to me like the prodigal son. And yet, reading this, I was back in the slurry pit that had held me captive for 47 months.

'The only way I managed to regain control of myself was by resolving that I would overcome all obstacles to win back the wings that belonged to my will,' wrote Gabriele d'Annunzio in *Notturno*, his extraordinary prose poem about regaining his eyesight after a plane crash. 'Against me stood the prognoses of science.' After nine months confined to bed in the darkness, racked by pain, almost entirely blind, he returned to life as a writer and even as a pilot, confounding the doctors who'd said he'd never see again.

When I read that Walton Centre brochure, I reached for the Neuroplastix workbook Michael Moskowitz had given me and flipped to the last page, where I'd highlighted half the words with a neon orange pen. My eyes went straight to a patch where the orange was darker because I'd gone over that line again and again with the pen until it tore through the paper and into my memory.

'The idea that persistent pain is inevitable and can only be managed is rejected,' it read. I breathed. The panic sank. I regained my control.

GETTING BETTER IS A GOOD THING

I felt purged and holy and ready for a new life.
Sylvia Plath, *The Bell Jar* (1963)

Am I cured, I asked. Am I cured am I cured am I cured.

I asked Michael Moskowitz, Ronald Kulich, Dan Carr, Herbert Benson, Dr Cuong and Jannie. I asked the ladies of Joshua Tree and the doctors of Lourdes. Because after four years of not trusting myself, it was hard to start now. Was I really cured, I asked them all, and if so, why?

'You've found your balance,' said Dr Cuong. He thought John of God might have helped me heal, but my own body had done the healing. It had lost its balance, but somehow in Brazil it had found it again.

Jannie, too, shrank from the C-word, but declared me 'pain-free'. I pressed – why am I pain-free? – and he said, 'No idea.' But Jannie wasn't just an interviewee; he was a psychologist who'd spent months analysing me during the depths of my pain, so I said to him, *why* – what did you notice in me three years ago that could explain what has happened?

'I always enjoyed working with you,' he pandered. 'You want to understand, and you'll try anything.' I thought of the flies dive-bombing me in Soweto as Thabiso and I broke our fast at a post-ceremony braai, congealed chicken blood tanning my face, my hair thickened with entrails.

'You engage with it,' said Jannie, 'but you're also critical. You don't just accept stuff. You say, "I don't want that because it doesn't work for me." You're stubborn – I like that. It never threatened me; it helped.' *Threatened*. It was the first time anyone had used that word.

I'd been sent to Jannie to learn CBT, of course, but had told him at my first appointment that CBT didn't work for me, and he'd listened. I had thought ours a natural patient-doctor relationship but hearing that word, and thinking back to the others, it suddenly occurred to me that maybe it hadn't been.

Had I threatened all those other doctors, I wondered? Had the neurologist felt threatened when I said his drugs were making me suicidal instead of pain-free? Had the anaesthetist felt threatened when I admitted the epidural nerve block hadn't blocked my pain? Had the problem, all along, been them and not me?

'I don't think any doctor wants to make anyone feel worse, but I think we do it all the time, and sometimes it's because we're crappy doctors, and sometimes it's because we've got something against women, sometimes it's because we've got something against women of a certain type, but all that stuff interferes with being a good healer. And a healer's a healer, whether they've got an MD degree or whether they're talking to their ancestors in Soweto.' Michael Moskowitz had said this, when I'd told him how replacing all those middle-aged men with Thabiso had made me think of my pain and myself in a completely new way.

I asked Jannie how, when I'd done everything the books advised – tried to observe my pain instead of pushing it away, be neutral towards it instead of hating it or cleaving to it – it had stayed, shrinkwrapped around me, but as soon as I'd followed Diego's advice and asked the entities to take it away, it had gone.

'Your brain is so powerful,' he said. 'Who knows? Maybe it released endorphins. Maybe there's something else, dynamics happening in that process that we just don't get. We shouldn't assume that we understand everything. We don't.'

I presented myself to Dan Carr as already cured, and asked how people like me did it. 'By a combination of behavioural and physical measures,' he said. 'And the use of whatever agents are needed to enable the person to become progressively more active, whether that's a drug, a nerve block or electrical stimulation.' Or a phalanx of entities, I whispered under my breath. 'The ones who are brought towards mobilisation again are the ones who are cured,' he said. That didn't tally with me, though, because although I was starting to mobilise again now – yoga, walking, navigating airports on foot instead of in a wheelchair – I hadn't done that until I was better. In Abadiania, when I wasn't sitting in the Current I was lying down to recover from it.

I told Ronald Kulich I was better, and asked if I was on the home straight. 'Yes,' he said, simply. He didn't seem surprised – sometimes people just got better. But why, I pushed. Why am I better? Was it Brazil, was it writing down my trauma, was it believing in myself? What's happened to me? *What happened?*

'I don't know,' he said. 'People get better. Sometimes.'

'Even after four years?' I said.

'Yeah.' He paused. 'But also people do things to get better, and they avoid doing things that make themselves worse. They don't have unnecessary surgeries which cause more scar tissue. They don't take medication which can cause GI problems or dependency. Or they mobilise their social supports or their vocational direction, or, you know...'

He looked at me. 'So, getting better is a good thing.'

'It's a great thing,' I said. But I still needed to know why.

He told me I'd shown resiliency, direction and an internal locus of control. Even though I'd flown around the world, telling people to do what they liked with my body, he said I'd been controlling the process. There was nothing he'd observed in me during our interview that might explain why the pain had arrived or why it had disappeared. When I asked what I could do to stop it coming back, he said, 'You're already doing it.'

Herbert Benson put it down to the Current – meditation, or the 'relaxation response', as he calls it. For him, I wasn't a phenomenon, because he'd witnessed similar events with patients who gradually learned that breaking their everyday thoughts could control the pain – and from there, they expanded the pain-free moments. 'The best explanation I have is that by doing away with the pathways that were plaguing you, there was no pain – it was a new learned behaviour,' he said. 'Some would argue that you could rewire pathways that were dominant in the pain experience. We know so little about this reinforcement in the brain, but perhaps a chronic pathway could be altered and sustained over a much longer period.' It made sense, except I'd only done five Current sessions and hadn't meditated since. Could that have been enough?

I went to Michael Moskowitz.

'I'd love to explore this for hours and hours,' he said. 'It's something I can't explain at all. It's fascinating.'

Had I neuroplastically changed my brain without realising? But of course.

'If you had back surgery and your back felt better, it wouldn't be because you had back surgery on your pain, it would be because the surgery fixed your structure well enough that it allowed the stimulus from your back to decrease enough for your brain to alter the way it was sending inflammatory chemicals down your back through the nerve endings, and as that whole loop started to fall apart, that's a neuroplastic change. Your brain's changed, your body's changed, and really it's neuroplasticity and somatoplasticity together, because really this is one thing. Your brain isn't separate from your body. It runs the whole show.'

We combed through every stage of the John of God process. The line in front of the Entity, the prescriptions and the herbs, the spiritual intervention, the 24-hour recovery, the Current and the breakthrough. I told him I'd thought John of God was a fake, maybe even the devil, but that suddenly, heavily, the change had pounced.

'Look, I don't know what happened, but *something* happened,' he said. 'The only thing I can think is that through your thinking "this is ridiculous" and setting the bar very low, when something happened, it was a shock to your system. And you sucked it up and kept doing it, and found something to counterstimulate your pain with. There's no reason for you to be better without something changing. It had to change.'

Maybe not believing it took the pressure off, I said.

'Maybe by resisting,' he said, 'when something *did* change it was clear that it wasn't because you'd been sucked in. And maybe when that change hit, it really grabbed you. And maybe, in that process, some process that's been going on for years just turned. And, you know, the Titanic turned slowly, but when it turned, it *turned*. Something changed, and it happened in your brain, and the way your brain perceived it all and reorganised itself turned this around for you.

'I don't believe in the last part of his name, the "of God" part,' he added. 'And I don't believe in entities. But I do believe John has some ability to help people heal, and he's got techniques that work for a lot of people. People keep flocking to him and some are walking away 80 per cent better, or even better than that. Yet I've known people who've seen him who think it was the most profound experience of their life, and they're still a mess!'

At our first meeting, he'd told me about the kind of patient who comes through his door, 'the elephant's graveyard of pain', as he called it: 'When everybody's been operated on and injected and stimulated and had pumps put in and everything else and it doesn't get them okay, they end up here.' He said his patients are in rough shape, have tried everything, 'John of God, blah blah blah blah blah.'

But why would John of God have worked for me where it hadn't for them?

I had several theories.

Perhaps it was the most boring explanation of all, a regression to the mean. It's a common explanation for why things like chiropractic and homeopathy often seem to work – your embarkation on alternative therapy happens to coincide with your body healing naturally. People just get better, as Ronald Kulich had said.

But I didn't think that made sense in my case, because a regression to the mean implies a gradual process – it's a regression, not a leap back to the mean, after all. And from what we know of the brain – of neuroplasticity, of what's fired is wired – it seemed unlikely that my brain had reset itself so suddenly. Pain from rheumatoid arthritis can burn out once the joints have been crippled, but pain circuits don't just burn out. Every second that they're firing, they're strengthening the connections; mine had fired for 1,464 days, and I could count the number of days they didn't fire, or hardly fired, on my fingers. To think that after so much conditioning – nerves coated with extra myelin to speed up the pain signals, synapses flooded by neurotransmitters, pain circuits swelling across my brain, eroding my coordination, empathy and memory – it would snap back from one second to the next, went against everything we knew about the brain.

Perhaps, as Moskowitz suggested, it was a simple neuro-plastic process. Asking the entities to take away my pain was, after all, very similar to his telling the brain to shut it off, calm things down. I sat through three long Current sessions using this technique – perhaps that was enough to see a difference, and perhaps when it made a difference, I kept doing it. Calm down, shut that off, please take it away. Two processes, same result – the only difference was whether I was pleading with entities or myself.

Perhaps, in a less delineated way, it was a simple placebo effect – 'The desire to be healed did heal; the thirst for a miracle worked the miracle,' in Zola's words. Conventional wisdom dictates that placebo responses can be recognised by their instant uptake and short-lasting benefits, but, as Ronald Kulich told me, that's being rewritten – they can last longer than thought, and studies are showing that they can create physical changes as well as just the mind's impression of them. A permanent placebo response was unlikely, but maybe it had lasted long enough for that neuroplastic rewiring to have taken place. Because it happens in the brain, pain can often be responsive to a placebo effect; though equally, of course, chronic pain patients are normally less receptive.

Perhaps, without realising, I had come to accept the pain. Perhaps Thabiso and her talk of suffering for a reason had kickstarted it, and perhaps in a contrary way, by asking the entities to take it away – throwing myself at their mercy – I was somehow accepting its presence. Perhaps by invoking the entities I had disassociated myself from the pain, something I hadn't done while trying to observe it. By asking them to relieve me, perhaps I'd reduced my somatic focus. I'd felt more fixated on my symptoms as I tried to work out whether they were disappearing with my prayers, of course, but maybe my brain had worked in a slightly different way, as contrary as its mistress. Perhaps that new, forensic attention had helped me get in tune with my body, in the same way that chronic pain patients are often asked to watch their movements in a mirror, literally showing the brain that there's no physical trauma in the hope that it'll reset their system.

Perhaps Thabiso had sparked some kind of existential experience. The early miracles of Lourdes, according to Ruth Harris in *Lourdes: Body and Spirit in the Secular Age*, were largely women who'd been written off by their doctors as hysterical taking charge of their health and declaring themselves cured – part mass hysteria, part placebo, part self-healing and part self-discovery. It's the same story in Salento, where the tarantate women would writhe and dance the pizzica for hours, sometimes for days; they stopped not when they sweated out the tarantula venom, but when they were ready to rejoin polite society.[35] Perhaps, after Soweto, I realised the full extent of the gaslighting – not just the doctors and medicine men, but the people who'd helped me too. In Abadiania, I even saw dear Kevin in a different light – his insistence that you could only be ill if you wanted to was not only upsetting; in a way, it was appropriating my body, too. I didn't want to be ill any more than I wanted to be depressed, and in Abadiania I realised that even those who'd helped me were no wiser than I was – that bigger boat would have to be mine and mine alone. Perhaps that realisation shook some scales from my eyes, and I began to trust the body of myself, six months after Mr Wong had told me to. Perhaps, like the women of Lourdes and Salento, I began to feel better as I listened to my body. Perhaps this was the internalisation of my locus of control.

Perhaps I had taken something from everyone who'd tried to heal me: Charmayne's unalloyed femininity, Kevin's belief, the nameless vicar's concern, Patrick's assurance, Jero Pura's kindness, Dr Good's tirelessness, Dr Cuong's support, the Stanley brothers' optimism, Samba El's quiet confidence, Richard Morse's faith, Mr Wong's empathy, Thabiso's love, John of God's charisma, the inspiration of all the sick and faithful I had seen and all the friends I had met – a gumbo that had come to the boil in Abadiania, made of all the ingredients I needed to heal.

Perhaps it had been the power of ritual: the solemn line to go in front of the Entity, the strict rules about the treatment and the Casa; the biblical 40-day ban on sex and healing post-intervention, and the taking of the passiflora tablets three times a day for months afterwards. The ban on pepper meant Abadiania was on my mind every time I ate. I was engaged in my recovery three times a day. Nine months without booze, rebirthing myself – as a concept, it had power.

Malidoma Somé, an elder of the Dagara tribe of Burkina Faso, has a theory that many of the problems of the modern world stem from a lack of community, that ritual is what holds a people together. Illness is a cry for help from our spirit, he posits in *Ritual: Power, Healing and Community*. Had my pain stopped because during my dark night of the soul in Abadiania I had time to listen to it, as Thabiso had instructed? Had I – who lived and worked alone – joined a community at the Casa? Perhaps.

Perhaps, like the army veterans with their paint pots, I had written the trauma out. Perhaps researching pain and writing about mine up there in my desert hermitage was the ultimate catharsis – because after that first, seismic tremor in Abadiania, the aftershock had come that morning in Joshua Tree. Perhaps my brain had been waiting for me to start writing before it flicked the switch. Perhaps I'd been holding on to my pain for four years because I wasn't working. Perhaps I'd clung on to it once I'd got the book contract, because I subconsciously panicked that if I got better I'd have nothing to write about.

Perhaps I was like those people who say they were fed up with online dating and reluctantly decided to meet one more person and what-do-you-know *he was the one!* I'd already decided that Brazil was going to be my last date with destiny, at least for a while – if it didn't work out, I planned to retreat home and think about acceptance. Perhaps that gave my subconscious the urgency to let things happen. Perhaps the potential humiliation of having to admit that I'd scoured five continents and still not found Him told me, get going, this has to be it. Perhaps it was my grandmother, my sangomic calling. Perhaps, perhaps, perhaps. I was willing to entertain all kinds of crazy possibilities, as long as it didn't mean examining the elephant in the room. Because the one 'perhaps' I couldn't quite bring myself to think about was the simplest of them all.

That perhaps on the fourth day in Abadiania, a phalanx of entities had performed a spiritual operation on me, and on the seventh day after that they had performed a healing, flicked a switch inside my head, and on the fortieth day – the day on which tradition said they fine-tuned their work – they had effected an incontrovertible cure.

'In 2015, I interviewed 110 people in this office,' Alessandro de Franciscis told me in the Lourdes Medical Bureau. 'They came to me to say they felt they were cured. Among these were people who were sort of disturbed, very tired, perhaps psychologically – I don't know. But I have retained, I have judged, *because I am a physician*' – I was amused by the constant insistence of medical authority from a man who led prayer meetings, welcomed bishops and had already shown me the clutch of saintly portraits he carried around in his wallet – '32 as being trustworthy. Stories that I think were, you know ... possibly real.'

Thirty-two miracles in one season, out of six million pilgrims – hardly astonishing. Still, it depended which ailments had been miracled. Show me an MS cure – which, supposedly, the shrine specialised in these days – and I'd be impressed.

He had asked all 32 to send in their medical files so he could investigate further, but as of 29 July 2016, not a single one had sent a thing.

'I've no way of proving it, but I think people come to my office as a way of thanking Our Lady, but they're not interested in proving that their cure is unexplained, nor willing to get into the annoying process of studying their cure which might one day be proclaimed a miracle. Do you see?'

The day before, when Kerry Jones had been telling me about miracles, she'd told me that she'd often witnessed little ones, but people chose not to report them. She thought it was probably because miracles were a private thing, she said, between the person and God. Someone being given one didn't want to be interrogated by doctors, called a fantasist by people who didn't believe, or fawned over by those who did. Also, they didn't want to tempt fate. I had expressed my surprise.

'Well, would you report it?' she had asked.

'Of course!' I had scoffed.

And there in Sandro's office – Virgin and Child looming over my left shoulder, four framed photos of him embracing Pope John Paul II on the wall above – I realised that of course I wouldn't report it. Did I want people to think I was mad?

I thought of Kevin's message – *you got your miracle!!!* – and my discomfort, my fear of tempting fate and doubt. The potential shame when it all unravelled.

I thought of Zee, hugging me goodbye at Johannesburg

airport, urging me not to talk to people back home about what had happened until I had processed it.

I had called Zee, as it happened, from my hermitage in Joshua Tree, one day when I was pushing myself towards a breakdown, going round and round in circles trying to unpick what had happened. And he'd told me a story he'd told me before, a tale that started with him wanting to die and ended with him wanting to live, with a cameo from the underworld in between.

'I remember telling you,' he said, 'that I never tell people that story. Because it was really real to me, and it really happened, and I don't need to convince anybody else that it happened. If anything, they're just going to try to convince me that it didn't.

'Once you've had an experience like that, it's not even important to try and prove it to anybody else, as long as it's real to you,' he'd said, his voice bouncing across oceans and continents, Johannesburg to Joshua Tree. 'You're the only one that counts. What matters most is that you need to believe what you're believing, you know? You need to believe what you're going through.'

I went to the grotto on my way out of Alessandro's office, the simple cave-turned-paved-chapel where, on 11 February 1858, Bernadette Soubirous had seen 'uo petito damizelo', a little lady, dressed in white and a ravishing smile. I still had concussion from the fall – vertigo, black spots sculling across my eyes, a piercing headache and a sore back. The line to enter the grotto and run your hand along its damp walls was about 300 deep, and this being Lourdes, there was no priority line for cripples. So I sat and watched instead.

Italian grannies wiping their hankies along the rock to extract the magic wetness. Teenage volunteers wheeling elderly people through its shallow recess. A slow-moving woman extricating an arm from a crutch to reach up and stroke an inch of rock nobody else had contaminated. The white dress and blue sash of the Carrara marble statue that perches in the niche – 'That's not her,' Bernadette was reported to have cried when it was unveiled. It wasn't me, either.

I went to find Kerry.

She told me about her son who'd been in intensive care for four months and survived against all odds. When he recovered, he gave thanks to Our Lady of Lourdes, not because she had saved him, but for giving him the strength to survive.

'We couldn't call that a miracle because he had the best medical care,' she said. 'It was a medical miracle, not a religious miracle.'

'Do you think "miracle" is overused?' I asked.

'Well, they actually try to refrain from using it these days,' she said. 'I don't know whether Dr Sandro told you but they don't call them miracles any more.'

'What do they call them?'

'Well, "inexplicable healings" is one of the definitions—'

'I like that,' I interrupted. 'I'm going to say that's what I have, an inexplicable healing.'

'Well, it's exactly that isn't it?' she said. 'You don't know how it happened. You just know that one minute you were ill, the next you weren't. It's an inexplicable healing.'

I thought, really, that's what Ronald Kulich and Michael Moskowitz and Jannie were all saying. We agree you're better, but we can't explain why.

'There's so much we don't know, isn't there?' Kerry was saying. 'There's so much in science that we can't explain, and maybe we were never meant to understand everything. Although we do all try.'

I told her about the people – friends, colleagues, strangers, interviewees, real experts and self-appointed experts – who'd told me just to accept the fact that I was better. But I couldn't accept it without knowing what had happened.

'Like, who am I even supposed to be thanking?' I said.

'Well it's dead simple to me,' she said. 'God decided you needed the help to get better and you got that help. I can accept that' – she saw me looking bilious – 'but that's what faith's all about, isn't it? Accepting the things you can't rationalise. That's an inexplicable healing to me.'

An inexplicable healing.

I needed a drink but I couldn't drink, what with the concussion and the John of God rebirthing pills, so I went to a bistro and had two jam-smothered crepes instead. Then I staggered back up the near-sheer hill, which Bernadette had trotted down that February morning on her way to collect firewood at the Massabielle cave. Past the Lourdes Wax Museum containing scenes from the lives of Bernadette and Jesus, past identical shops selling Lourdes mugs and towels and statues and water features, hologram Christs which seemed to wink, pens which Virgin Marys poledanced up and down as you wrote, mints made with grotto water. I hauled myself up to the apartment I had rented overlooking Lourdes Castle, and lay in bed as the flat spun around me.

I lay there for the best part of two days, waiting for the spots to retreat from my vision, for the drill in my head to switch off, wondering – for my somatic focus remained strong – whether this really was concussion or if my brain was slowly bleeding out. I read the testimony of Jean-Pierre Bély, a wheelchair-bound MS patient who was inexplicably healed in 1987. As a devout Catholic, he'd known better than to beg for a miracle, and had gone to Lourdes asking only for what the Lord had in store. During the blessing of the sick ceremony – the procession I'd watched roll into the underground church and had walked away from, slightly sickened – he felt 'as if he'd been whisked off in a dream'. Back in his dormitory – for in Lourdes, the malades sleep in dorms, not individual rooms – he heard a voice: 'Lève-toi et marche!' Get up and walk!

'I stay there, sitting down, trying to understand what just happened to me,' he wrote in his testimony. 'Why me and not another, sicker than me?' Out of respect to the others, he said nothing till he got home, when he walked up the steps of his house and into his life again. Tests confirmed he was completely cured.

Jean-Pierre Bély was recognised as an inexplicable healing in 1999. Until his death – in 2005, of causes unrelated to MS – he acted as unofficial ambassador for Lourdes (there was nothing else to do, really, because having been signed off as disabled for life, he could never be declared fit for work again). He was a believer well before his healing, but even he was reluctant to report his miracle.

'I wasn't much inclined to enter into this long and difficult process,' he wrote. 'The procedure lasted 11 years, 11 long years of exams, of meetings, of medical reports, of checks. A real obstacle course... Every time I was tempted to call a halt to it, the thought came to mind that I didn't have the right, because this token did not belong to me.'

I thought of my fellow COPE victims. This token did not belong to me.

On the third day, I asked Jenny Klimiuk what had happened to me.

'Umm, I don't know,' she said. 'It's interesting because you had that very sudden thing which a lot of people don't always experience.'

She looked at me.

'And you said you didn't feel better at all up to that point, is that right?'

I'd had my moments, I said, and I had always tried to make them into something, but they would always go.

'And you're asking everybody what they think? If someone came to me and asked me that, I would say I thought that was miraculous,' she said breezily and the M-word caught in my throat.

'You're the first person who's said that,' I said quickly, hoping she'd take it back.

'Really?' said Jenny.

'All the other doctors said, "I don't know",' I said, daring her to retract it because she, of course, was a doctor, too. 'Someone said it was regression to the mean.' We looked at each other.

'You really would think that?' I said in a small voice.

'Yes, definitely,' she said. 'From everything you've said and the experience that you had, yeah I would definitely say that. I'm interested that nobody else has said it.'

Another doctor from her pilgrimage, Claire, sat down beside her.

'That's my – that's how I honestly feel,' said Jenny.

'I'd better start being more devout then,' I said. 'Haha!' They laughed awkwardly.

And a memory I'd tried to bury suddenly bounced up like Baron Samedi from the grave: of the first weeks after I'd left Abadiania, when I was feeling so much better but could also feel the travel and the work and the stress and exhaustion making me worse, dragging me back to the Julia I'd come to know. I remembered the crystal I'd set beside my bed, and the picture of Dr Augusto de Almeida I'd slipped into my bag, and the blessed water I was carrying around with me (because blessed water was like yeast, you could dilute it with one part blessed to one part normal water, and it would automatically bless the normal water – at least, that's what John of God said), and the thanks that I'd say each night and every morning.

I wasn't sure when I'd stopped doing all that, but at some point in London, in grief, it had all been put away.

'I was for a bit,' I said quietly. 'Being all devout. But so many people were saying it's the placebo effect.'

'But the most important thing is what you think, not what someone else thinks,' said Claire. 'And if you think it was that, then that's what it was. For some things, you can't scientifically prove whether it's happened or not, and the most important thing is what the person it's happened to thinks. That's the only thing that's relevant.'

She talked about the idea of the doctor herself being a drug – an idea that went back to Hippocrates, 'until recently ... the physician's most important tool', according to Herbert Benson. 'It's absolutely true,' Claire said. 'Sometimes people come to see a doctor, and you basically haven't done anything but listened, yet they're healed.'

It was the placebo effect again – remembered wellness – or maybe it was the mind-body link, finding your balance, or even neuroplasticity, but ultimately it didn't matter. All that mattered was getting better.

'All we're interested in really, as doctors, is making people feel better,' said Claire. 'Just remember that what works for one person might not work for someone else.' Jannie had said a similar thing: 'Some interventions work for some people.' Don't go sending people to Brazil, he meant, but sending people to Brazil would be taking what had happened to me too lightly. It may have happened in Brazil, but it had started elsewhere. Good and bad, I'd taken something from all my experiences, right from my first diagnosis.

If I could lose the connotations, I realised, saying goodbye to Jenny and Claire, I liked the idea of a miracle because nobody could take that away from me, not even my brain. A miracle was for life. It couldn't slip away.

The Salford Diocese was going to take part in the procession of the Blessed Sacrament later – the one that had made me feel queasy and delivered Jean-Pierre Bély his inexplicable healing. It was where many healings took place, and Jenny thought I should go. I said I was too concussed. But when I got back to the flat, I thought, I can't go to Lourdes without seeing the blessing of the sick. I hadn't been to the church, I hadn't set foot in the grotto, I hadn't seen Bernadette's solitary rib in its reliquary; I hadn't done anything, this time, except walk into a wall, spend two evenings in hospital, and wonder how Ryanair would repatriate me if I died of a brain haemorrhage.

So at 5pm I followed the crowds into the basilica of St Pius X, an underground spaceship held up by whalebone arches, where the priests arrived to a literal fanfare and a screen beside the altar streamed a live feed from the grotto.

Row upon row of hard benches fanned out ahead of me – there were no creature comforts here, even in worship. I crept nearer the altar, where there was a clutch of pews with backs. Token malades – because although on a personal level, pilgrims were treated as people, to the church they were still The Sick – were drawn up at the front of each section, facing the altar.

Jean-Pierre Bély had been anointed, he wrote in his testimony, but today there was no anointing – just the holy wafer, spotlit in a gold case, processed around the congregation by a group of priests so dramatically that my neighbour began to film it on his mobile phone.

They walked up through the middle of the main aisle and snaked round the sides. They turned to every block of seats at every angle, brandishing the Blessed Sacrament at us. The congregation bowed their heads and crossed themselves. I thought of Jean-Pierre Bély, and of Zola.

The Blessed Sacrament was on its second turn, winding back towards the altar, when I saw him amongst the malades. It approached from behind but he could feel it coming, as everyone in the room could feel it, even I could feel it, because the atmosphere was bristling with hope and the Blessed Sacrament was like a magnet, bending us towards it like iron filings. He was in a wheelchair with a rug over his knees, and as the Blessed Sacrament went by, he heaved himself onto his feet, shaking with the struggle. I caught my breath.

Images raced through my brain: of Patrick, circling his finger at me, of John of God flinging people's crutches asunder, of Jean-Pierre Bély sauntering up the steps of his home. The women of early Lourdes uncoiling from their chairs and following the holy wafer, Zola's heroine, Marie de Guersaint, leaping up – inexplicably cured, or maybe not so inexplicably, according to the novel, which puts it down to the power of the mind.

Lève-toi et marche! Get up and walk!

As the Blessed Sacrament moved on, he struggled back down.

COMPLETELY NORMAL

The Lourdes miracles can neither be proved or denied.
Emile Zola, *Lourdes* (1894)

Before I went home, I played my brain scan.

There were two of them, both taken in Lourdes, one the night I slammed my head into the wall, and one the following evening, when I was still concussed and the doctor wanted to be sure I was okay.

At least, he said he wanted to be sure, but by the time I looked at the scans, I realised he had probably been sure all along, and just wanted to reassure me.

I had known he was a different kind of doctor from the moment he walked in. He was the polar opposite of the one the night before.

Instead of looking harried, he swept in with a business-like rush. He made eye contact as he said hello, as if I were a person not a patient. He'd started in French and so I'd tried to continue, telling him how I had *tombéed* yesterday, scrabbling around for my schoolgirl vocabulary. 'Je suis désolée,' I said, regressing to the sixth form. 'Mon français c'est affreux!'

'Je le trouve charmant,' he said, looking up from his notes with a genuine smile, and I thought, this is the real miracle of Lourdes, a doctor who realises I'm a human being.

Of course, when it became clear that his impeccable English was leagues ahead of my French, we switched languages, but he did it so daintily I didn't feel a bruise.

I explained I wasn't a hypochondriac, that I hadn't wanted to come back, but the doctors at the grotto had insisted. I gave him my medical history: hypermobility, easy bruising,

EDS, POTS. I said confusedly that I'd had chronic pain for four years and I thought it was gone but was concerned this might resurrect it – because I could hear the thrum of my mustang's hooves, already feeling for its old paths – and as I said it, he scrunched up his face with such empathy that I thought I might cry.

When they'd told me at the grotto that I had to go back, my Pavlovian response to hospitals and doctors had started up: balloon expanding in my throat, bats circling in my stomach, hyperventilation, tears. Now I was starting to wonder if I'd been sent back for a reason, to see how it should be.

I was concerned because I was alone, I said – I wasn't with a pilgrimage, nobody would know if my brain bled out in my sleep and I never woke up. The night before, I'd locked the door but taken the key out in case I died and my landlady had to come in to retrieve my body.

What on earth are you doing in Lourdes alone, he asked – are you a pilgrim or a tourist? When I told him why I was there, he asked if I'd been to the meeting that week about the case of the person who appeared to have been cured – of MS, he thought, though he wasn't sure because he hadn't gone.

You, the A&E doctor, go to meetings about miracles, I screeched, *bouleversée* (another integral word in my French vocabulary).

Of course, he said with a Gallic shrug, as if only the concussed could find that strange. He tested my reflexes, my eyes and my strength, made me puff out my cheeks to check I wasn't lopsided and follow his finger around the room. And then he said, I think everything is fine, but would you like another CT scan, just to be sure?

Yes, I said, yes please, because Kerry had drawn me a diagram of a late-starting brain haemorrhage and it was etched onto my eyeballs.

He made a phone call in front of me, explaining the situation, and I heard he was taking it seriously – vertigo and vision impairment after a head injury – not putting me down.

He explained that there was no radiographer on duty at Lourdes so it would be emailed to someone in some central French hospital, but he was calling them to flag it up and to make sure they compared it to the previous night's scan.

And then we talked miracles.

He didn't think they were ridiculous. He didn't think it was dangerous to talk about them, or to lure people to Lourdes in search of one.

'This is hope, makes you live, maybe tomorrow can be better,' he said. 'When you have faith in something it makes you maybe stronger and then you can overcome things until the next thing, the big thing.

'You know,' he said. 'This is life.'

'So if you had a patient who wanted to try the piscines, you wouldn't think they're stupid?' I asked, baffled. I thought of the foot specialist dealing with the neuritis of my sural nerve. It had inexplicably healed and he couldn't think why, and when I'd mentioned Patrick he'd snorted, 'I hope you're not paying him too much.' Of course, I'd paid less to see Patrick and spend three days in Vienna than I had for two 30-minute sessions in his Mayfair office.

'Why would I say it's stupid?' said the doctor. 'This is very judgemental. You can say, "Okay, here is what science today can offer." You can either help or not. If you cannot help, you've tried everything, yes, you can go. Go. Why would I say no? Maybe I would not go for myself, but I cannot prevent someone from going, or say to someone, "Don't go". We can all be together with different beliefs.'

You have to accept you already have a diagnosis, Julia, and the pain might never go away.

'This is stupid,' said the doctor. 'I mean, look. What you are now shows your doctors to be wrong.'

It's just a flare-up.

'When it comes to science, we can say, "Our reasonable expectation is this." But there are things that I do not know today. There are so many things! Maybe we know 10 per cent. That means there is 90 per cent to discover.'

Don't be so angry.

'One must have some humility and say, okay, I know things but what I am sure I know is that I do not know everything.'

You're hurting the group.

'So, okay, if I don't know or if I cannot help, maybe someone else can help, and if it's a belief in miracles, in a religion, in holy things, why not? Why not?'

It's okay to be depressed.

'Yes, science can help, can help in many things, but it can also be very – how you say, *impuissant*?'

'Powerful?'

'Non non non, the opposite. And if it cannot help in a particular situation, you turn to something else that might help. And this is hope.'

'Hope is important.'

'It is very important.'

'That's what keeps us going.'

'Yes, in every aspect of life.'

'Yeah.'

'If you have no hope that tomorrow will be better...' he laughed, drew a finger across his throat and went, *splat*.

'Well, exactly,' I said.

'What is really funny about doctors,' he said – and a bell rang in the background, calling him for something more urgent than a discussion about miracles, maybe to perform a miracle of his own – 'they have an ego that is so inflated, that is so big, that they have the impression they know everything.'

Think of a job you've always wanted to do that doesn't involve your hands.

'We have to be very careful about this. We know many things, but we are far from what we still need to know.'

There's no way this drug can be making you suicidal.

'And what you'll know in five years' time,' I said, and he said, 'Yes, yes!'

If you only stop worrying, you'll be absolutely fine.

'There are so many things to discover, and even our ways of doing things sometimes turn out to be not so effective or so good. We keep on discovering things.'

He stood up.

'So it is evolving and let's be humble and think that tomorrow can bring us a lot of things, instead of thinking, oh I know everything, don't go there, don't do this. I mean, of course there are things we know of, but we cannot ... I mean, for disease, "Don't go to see Lourdes, you won't get anything from this..."' He blew a little raspberry. 'I don't know, I don't know. Probably not, but if there's a tiny, tiny, tiny possibility ...'

'If it doesn't hurt you,' I said.

'Yes, it doesn't hurt you,' he said. 'And people are ... you know, life is so dear to the human being. They will do everything just to stay alive.'

'Stop,' I said. 'You'll make me cry.' But I was already crying.

The night before, they had dumped me on a trolley in the corridor for five hours as I drifted in and out of consciousness, hallucinating the face of Bernadette onto a girl in shorts and dreadlocks as she paced the corridor. But tonight, he let me stay in the little private room to read my book and charge my phone, as civilised as I'd always imagined a French hospital might be. Then he came back in, grinning.

'It's all fine,' he said. 'Your brain is completely normal.' He'd made a copy of the report, and went over it with me to make sure I could understand the French. I thought, in England no one has been this assiduous even when I'm paying them £300.

Your brain is completely normal.

The next day, I went back to collect the scans, two CDs inscribed with 'Centre Hospitalier de Lourdes' and filed in a pink envelope. I told them Dr Good would need them, but that was a lie. I needed them to meet my nemesis of the past four years.

I played the first, which was actually the second, the one that the kind doctor had gone over with me.

I was expecting stills but it was more like a video, delicate slices of my brain running into each other, from my spinal cord to the top of my head.

TECHNIQUE: *CT scan of the skull and contents, without injection of a contrast agent.*

My brain ebbed and flowed, each picture dissolving into the next as if it were breathing. Here was the round, solid spinal cord, here was the nose I'd hated for three decades, a long bony beak. There were my eyes, quivering like jelly. And here was my brain, my completely normal brain. Maybe I could make out the lobes, right at the bottom, and there, imperceptible, was the dividing line between the hemispheres, but mostly it just looked slate grey and dense, with its thick, white corona of bone. Unremarkable. Completely normal.

RESULTS: *Absence of subdural or epidural haematoma. No signs of cerebral contusion. No signs of ischemic or haemorrhagic stroke.*

Within that dense grey cloud were neurons blazing, neurotransmitters arcing across 1000 trillion synapses, millions of networks being made and broken as the CAT scan sieved through it.

No sign of extradural haemorrhage or of venous thrombosis. No midline shift.

Somewhere towards the bottom was my timorous amygdala, seat of my pain and outgoing governor of my body after its four-year term. Somewhere above it was my insula, dripping soothing GABA (my favourite neurotransmitter) onto the amygdala in a bid to calm it down. It's okay, I'd told my brain, lying there in the CT doughnut; nothing's wrong, this isn't as bad as an MRI and you'll never be in here again – calm down. Somewhere above my eyes was the orbital frontal cortex, finally reclaiming its areas of empathy, emotion and decision-making.

> No *intracranial expansive process. No anomaly of the paranasal sinus.*

And as the scan rose up, a face emerged like a will-o'-the-wisp: shadows in the lobes flickering into life that made a smiley face turn into a scowl turn into an expression of shock and then a giant grin as the pictures flicked past, and I had an urge to call it a sly little shit, berate it for what it had done to me, tell it how it had nearly finished us both, but I looked at it – its impish grin created from some cavities, maybe, or lighter matter, or just a trick of the camera – and then I smiled back.

> CONCLUSION: *Satisfactory examination with no traumatic cerebral abnormality.*

You are completely normal, I whispered to it.

I put the CD back in its pink envelope. I didn't need to play the other one.

Afterword

*I had known the pain, and survived it. It only
remained for me to give it voice, to share it
for use, that the pain not be wasted.*
Audre Lorde, *The Cancer Journals* (1980)

'Write what you like as long as it's true,' said John of God, or
whichever entity was possessing John of God that last time I
saw him. So this is my truth.

When I started this book – after Kevin, before Patrick – it
was a means to an end, a foolproof way to flush out The
One, the real miracle worker. It didn't matter to me whether
he – because I, too, had Yentl Syndrome, and always assumed
The One would be a he – was a doctor or a faith healer,
an ancient medicine man in the mountains of China or a
top-brass neuroscientist. I wasn't disavowing all medicine – I
think medicine is great. I just knew that the current medical
setup for pain in the UK wasn't working for me. More than
that; it was killing me.

I'd assumed that once I signed the contract, everyone
would want to talk to me and I could pick and choose my
miracle. I was wrong.

As I progressed – the travel, the interview rejections, the
treatment failures – it occurred to me that maybe I wasn't
going to find Him, and that thought was unbearable. I
postponed the book deadline twice – unable to write it
physically, but also mentally. It would have to become a
book about acceptance, I realised, but I didn't want to write
a book about acceptance, because acceptance was failure,
and I feared that putting my failure into print would sound

my death knell. It was something I was grappling with as I boarded the plane to Brazil.

I don't know what happened, and I don't know why or how it happened. But I know something happened while I was in Abadiania, and I know it was seismic and lasting. It didn't just turn my Titanic, as Michael Moskowitz would say; it peeled it off the iceberg, plugged up the hole and set it back on course.

It was life-changing however you look at it, whatever you think happened, because it meant that everything my doctors had told me about my condition was wrong.

But then, I think they've got chronic pain all wrong. I think our doctors are currently sentencing up to half the British population to life in pain – whether that's relentless pain, persistent pain, pain that migrates round the body as they chase it with operation after operation, or pain that submits, at first, to medication, but then comes roaring back, stronger than before.

I think telling us to accept it, to manage our pain and our lives around it, is the wrong approach because it strips us of our hope, and hope is what every one of us needs in order to put one foot in front of the other.

And I think they're wrong to say that pain doesn't kill you, because one look at the suicide rates will show you that it does.

I think the way we treat pain in this country should be a national disgrace, but because we can't really understand it – like my cousin, who couldn't fathom that I could be talking, eating, drinking while fire ants raced up and down my arm and a palette knife cleaved my vertebrae apart – we shove it under the carpet and try to tread it down. And I know that doesn't work.

I think the link between body and mind is Olympian strong and it doesn't help anyone when sceptics dismiss it or write off the placebo effect as something shameful or embarrassing.

I don't believe there exists a panacea for pain – not

336

neuroplasticity, not genetic testing, not precision-targeted medicine. I don't believe entities are necessarily the answer, nor ancestors, nor qi reserves. I certainly don't think anyone should be rushing to John of God thinking he's going to wave a magic wand at them, whether it's for pain or for anything else. What works for one person doesn't work for another – Kevin gave me my life back, but did nothing for a friend of mine's back pain. I believe that when it comes to reprogramming your errant brain, you have to find what works for you. But I know that you can.

If you're reading this and you have pain, know that your pain is real and it's not your fault. It's not because you have a pain personality or because you ate too many cakes, because you're angry or because you cry a lot for the life you've lost.

You are not to blame for your illness. Sometimes people will say you are because they can't explain it, because they feel powerless, or because it makes them feel safer and more in control. But you don't get cancer because you repressed your emotions, you don't have a stroke because you're not in tune with your higher self, you don't grow a lesion on your brain because you secretly want to. You didn't choose pain, either. And if someone says that you did, it reveals more about them than about you.

If someone doesn't cure you, it's not your fault. Never let anyone tell you otherwise.

Never let anyone make you feel bad if you don't respond to something that works for others, because every body is different and every brain is different. CBT works for 80 per cent of people, they say, but it didn't work for me. Acceptance is the cornerstone of bettering your pain, they write, but I couldn't accept it, and still I got better. You know your body best, and only you can feel its ebbs and flows. Don't take anything as gospel; play around and see what works for you. You will find something, if you can only hold on. Keep going, as my Swedish Kate Middleton would urge us every day in the Current. The wound is where the light goes in.

337

And when it does go in, let it in. Accept it and work it out and work on it until it stays.

It was in Boston, the medical capital of the world, that I accepted my inexplicable healing. I had planned to go there to find an answer, and by the time I boarded my flight I had found my answer and just needed an explanation, and then when I got there and listened to the lectures about pain at Harvard Medical School, and talked to eminent doctors about the history of pain and the future of pain and the current best practice for pain, I realised that I would never get an explanation, but also that I didn't really need one.

Waiting between interviews one day, I parked on Boston Common and walked up Boylston Street where two pressure cooker bombs had exploded in April 2013 near the finishing line of the Boston Marathon. There was no memorial; just photos of the victims and a single trainer tied to a nondescript tree at one of the sites. The mangled pavement beside it had been filled in with a concrete block, and unofficial tributes graffitied onto it with marker pen were fading to nothingness. People were walking past clutching shopping bags and mobile phones. Nobody stopped. Nobody went around the concrete block; they walked over it. The scar was there, and it would always be there, but life carried on, on Boylston Street, because people were choosing to carry on. I would never get back my four lost years, and I would see them every time I looked in the mirror – in the grey hairs and frown lines that the pain had delivered me, in the jowls that had crept up on me as I ate to forget. But I could choose to carry on.

Ronald Kulich was the last of my interviews. He had agreed I was cured, and I hadn't expected him to say that, and so I had hovered round him, not wanting to go, even as our interview had finished and he'd ushered me into the corridor. 'You're already doing it,' he'd said, when I'd asked what I could do to nail my recovery, and now I stood there as if he'd sprayed perfume into the air, unable to leave until it settled on my hair and soaked through my pores.

Goodbye, he said three times before I walked out, past a thin, white sixtysomething, back stiff, legs held apart, the stance of someone who's found their comfort and daren't let it go. He watched me pass with a look I knew well – terror mixed with a pinch of hope. His wife held his arm, looking concerned: reinforcing his pain, the textbooks would say. I smiled at them and walked out, across the corridor to the toilet, and I pulled the lid down and sat there with my head on my knees and let the tears roll out.

I was scared to leave, in a way, in case it broke the spell, but eventually I hauled myself up and took the lift down. I stood there for a second, not quite daring to move. A young man in scrubs and a woman in a sensible dress – a registrar, I decided, from her demeanour – manoeuvred past me to reach the lift I was blocking. We smiled at each other: blank smiles, professional smiles, hospital smiles.

And then I pumped some antibacterial gel on my hands and walked out of their world and into mine. It was Monday 27 June 2016, 1,504 days since the pain had arrived, and this time, it really was over. I had done it. I hope you can do it too.

Acknowledgements

It was surprisingly easy to write this book, but often unbearable to live. Thank you to everyone who put up with me during my lost years – I know it wasn't easy.

I had an extraordinary amount of support with this book, and am hugely grateful to everyone who helped me shape it. Where to start?

Huge thanks to all those who gave me their time and expertise. Even if your contributions were lost in the edit, everything you told me informed what I wrote, and I am so grateful – particularly to Prof Robert Lemelson, Dr Cheryl Louw, Lucy from Denver and Frank Pellett in Salt Lake City. Ryan Kingsbury, Paige Figi and Jesse and Joel Stanley – you were the first to agree to be interviewed and I can't thank you enough for getting the ball rolling. Thank you to everyone at Realm of Caring who shared their stories with me.

An extraordinary number of people gave their time and energy into helping me plan trips and make introductions: Mikey Adekunle Abegunde, Julia Barber, Julie Bell, John Bowker, Catherine Crawley, Olivia Cruz Ramonet, Mary Daley, Chiara di Giorgio, Laurence Donaghy, Cynthia Drescher, Allison Duck, Jean-Paul Duvivier, Dawn Emery, Chris Farmer, Eva Fisher, Daniel Hayward, Jennifer Hoogewerf-McComb, Jason Huque, David and Barbara Keith, Folarin Kuku, Jas Lehal, Lori Miller, Elizabeth Pierre-Louis, Bertus Louw, Sarah O'Kane, Giulio Siena, Kate Simon, Jin Shiwei and Andrew Sutton, Natalie Trice, Clementine Wallop, Louise Whitworth, Salvo Xerri, Jacqui Labrom, Jean Sacra Sean Roubens (Serge) and Geffrard of Voyages Lumières, Shradha and all at the Samarpan Foundation,

Katie Dingle, Victoria Hall and Nicky Hallows of Nute Veterinary Surgery. Josh Neicho and Don Levett – I won't hold it against you. Thank you all for your logistical generosity, and apologies for any names I've left out.

To my army of Amazonian transcribers, of both interviews and notes: Allie Dickinson, Elizabeth Rushe, Jamie Constance and Steph Towan, Noor Al-Samarrai, Ashley Steves. Thank you so much for never (as far as I know) blanching.

My medical advisors who answered my idiot questions with immense grace and fact-checked my unscientific prose – any remaining errors are on me. Thanks to Stephen Adcock, John Lee Alan, Melissa Ford, Chris Howarth and Charles Stillman. Charlie Wilson translated my French brain scan.

To all the professionals who fact-checked things for me and gave me their take on what I was seeing: Tim Waters for botany advice, Fiona Chow (and parents) on herbal tea, Charles Gittins, Joseph McAuley and Mark Thakkar for grammar pedantry and linguistics, Jo Joyce for legal stuff, Eileen Smith on Brazilian Portuguese, Scott Roeben and Elena Ray for your soft-lense skills. Special thanks to Lilit Marcus for a feminist reading list that focused my direction and radicalised me via Kindle, and the super-sub Don Connigale.

Many people showed incredible generosity of resources – without which I'd never have been able to complete this. Thank you so much: Bailey Claire and Carl Schmidt of Capitol Hill Mansion in Denver (not the B&B described in the book), LUX Lijiang, Two Bunch Palms in Desert Hot Springs, Rowan Bouwer at Glen Afric Lodge, and Ajay Goyal at Zening Cyprus, for your generosity. Iluh and Ketut of Villa Rumah Surga in Ubud – I miss you.

When I had nowhere to write apart from a shed that rained on the inside, these people gave me shelter. Thanks to John Schuster and Clea Benson of the Modernist Cabin in Joshua Tree, Bev and Geoff Munsey of Knighton Farm in Exmoor, and Marcello Murzilli of Eremito in Umbria for your generosity. Being able to work in a place of peace changed everything for me.

Jessica Barrett, Luke Blackall and Francesca Hornak: you probably won't remember the day I was venting at you about what my life had become, and one of you suggested I write about it – but I do. Sophie Buchan, who pushed me to write, insisted I should and could do this, and hung around for the fallout. I'm still undecided whether this is a thanks or a thanks for nothing, but either way, this is on you four.

To those who were generous enough to read the initial beast of a manuscript and give insightful and honest feedback: Beth JoJack, Sue Carthew, Jude Randall, Claire Dodd, John Morphew, Karen Silver, Stephen Adcock.

Thank you Ed Wilson, my agent, who took me on when I was completely pain-brained, and believed in this from the start. Thank you Bea Hemming for seeing the potential in it and supporting me well past the point you needed to – I will forever be grateful. Thank you to my editor Jenny Lord for seeing the wood for the trees and showing me how to trim an obese first draft to merely chubby. Thank you to Becca Allen, Elizabeth Allen, Cait Davies, Katie Espiner, Holly Harley, Jennifer Kerslake, Maddie Mogford, Alan Samson and Paul Stark at W&N.

Every time I thought I couldn't do this, someone stepped in to tell me I could and should, normally without realising the effect they had. Thank you for taking an interest: Kate Adams-Dobos, Kelly Eroglu, Jennifer Fenner, Micaela Scapin, Christopher Storey, Lucie Lamster Thury. Sue Carthew – you've been like a second mother. Christine Williams and Made Reni, I'm sorry I didn't finish in time.

For pastoral support at various points: Ravneet Ahluwalia, Tim Ayles, Theresa Boggan, Janine Clagett, Oriana Fox, Duncan Harris, Alex Heybourne, Tony Horkins, Johnny Jones, Missy Krehbiel, Mike Lanning, Léa Shu, Sheryl Long, Marc Meltzer, Gillian Nicholls, Nancy Nishihira and Alex Pontois, Nick Randall, Michelle Rodriguez, 'Tommaso', Thula 'Zee' Cube. For murdering my writer's block: Wanita

Holmes. For hand-holding through the publishing labyrinth: Chris Beanland, Damian Barr, Rob Cowen, Matt Greene, Ruth Fowler, Laura James, Belinda Jones, Laura Tait, Andy Barr of Belgravia Books and Anna Davidson of the Wadebridge Bookshop.

Thank you to all those I met on the way. Gabriele d'Annunzio and the Libreria Acqua Alta for *Notturno*, Padre Adriano Campesato for our chats in San Francesco della Vigna, San Salvatore in Lauro for a bloodied glove. My mentor Norm Clarke, who has taught me so much.

Special thanks to those who supported me professionally while I was ill and struggling, and didn't cut me off when I filed late: Frank Barrett, Katie Bowman, everyone at National Geographic Traveller. Laura Chubb and Dave Maclean at The Independent for taking a chance on a four-year career break.

'Dr Good' and Stephen Adcock (again) – you are the best ambassadors the NHS could hope to have. Dr Cuong, Stella Durnall, Jannie Van Der Merwe – thank you. Michael Moskowitz – thank you for telling me I had something worth saying. It meant a lot. Dr Fouad Cheddadi – your kindness still brings me to tears. Thank you so much.

Kevin Ackad: thank you forever for saving my life.

To everyone featured in the book, thank you so much for your time and expertise – even if we didn't agree, you gave me a new perspective. To those who gave me hope or opened my eyes, thank you. Thabiso Siswana: thank you for your friendship. Richard Morse and Jenny Klimiuk: for changing my world order.

To everyone who contacted me after I first wrote about this – you are all in my thoughts and I wish you all the luck in the world.

Finally to my mum, for literally everything.

Notes

PERFECT STORMS

1 Fayaz A, Croft P, Langford RM et al., 'Prevalence of chronic pain in the UK: A systematic review and meta-analysis of population studies', *BMJ Open*, 2016; 6.

PEELING OFF THE LABELS

2 Bairey Merz CN, 'The Yentl Syndrome and gender inequality in ischemic HD', *Cardiology Today*, August 2011.

3 Park SM and Bairey Merz CN, 'Women and Ischemic Heart Disease: Recognition, Diagnosis and Management', *Korean Circulation Journal*, Jul 2016; 46(4): 433–42.

BAD BALIANS

4 Finniss DG, Kaptchuk TJ, Miller F, Benedetti F, 'Placebo Effects: Biological Clinical and Ethical Advances', *Lancet*, 20 Feb 2010; 375 (9715): 686–95.

5 Klein AS and Forni PM, 'Barbers of Civility', *Archives of Surgery*, 2011; 146(7): 774–7.

FOURTEEN TIMES MORE LIKELY TO

6 In June 2017, the *Washington Post* published an article about a Missouri family, all on disability benefits, praying for the 'right' diagnosis for 10-year-old twins so they could be the fourth generation to be diagnosed as disabled in that family.

7 Singhal A, Tien YY, Hsia RY, 'Racial-Ethnic Disparities in Opioid Prescriptions at Emergency Department Visits for Conditions Commonly Associated with Prescription Drug Abuse', *PLoS One*, 8 Aug 2016; 11(8).

JUST ANOTHER MEDICINE

8 Another theory is that Evita may have been lobotomised on her husband's orders, in order to control her behaviour towards the end of her life.

SOMETHING PRETTY

9 Kappesser J and Williams AC de C, 'Pain Estimation: Asking the right questions', *Pain*, 148; 184–7.

THE WORLD'S MOST FAMOUS MEDICINE MAN

10 Goldman N, Chen M et al., 'Adenosine A1 receptors mediate local anti-nociceptive effects of acupuncture', *Nature Neuroscience*, Jul 2010; 13(7): 883–8.

11 Harris RE, Zubieta JK et al., 'Traditional Chinese acupuncture and

placebo (sham) acupuncture are differentiated by their effects on μ-opioid receptors (MORs)', *NeuroImage*, Sep 2009; 47(3): 1077–85.

12 Sun Y, Gan TJ et al., 'Acupuncture and related techniques for postoperative pain: A systematic review of randomized clinical trials', *British Journal of Anaesthesia*, Aug 2008; 101(2): 151–60.

13 Napadow V, Kettner N et al., 'Hypothalamus and amygdala response to acupuncture stimuli in carpal tunnel syndrome', *Pain*, Aug 2007; 130(3): 254–66.

RIDING THE ROLLERCOASTER

14 YouGov poll, 6 March 2015. 74 per cent of respondents thought chiropractic was effective, 68 per cent osteopathy, 66 per cent acupuncture, 51 per cent herbal medicine, down to 3 per cent astrology.

15 Spence DS, Thompson EA and Barron SJ, 'Homeopathic treatment for chronic disease: A 6-year, university-hospital outpatient observational study', *Journal of Alternative and Complementary Medicine*, Oct 2005; 11(5): 793–8.

PRIEZ POUR NOUS

16 USA Today/ABC News/Stanford University Medical Center poll, May 2005. More than half the respondents used prayer to control pain; 90 per cent said it worked 'well', 51 per cent 'very well'. For painkillers, the response rate was 89 per cent 'well', 51 per cent 'very well'.

17 Eltaiba N and Harries M, 'Reflections on Recovery in Mental Health: Perspectives from a Muslim Culture', *Social Work in Health Care*, 2015; 54(8): 725–37.

18 Jim HSL, Pustejovsky JE et al., 'Religion, spirituality and physical health in cancer patients: A meta-analysis', *Cancer*, 1 Nov 2015; 121(21): 3760–8. The study didn't look at recurrence or survival rates.

19 Vespa A, Jacobsen PB et al., 'Evaluation of intrapsychic factors, coping styles and spirituality of patients affected by tumours', *Psychooncology*, Jan 2011; 20(1): 5–11.

20 Tsai TJ, Chung UL et al., 'Influence of religious belief on the health of cancer patients', *Asian Pacific Journal of Cancer Prevention*, 1 Jan 2016, 17(4): 2315–20.

THEY CAN KILL US

21 Chinua Achebe, 1958.

TEMPLE TO THE SICK

22 Kelley JM, Kraft-Todd G et al., 'The Influence of the Patient-Clinician Relationship on Healthcare Outcomes: A Systematic Review and Meta-Analysis of Randomized Controlled Trials', *PLoS One*, 2014; 9(4): e94207. The systematic review looked at 13 studies of the patient-doctor relationship and selected those studying chronic illness with measurable symptoms. In most of the trials the professionals either delivered their normal standard of care or underwent patient interaction training – anything from making more eye contact to goal-setting.

23 Prescriber attitudes significantly affected treatment outcomes for anxiety

and depression in one study; another showed 80 per cent of schizophrenic patients improved with increased attention from care-givers.

24 Middendorp M, Kollias K et al., 'Does therapist's attitude affect clinical outcome of lumbar facet joint injections?', *World Journal of Radiology*, 28 Jun 2016; 8(6): 628–34.

25 NHS figures, August 2016. The same month, the BMA suggested GP appointments should be increased to 15 minutes.

26 Morris PA, 'The effect of pilgrimage on anxiety, depression and religious attitude', *Psychological Medicine*, May 1982; 12(2): 291–4.

27 Goldingay S, Dieppe P and Farias M, ' "And the pain just disappeared into insignificance": The healing response in Lourdes', *International Review of Psychiatry*, Jun 2014; 26(3): 315–23.

AN UNSTOPPABLE PROCESS

28 Uttley L, Scope A et al., 'Systematic review and economic modelling of the clinical effectiveness and cost-effectiveness of art therapy among people with non-psychotic mental health disorders', *Health Technology Assessment*, Mar 2015; 19(18): 1–120, v–vi.

29 Interview with Prof 'Janet Williams', June 2016.

30 McCracken LM, 'Learning to live with the pain: Acceptance of pain predicts adjustment in persons with chronic pain', *Pain*, Jan 1998; 74(1): 21–7.

31 Flor H, Fydrich T et al., 'Efficacy of multidisciplinary pain treatment centers: A meta-analytic review', *Pain*, May 1992; 49(2): 221–30.

32 Tyson JE, Furzan JA et al., 'An evaluation of the quality of therapeutic studies in perinatal medicine', *The Journal of Pediatrics*, Jan 1983; 102(1): 10–13.

33 Olsen O, Middleton P et al., 'Quality of Cochrane reviews: Assessment of sample from 1998', *BMJ*, 2001; 323.

34 There are free explanations and exercises on Michael Moskowitz's website, neuroplastix.com, but I'd suggest buying the workbook ($50) because it lays out the science so clearly.

35 Even today there's a swish hotel in Puglia, Borgo Egnazia, that offers female-only courses in the *pizzica*, designed to help them embrace their womanhood.

PERMISSIONS ACKNOWLEDGEMENTS

"Ieri ho sofferto il dolore" by Alda Merini. From *Fiore di Poesia*, Einaudi, Turin, 2014; Audre Lorde: *The Cancer Journals*. Quotes by permission of Aunt Lute Books. www.auntlute.com; *Go Tell it on the Mountain* by James Baldwin. Used by permission of the James Baldwin Estate; *Giving up the Ghost* by Hilary Mantel. Reprinted by permission of HarperCollins Publishers Ltd © Hilary Mantel 2003; *Wide Sargasso Sea* by Jean Rhys (Andre Deutsch 1966, Penguin Books 1968, Penguin Classics 2000). Copyright © Jean Rhys, 1966. Introduction copyright © Andrea Ashworth, 2000; *The Death of Ivan Ilyich & Confession*, Leo Tolstoy tr. Peter Carson. Reprinted by permission of Liveright; *I Love Dick* by Chris Kraus. Reprinted by permission of Serpent's Tail © Chris Kraus 1997; *Pain Woman Takes Your Keys* by Sonya Huber, University of Nebraska Press, 2017. Reprinted by permission of Sonya Huber; *Sharp Objects* by Gillian Flynn, Orion, copyright © Gillian Flynn 2006.